Proceedings of the International Collaborative Effort on Injury Statistics Volume I

From the CENTERS FOR DISEASE CONTROL AND PREVENTION/National Center for Health Statistics

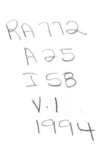

U.S. DEPARTMENT OF HEALTH AND HUMAN SERVICES
Public Health Service
Centers for Disease Control and Prevention
National Center for Health Statistics

Hyattsville, Maryland
March 1995
DHHS Publication No. (PHS) 95-1252

Preface

On May 18-20, 1994 the National Center for Health Statistics (NCHS) convened the first symposium of the International Collaborative Effort (ICE) on Injury Statistics. This symposium was co-sponsored by the National Institute of Child Health and Human Development (NICHD), National Institutes of Health.

The mission of the Injury ICE is to identify the problem(s) and propose solutions aimed at improving the quality and reliability of international statistics related to injury. In order to achieve the maximum benefits for participating researchers, the symposium brought together leading researchers from the United States and from 13 other countries to address the multiple issues related to the comparability of injury data.

The members of the ICE on Injury steering committee are from: the NCHS, Lois A. Fingerhut, Bob Hartford, Harry Rosenberg, Sue Meads; the National Center for Injury Prevention and Control (NCIPC), Lee Annest; the NICHD, Mary Overpeck; the Johns Hopkins Injury Prevention Center, Gordon Smith; and the WHO Working Group on Injury Surveillance and the Consumer Safety Institute in Amsterdam, Netherlands, Wim Rogmans.

This volume contains the papers presented at the symposium as well as the deliberations that took place in the various workshops.

Acknowledgments

Overall responsibility for planning and coordinating the content of these Proceedings was assumed by Lois A. Fingerhut, Special Assistant for Injury Epidemiology, Office of Analysis, Epidemiology and Health Promotion, and Bob Hartford, Deputy Director, Office of International Statistics, National Center for Health Statistics.

Many thanks to the individual authors and workshop chairs for their contributions to this volume. Each of the presentations is included as submitted by the respective authors. Individual comments should be addressed to them.

Publications management was provided by Thelma Sanders.

Participants

Interests are included after the address for those who provided the information.

*Anders Àberg
Principal Administrative Officer
Centre for Epidemiology
National Board of Health and Welfare
S–106 30 Stockholm
SWEDEN

Interests: Surveillance, data analysis

*Duane Alexander, M.D.
Director
National Institute of Child Health and Human
    Development
Building 31, Room 2A03
Bethesda, MD 20892

Jean Athey, Ph.D.
Director
Injury Prevention and EMSC Programs
Maternal and Child Health Bureau
Room 18–A–39
5600 Fishers Lane
Rockville, MD 20857

Tim Baker
621 North Washington Street
Baltimore, MD 21205

*Vita Barell
Head, Health Services Research Unit
Ministry of Health
The Gertner Institute
The Chaim Sheba Medical Center
Tel Hashomer 52621
ISRAEL

Interests: Injury surveillance; emergency room
    information systems; Trauma registries; outcome
    evaluation; Registry of effective prevention
    programs; consumer product safety programs

*Henning Bay–Nielsen, M.D.
Syndhedsstyrelsen
National Health Council
P.O. Box 2020
1012 Copenhagen
DENMARK

Les R. Becker
Evaluation Manager
Division of Injury and Disability Prevention and
    Rehabilitation
Department of Health and Mental Hygiene
State of Maryland
201 West Preston Street
Baltimore, MD 21201

BECK103W@WONDER.EM.CDC.GOV

Interests: Program Evaluation and data
    needs;E–Coding;GIS

*Gerry Berenholz
Berenholz Consulting Associates
27 Locke Lane
Lexington, MA 02173

Interests: ICD–9–CM all disease, injury and
    external cause codes; Coding rules and
    guidelines; Perform coding validations and
    analyze coded information; insurance billing
    processes and DRG reimbursement

*Lars Berg, M.D.
Research Unit in Primary Health Care
Tibro Health Center
S–543 81 Tibro
SWEDEN

Interests: Surveillance, linkage, database design

Kathie Binysh, M.D.
Senior Medical Officer
Department of Health
Room 527
Wellington House
133–155 Waterloo Road
London SE1 8UG
ENGLAND

Ruth Brenner, M.D.
NICHD
6100 Executive Blvd. Room 7B03
Bethesda, MD 20892

Bill Carl
Injury Prevention Unit
Minnesota Department of Health
717 SE Delaware Street
P.O. Box 9441
Minneapolis, MN 55440–9441

Interests: Suicide, child mal–treatment, sports
   injury

*Erich M. Daub
Injury Prevention Program
Baltimore County Dept of Health
One Investment Place, 10th Floor
Towson, MD 21204–4111

Interests: Surveillance (intentional/unintentional);
   coding; mapping/geog.; Prevention

John Delargy, M.D.
Consumer Safety Unit
10/18 Victoria Street
London SW1H 0NN
ENGLAND

Interests: Home and leisure accident prevention,
   Special Studies

Alan Dellapenna
Injury Prevention Specialist
Phoenix Area IHS
3738 N. 16th Street, Suite A
Phoenix, AZ 85016–5981

*Patricia C. Dischinger, Ph.D.
University of MD at Baltimore
MD Institute for Emergency Medical Services
National Study Center for Trauma
22 South Greene Street
Baltimore, MD 21201

Benjamin C. Duggar
Center for Health Policy Studies
9700 Patuxent Woods Drive, Suite 100
Columbia, MD 21046

John H. Ferguson, M.D.
Director, Office of Medical Applications of
   Research
Office of the Director
National Institutes of Health
Federal Building, Room 618
Bethesda, MD 20892

Samuel Nana Fourjuoh
Center for Injury Research and Control
200 Lothrop Street – Room NE–560 MUH
Pittsburgh, Pa 15213

*Birthe Frimodt–Moller, M.D.
Syndhedsstyrelsen
National Health Council
P.O. Box 2020
1012 Copenhagen
DENMARK

Interests: Cclassifications, surveillance, utilization
   of injury data for prevention

*Sue Gallagher
Children's Safety Network
Education Development Center, Inc.
55 Chapel Street
Newton, MA 02160

E– mail: SUSANG@EDC.ORG

Interests: ED surveillance, coding, minimum data
   sets, child and adolescent injury prevention,
   evaluation

*Herbert Garrison, M.D.
Center for Injury Research and Control
University of Pittsburgh, MUH, Rm. NE–560
200 Lothrop Street
Pittsburgh, PA 15213–3170

Rosa Gofin, M.D.
Department of Social Medicine
Hadassah School of Public Health and Community
   Medicine
P.O.B. 1172
Jerusalem 91010
ISRAEL

Interests: Injury surveillance;Outcome of
   Injuries;Prevention program evaluation

Cathy Gotschall
National Children's Medical Center
Washington, DC 20010

*Yossi Harel, Ph.D.
Head, Medical Sociology Program
Bar Ilan University
Ramat Gan, 52900
ISRAEL

Interests: Childhood and adolescent injury; risk
    behavior; psychosocial cross–national
    comparisons; survey methodology in injury
    research

*Keith D. Harries, Ph.D.
Chair
Department of Geography
University of MD
Social Sciences Building, Room 211
5401 Wilkens Avenue
Baltimore, MD 21228–5398

Joan Harris
National Highway Traffic Safety Administration
400 Seventh Street, SW
NPP–32
Washington, D.C. 20590

*James Harrison, Ph.D.
National Injury Surveillance Unit
Mark Oliphant Building
Laffer Drive, Science Park
5042 Bedford Park
AUSTRALIA

E-mail: NIJEH@FLINDERS.EDU.AU

Interests: Minimum data set for injury
    surveillance;Improved mortality surveillance,
    (through work with coroners);Technical aspects
    of inpatient morbidity (standards; definitions;
    achieving state to state comparability; etc.);
    Emergency room surveillance; Linkage (esp. of
    police and hospital data for road injury); Severity
    measures; Injury information reporting
    methods(how to get the information to the right
    people, in useable forms); Special purpose injury
    registers (spinal cord injury); Monitoring national
    injury targets.

*Michael Hayes, Ph.D.
Project Director
Child Accident Prevention Trust
Clerks Court, 4th Floor
18–20 Farringdon Lane
London EC1R 3AU
ENGLAND

*Yvette Holder
PAHO/WHO Caribbean
Caribbean Epidemiology Center (CAREC)
P.O. Box 164
16–18 Jamaica Blvd.
Port of Spain
TRINIDAD

Interests: Surveillance, injury economics; quality of
    data

David H. Janda, M.D.
Director
Institute for Preventative Sports Medicine
P.O. Box 7032
Ann Arbor, MI 48107

Interests: Sports Injuries/Prevention

Lt. Col. Bruce H. Jones, M.D.
Chief, Occupational Medicine Division
U.S. Army Research Institute of Environmental
    Medicine
Natick, MA 01760–5007

Arthur L. Kellermann, M.D.
Emory University
School of Public Health
Center for Injury Control
1462 Clifton Road, NE
Atlanta, GA 30322

Eileen Kessler
U.S. Consumer Produce Safety Commission
Washington, DC 20207

Interests: Injuries and deaths (unintent.,
    intent.);surveillance systems;in–depth
    investigation of injury events

*Jess Kraus, Ph.D.
University of California, Los Angeles
School of Public Health
10833 Le Conte Avenue
Los Angeles, CA 90024-1772

*John Langley, Ph.D.
Director, Injury Prevention Research Unit
University of Otago Medical School
P.O. Box 913
Dunedin
NEW ZEALAND

*Jean A. Langlois, ScD
National Institute on Aging
Gateway Building
7201 Wisconsin Avenue, Suite 3C–309
National Institutes of Health
Bethesda, MD 20892

Ilana Lescohier, Ph.D.
Assistant Director
Harvard Injury Control Center
Harvard School of Public Health
718 Huntington Avenue
Boston, MA 02115

*Andre L'Hours
Strengthening of Epidemiological and Statistical
    Services
World Health Organization
1211 – Geneva – 27
SWITZERLAND

*Johan Lund
Director
Norwegian Safety Forum
P.O. Box 2473, Solli
N–0202 Oslo
NORWAY

Ronald Maio, M.D.
University of Michigan
Section of Emergency Medicine
Taubman Center, TC–B1354–0303
1500 East Medical Center Drive
Ann Arbor, MI 48109–0303

Interests: Motor Vehicle Injury (Regional variation
    and Medical care outcome), Alcohol and Injury;
    Injury Control; Injury Severity Scoring/Scaling

*Sue Mallonee
Director, Injury Program
Oklahoma State Department of Health
Injury Epidemiology Division
1000 NE 10th Street
Oklahoma City, OK 73117–1299

Interests: Injury Surveillance, epidemiology and
    program evaluation data linkage

Elizabeth McLoughlin, ScD
Director, San Francisco Injury Center
San Francisco General Hospital
Building 1, Room 400
San Francisco, CA 94110

Interests: Domestic violence, helmet laws,
    cigarettes and fatal fires

Angela Mickelaide
Safe Kids Campaign
111 Michigan Avenue, N.W.
Washington, DC 20010–2970

Nancy Macrina
The University of Alabama at Birmingham
School of Medicine
403 Community Health Services Building
Birmingham, AL 35294

Interests: Rehabilitation, E–coding, head injuries

Ted Miller, Ph.D.
NPSRI
8201 Corporate Drive
Landover, MD 20785

Martha Moore
Department of Health and Social Services
Emergency Medical Services
PO Box 110616
Juneau, Alaska 99811–0616

Interests: Surveillance, data linkage, utilization of
    injury data for prevention

*Mary Overpeck, Dr.P.H.
Epidemiologist
NICHD
6100 Executive Blvd. Room 7B03
Bethesda, MD 20892

Victoria Ozonoff, Ph.D.
Director of Health Resources Statistics
MA Department of Public Health
Bureau of Health Statistics and Research
150 Tremont Street
Boston, MA 02111

Juana Palma–Ulloa
Health Situation Analysis Program
Pan American Health Organization
525 23rd St. NW
Washington, DC 20037–2895

Donna Pickett
American Hospital Association
Central Office on ICD–9–CM
840 North Lakeshore Drive
Chicago, IL 60611

Louis Quatrano, Ph.D.
Chief
Center for Rehabilitation Medicine
Room 2A03
NICHD
Building 6100
Bethesda, MD 20892

Michael Rand
Bureau of Justice Statistics
633 Indiana Avenue, N.W.
Washington, DC 20531

Interests: Intentional injury, firearm injury, mortality

Susan Reed
Department of Veterans Affairs
810 Vermont Avenue, NW
Washington, DC 20420

Edna Roberts
Pan American Health Organization
525 23rd St. NW
Washington, DC 20037-2895

Interests: Comparability of international statistics (Mortality and morbidity); minimum data sets; indicators

*Ian Rockett, Ph.D.
Department of Health Leisure and Safety
University of Tennessee at Knoxville
1914 Andy Holt Avenue
Knoxville, TN 37996-2700

Interests: Ssurveillance, mortality, data linkage

*Wim Rogmans, Ph.D.
Consumer Safety Institute
P.O. Box 75169
1070 AD Amsterdam
THE NETHERLANDS

*C.J. Romer, M.D.
Chief, Injury Prevention Program
World Health Organization
20, Avenue Appia
1211 Geneva
SWITZERLAND

Cleone Rooney, M.D.
Office of Population Censuses and Surveys
Medical Statistics Division
10 Kingsway
London WC2B 6JP
ENGLAND

Interests: Comparability and accuracy of mortality data; suicide; international comparisons – cure and prevention; record linkage and followback

Beatrice Rouse, M.D.
Substance Abuse and Mental Health Services Administration
16–105 Parklawn Building
5600 Fishers Lane
Rockville, MD 20857

phone–301–443–8005
fax 301–443–9847
BROUSE@AOA2.SSW.DHHS.GOV

Interests: Injuries and deaths associated with substance abuse, mental disorders, and violence; epidemiology; and methodological issues such as classification and coding rules and guidelines.

Carol W. Runyan, Ph.D.
Director, IPRC
University of North Carolina
Chase Hall - CB 7505
Chapel Hill, NC 27599-7505

*George Rutherford, M.S.
U.S. Consumer Product Safety Commission
Epidemiology
Washington DC 20207

Interests: Unintentional injuries

Sue Ryan
Chief
Emergency Medical Services Division
National Highway Traffic Safety Administration
400 Seventh Street, SW
Washington, DC 20590

Interests: Out–of–hospital data, data linkage, GIS

Nancy Rytina
Division of Hazard Analysis
U.S. Consumer Product Safety Commission
Washington DC 20207

*Peter Scheidt, M.D.
Director
Department of General Pediatrics
National Childrens Medical Center
111 Michigan Avenue
Washington, DC 20010

Robert Schwartz, M.D.
Department of Medicine
Hartford Hospital
80 Seymour Street
Hartford, CT 06115

Interests: Ed surveillance; Documentation issues
    (data acquisition); Computers in medicine
    (computer based patient record); the clinician as
    injury prevention specialist

*Greg Sherman, Ph.D.
Chief, Diseases of Infants and Children Division
Health Canada
46–LCDC Building
Tunney's Pasture
Ottawa ON K1A OL2
CANADA

Interests: GIS, data analysis, database
    design/linkage

*Gordon Smith, M.B., M.P.H.
Associate Professor
The Johns Hopkins University
Injury Prevention Center
624 North Broadway
Baltimore, MD   21205

*Richard J. Smith, M.S.
Injury Prevention Program Manager
Indian Health Service
610 Twinbrook Plaza Suite
12300 Twinbrook Parkway
Rockville, MD 20852

*Lorann Stallones, Ph.D.
Associate Professor
Colorado State University
Department of Environmental Health
B120 Microbiology Building
Fort Collins, CO 80523

E–mail:
    LSTALLONES@VINES.COLOSTATE.EDU

Interests: Rural/farm injuries (intentional and
    unintentional); GIS

*David Stone, Ph.D.
Public Health Research Unit
University of Glasgow
Greater Glasgow Health Board
1 Lilybank Gardens
Glasgow G12 8RZ
SCOTLAND

Interests: GIS, data analysis, database
    design/linkage

*Leif Svanstrom, Ph.D.
Karolinska Institute/ Kronan Health
Centre, Department of Social Medicine
17283 Sunbyberg – Stockholm
SWEDEN

Alvin R. Tarlov, M.D.
The Health Institute
New England Medical Center, Box 345
750 Washington Street
Boston, MA   02111

Roger Trent , Ph.D.
Chief, Injury Surveillance and Epidemiology
Emergency Preparedness and Injury Control
    Program
601 North 7th Street
PO Box 942732
Sacramento, CA 94234–7320

Internet RTRENT@HW1.CAHWNET.GOV

Interests: Injury surveillance; central nervous
    system trauma; drowning; violence

Ann Trumble, Ph.D.
Epidemiology Branch
Room 7B03
National Institute of Child Health and Human
    Development
Building 6100
Bethesda, MD 20892

*Anne Tursz, M.D.
Scientific Director
International Children's Center
Chateau de Longchamp– Bois de Boulogne
F 75016 Paris
FRANCE

Interests: Childhood injury; long term
    consequences of injuries; sports related injuries

Elinor Walker
Health Science Administrator
Agency for Health Care Policy and Research
Division of Technology and Quality Assessment
Center for General Health Services Extramural
    Research
2101 East Jefferson Street
Suite 502
Rockville, MD 20852–4908

*Patricia F. Waller, Ph.D.
Director
University of Michigan Transportation Research
    Institute
2901 Baxter Road, Room 154
Ann Arbor, Michigan 48109–2150

*William Walsh
Director
National Center for Statistics and Analysis
National Highway Traffic Safety Administration
Room 6125
400 Seventh Street, SW
Washington, DC 20590

Harold B. Weiss
Center for Injury Reduction and Control
Division of Emergency Medicine
MUH–Room NE 560
3459 Fifth Avenue
Pittsburgh, PA 15213–3241

E– mail: WEISS@VAXA.MUH.UPMCEDU

Interests: Surveillance, emergency department

Diane Willard
American Medical Association
515 North State Street
Chicago, IL 60610

*Pnina Zadka
Director, Health Division
Central Bureau of Statistics
Hakirya–Romema
PO Box 13015
Jerusalem 91130
ISRAEL

Interests: Mortality, morbidity, coding, data linkage

Craig Zwerling, M.D., Ph.D.
Deputy Director
Injury Prevention Research Center
University of Iowa
100 Oakdale Campus, #126 AMRF
Iowa City, IA 52242–5000

Centers for Disease Control and Prevention

CDC participants, on pages 14–15, are not alphabetized.

*David Satcher, M.D., Ph.D.
Director
Centers for Disease Control and Prevention
1600 Clifton Road NE
Atlanta, GA   30333

From the National Center for Health Statistics:
6525 Belcrest Road
Hyattsville, MD   20782

Office of the Director
*Manning Feinleib, M.D., Dr.P.H.
Director

Office of International Statistics
*Robert Israel, Associate Director
*Bob Hartford, Ph.D., Deputy Director
Paul Ahmed
*Jacqueline P. Davis
Sam Notzon, Ph.D.

Office of Analysis, Epidemiology and Health
   Promotion
Jacob J. Feldman, Ph.D., Associate Director
*Lois A. Fingerhut, Special Assistant for Injury
   Epidemiology

Interests: Childhood injury, injury resulting from
   violence; cross–national comparisons

E–mail: LAF4@NCH07A.EM.CDC.GOV

   Division of Epidemiology
Jennifer Madans, Ph.D., Director

   Division of Heath and Utilization Analysis
Harold Lentzner, Ph.D.
Deborah D. Ingram, Ph.D.
Laura E. Montgomery

Interests: Child health, family violence,
   socioeconomic indicators

   Division of Health Promotion Statistics
John F. Seitz, Ph.D.

Office of Vital and Health Statistics Systems
   Division of Vital Statistics
   Mortality Statistics Branch
*Harry Rosenberg, Ph.D., Chief
Hsiang–Ching Kung, Ph.D.
Jim Spitler

Division of Health Care Statistics
Edward W. Bacon, Ph.D., Director

   Morbidity Classification Branch
Sue Meads, Chief
Perianne Lurie, M.D.

   Hospital Care Statistics Branch
*Brenda Gillum

Interests: Childhood Injury Prevention; Coding
   Issues;Computerization of coding systems

   Division of Health Interview Statistics
Peggy R. Barker

Office of Planning and Extramural Programs
Gail F. Fisher, Ph.D., Associate Director

Office of Research and Methodology
Chuck Croner

Office of Data Processing and Services
Sandy Smith, Public Affairs Specialist

**From the National Center for Injury Prevention
   and Control**
4770 Buford Highway
Atlanta, GA   30341 (Mailstop F36)

Office of Statistics, Programming and Graphics
*Joseph L. Annest, Ph.D., Director

Interests: Mapping, injury statistics, firearm
   injuries, coding, injury surveillance

Division of Unintentional Injury Prevention
Terry Chorba, M.D.
Julie Russel, Ph.D.
Interests: Motor vehicle related injury prevention,
   data linkage, childhood injury prevention

Division of Violence Prevention
*Ken Powell, M.D.

Division of Acute Care, Rehabilitation Research,
and Disability Prevention (Mailstop F41)
Rick Waxweiler, Ph.D., Acting Director
*Dan Pollock, M.D.
David Thurman, M.D.

From the National Center for Environmental Health
Atlanta, GA 30333 Mailstop F35

Division of Environmental Hazards and Health Effects
Roy T. Ing, M.D.

Surveillance and Programs Branch
*Gib Parrish, M.D., Chief

From the National Institute for Occupational Safety and Health
*Nancy Stout, Ed.D.
Chief, Injury Surveillance Section
Division of Safety Research
944 Chestnut Ridge Road
Morgantown, WV 26505–2888

E–Mail NAS5@NIOSR1.EM.CDC.GOV

Interests: Occupational safety/injury; automated coding software; child labor

* **Co–Author of paper or Co–Chair of workshop**

Contents

Coding Issues

Workshops

Closing Remarks

Keynote

David Satcher, M.D., Ph.D.

I am delighted to be with you as a part of this very important conference. I am sorry I am not going to be able to spend more time with you, because I think it is going to be an exciting and precedent–setting meeting.

I don't know whether it is better to speak early in the morning or late at night. I guess I had one of my worst experiences at an evening speaking engagement. I spoke once after dinner where they had had a cocktail hour before dinner. When I got up to speak, I said, "I have only about 10 minutes here and I just don't know where to start. A guy in the back of the room said, `Well, why don't you start at the ninth minute?' So, I'm not going to ask you where I should start. I am delighted to be here and I appreciate your accommodating my crazy schedule.

On behalf of the Centers for Disease Control, I am very pleased to welcome you to this very important conference—especially our international guests. I think it makes a very important point that we are here together to collaborate on the issue of health statistics. Collaboration has solved many of the world's greatest health problems.

CDC, throughout its history, has recognized health as a global issue and has stayed focused on the vision of Healthy People in a Healthy World. Nowhere has that been illustrated better, I think, than in the area of infectious diseases and our global efforts in immunization. The eradication of smallpox in 1977 was a historic international milestone. In fact, today we are very close, working with our partners throughout the world, to eradicating polio. So, the time is right for us to come together internationally to look at the issue and the value of injury statistics.

I want to thank Manning Feinlieb and the members of the National Center for Health Statistics for organizing this ICE. One of the responsibilities of NCHS through the Office of International Statistics, is promoting international collaboration in the field of health statistics.

This international collaborative effort is one of several ways that NCHS accomplishes its important tasks. These efforts are designed to bring together researchers from several countries and the United States to study common problems and to arrive at results that will be mutually beneficial.

The goal of the ICE on injury statistics is to improve the quality, the reliability and the comparability of international statistics on injury. The ICE recognizes the need for worldwide collaborative approaches and the reliance upon data to direct prevention efforts.

Let me tell you what I think this meeting can accomplish. Many agencies and programs represented here today are critical to our success. This symposium represents the need for cooperation and collaboration within, as well as among, countries.

The U.S. federal agencies with key roles in the collection, analysis, and dissemination of injury data, are joined by state and local governments, as well as representatives from many of the primary research centers across the nations, such as the directors of injury prevention research centers.

This is a tremendous opportunity, bringing together a wealth of expertise. The organizers of this symposium have taken on a very important task, and I commend them.

By focusing on what has proven to be successful, here in this country and in other countries, and equally important, by avoiding those things that have not proven to be worthwhile, our efforts can be combined, our knowledge compounded, and our success rates maximized.

This symposium is only the first step in this ICE. During this meeting, we will develop our plan for future research and action. We will widely circulate the proceedings of this symposium, which will illuminate the problems and limitations, as well as a successful and innovative approach to provide the needed statistics for injury prevention.

You were all invited to be here because of your contributions and your expertise and your devout interest in the broad arena of injury prevention and injury statistics. We are here to share our collective knowledge so that we can achieve the ultimate goal of reducing the toll that injuries take throughout the world.

I want to relate what you are doing here to the priorities which we have been establishing at CDC. We call our priorities evolving priorities, because we recognize the rapidity of change taking place, not only in our country, but throughout the world. Because of this rapid change, CDC must remain vigilant in monitoring changes, challenges and opportunities.

As I mentioned before, our vision is that of Healthy People in a Healthy World through Prevention. It is clear to me that, in order for us to achieve this goal, we must have priorities that are relevant and evolving. As the world evolves, so should our priorities.

I know that the areas that we have identified as priorities match many of the public health and prevention priorities identified by other nations. We have grouped our priorities into four major categories which I will discuss, with particular emphasis on injury prevention and the important role of data in each of these priorities areas.

The first priority area for CDC in 1994 is to strengthen the essential public health services—we call these the core public health functions. These are especially important during this era of health care reform discussion in our country, as we try to fix the health care delivery system that we all agree is in such great need of fixing.

Clearly, this is a starting point—to look at the core functions of public health. We must articulate a vision of public health that is broad and comprehensive. That vision must be clear enough for us to speak not only to local and state health departments, and to our colleagues internationally, but to communities at every level. For us to really carry out these essential services of public health in the 1990's, we need the cooperation of people in communities everywhere, at every level.

From this vision, core public health functions are defined. In addition to the traditional areas of public health, such as infectious diseases, we have added lifestyles and environmental influences. They affect the quality of life in ways unimaginable until just a few years ago.

Violence, for example, is now a major public health issue, amenable to the research and intervention that public health disciplines can provide. That is true, not only in this country, but in other countries as well. In December, I had an opportunity to visit an injury control program that our field epidemiology training program has established in Cairo, Egypt. I saw the impact that that program is having on injury prevention in Egypt.

A year ago, in May, I attended my first World Health Assembly as a U.S. delegate. I remember some of our colleagues from sub–Saharan Africa pointing out how the glamorization of violence on TV and in the movies in the United States is having an extremely negative impact on our teenagers. The global aspect of this issue is very clear.

The next thing we have to do is to develop a social marketing strategy. We must frequently relearn the lesson that an ounce of prevention is worth a pound of cure. We must constantly communicate that message in a way that is appropriate, meaningful, and effective to the various audiences that we reach—from the public, to the policy makers, to the health providers. We are especially encountering that lesson in some of our programs today.

Our biggest task is to develop strategies to turn knowledge into behavioral change. There have been many successes in the arena of injury prevention. We know some of those successes, especially in motor vehicle accidents. From 1968 to 1991, motor vehicle deaths decreased by 21 percent in this country, while deaths from violence increased by over 60 percent. We have also had success in the use of bicycle helmets, which are 85 percent effective, and have made a measurable difference, not only in terms of injuries, but also in terms of cost savings.

Within this priority of strengthening the core functions of public health is the development of a nationwide health information and surveillance system. That system must be capable of producing information wherever and when it is needed. Information that is standardized is especially important for injury prevention.

We can also strengthen our national systems through international collaboration and exchange. Two weeks ago, the National Center for Infectious Diseases issued a report—which I hope you have seen—on emerging infections. The first recommendation in that report was to develop strong surveillance systems throughout the world to really get a handle on infectious diseases, particularly the new and emerging infectious diseases. So, utilizing surveillance systems is no longer critical just nationally, but internationally, as well.

Our second priority at CDC is to develop, maintain, and enrich our capacity to respond to urgent threats to health. What are some of these urgent threats to health that we are concerned about? This priority includes such urgent threats as the new and emerging infections which I have mentioned, environmental toxins, where we are heavily involved, work place hazards, and injuries.

We can use statistics from the United States to illustrate some of our concerns. While specific problems vary from country to country, and we each have different priorities, injury is an urgent threat in every country. For example, in this country, we have 150,000 deaths per year from injuries, nearly 3 million hospitalizations, 31.5 million visits to the emergency room, which means more than one third of visits to the emergency room in this country are due to injuries. These injuries are both intentional and unintentional.

We are having a real problem with our young people—teenagers—in terms of violence. Since 1985, deaths from violence among teenagers in this country have increased by 77 percent.

Injuries are a leading cause of death in this country, for the population from ages one through 44. When it comes to the cause of potential years of life lost in this country, no cause of death even comes close. Injuries are way out front.

At least 10 million people suffer traumatic injuries on their jobs each year in this country. During the last decade, over 60,000 Americans died from workplace injuries. And the cost of injuries is escalating. The impact of injuries on health care services and the ability to provide care costs our economy more than $83 billion a year.

Now, we must develop the capacity to respond to these urgent threats. When it comes to infectious diseases, obviously we must have the capacity to immunize.

We also must have laboratories and qualified facilities and personnel. In order to respond to the injury problems, we must also be able to monitor. We must have domestic and international emergency response teams. We must have global networks for disease detection, and violence and injury prevention programs globally.

CDC's National Center for Injury Prevention and Control, was created just two years ago, to emphasize the importance of injury prevention, along with CDC's long standing programs in the prevention and control of infectious and chronic diseases. Worldwide, CDC has collaborated with four other nations, to prevent and control injury and disease, by the establishment of our field epidemiologist training program. CDC is committed to training—I want those of you who are visiting, especially, to know that. We are committed on an international basis.

Certainly, the most effective program in CDC's history has been the epidemiology intelligence service. We have trained more than 2,000 people who are leaders in epidemiology and prevention throughout the world. And we are committed to working with other countries to develop epidemiology and training programs, along with the 12 that you already have participated in. We look forward to working with some of you in this arena.

CDC's National Institute for Occupational Safety and Health (NIOSH) is an important partner in injury prevention in the workplace. NIOSH has developed a surveillance system for collecting information on fatal workplace injury in every state across the nation. The Institute has just released a document analyzing the data from 1980, which provides the most comprehensive statistics to date on the magnitude and nature of the problem, the potential risk factors, and the industries and occupations in this country at greatest risk. The data provide the foundation for the next decade of research and prevention efforts, aimed at reducing fatal injuries to workers in this country.

So you can see that our second priority—responding to urgent health threats—is a very important one, as you can see, and I think quite relevant to the work we are going to be discussing in terms of injury statistics at this conference.

The third priority at CDC is to develop a nationwide prevention network and program. First, we must determine the opportunities for prevention. Data on injuries are helping to formulate those prevention messages, as well as to implement our prevention strategy. We have 25 programs now in 19 states, dealing with injury prevention. But we must develop local, state, national, and international partnerships, if we are to be successful in our injury prevention programs.

We must ensure work force diversity to be responsible to the diverse needs of this nation, but also of the world. We are, by definition, a diverse group at this ICE symposium. And from that diversity comes an enormous opportunity to learn and advance.

We must implement prevention strategies in many areas, such as AIDS, where we have a major strategy now in this country called the Prevention Marketing Initiative, which is having a significant impact.

Statistics are helping to develop, implement, and evaluate prevention strategies. So, as we implement prevention strategies throughout the country, we must have the monitoring systems and we must have the data bases, to assess what works and what does not work.

It is not enough to develop good programs. We have spent billions of dollars on programs in this country, often without really knowing whether the money was well spent, and sometimes finding out 10, 20 years later, that they were not effective. We have done that in clinical medicine. We can't afford to do that in the future, and we certainly can't afford to do that in our arena.

As I said earlier, a recent report from NCHS shows that deaths from firearms may soon exceed deaths from motor vehicle crashes as the leading cause of injury mortality in the country, because of what has happened over the last 10 to 15 years. Already, in seven states in this country, deaths from firearm injury equal or exceed deaths from motor vehicle crashes. This fact reflects two changes. For the past two decades, motor vehicle mortality has been declining, while violent deaths have been rising.

Public health, law enforcement, citizens groups, educators, individuals, have united to bring about the decline in motor vehicle crashes. And there is a lot we can learn from that success.

How did it happen? How have we been so successful in terms of motor vehicle accidents? We have designed safer cars in this country. We have built better highways. We have had fewer alcohol– related deaths, although we still have too many. And we have promoted seat belt use. All have contributed to this reduction.

We are now bringing in a similar coalition of concerned officials and citizens, to address gun– related violence. We need to know where to intervene. The CDC funded work led by Art Kellerman, who is here with you, and his colleagues, published in the New England Journal of Medicine last year, shows what happens when a family purchases a gun and brings it into the home. In part the study showed that rather than confer protection, guns kept in the home are associated with an increase in the risk of homicide by a family member or intimate acquaintance. This is a good example of the kinds of information we need documented scientifically in order to get a handle on this problem.

I spoke on this problem the other day at the National Press Club after Senator Bradley had recently said that ultimately the violence problem is not going to be solved just in Washington, but in our communities and in our homes. And believe me, we have a long way to go in our homes, where children still have access to firearms, and often find them when parents and grandparents are away.

Our fourth CDC priority is women's health. I can tell you that the issue of women's health as a priority, is not just a CDC priority, but a top priority throughout the Department of Health and Human Services. First of all, this priority acknowledges years of neglect in this area, and that neglect also applies in the area of prevention as evidenced by the fact that AIDS is spreading fastest among women in this country.

I attended the Eighth International Conference on AIDS in Morocco, for the African continent in December. It was a little frustrating, because there is so much bad news, as you know. On the plane back, I was reading a UNICEF assessment of AIDS in Africa. The report said that perhaps the single most important factor that could curtail the spread of AIDS in Africa would be the empowerment of women there, especially in the areas of sexual relationships and family relationships.

To a lesser extent, I believe, the same issue relates to health in this country, where women play such an important role in the health of the family, and yet often are not empowered to make a difference in their own health status, let alone their family's.

AIDS and other STDs such as chlamydia still account for about 150,000 cases of infertility in women each year. CDC has demonstrated the ability to significantly impact the problem, using a model in four states in the country, which we now hope to take to the rest of the country.

Domestic and workplace violence are also problems that pose serious threats to the health of women. Homicide is the leading cause of death for women in the workplace in this country. Domestic violence often leads women to the emergency room and, according to our data, during these visits to ER's, domestic violence often is not even diagnosed or reported.

We have established these four priorities, and we have identified cross– cutting issues that relate to all of these priorities. In order to accomplish our goals, we are adopting some new approaches.

I want to reemphasize the importance of new partnerships, if we are going to be successful. When I say new partnerships in this country, of course, we recognize that our relationships with local and state health departments, schools of public health, and preventive medicine programs remain critical.

We have also recognized that, if we are going to be successful in our prevention of AIDS and violence, we must develop some new partnerships. So, we are looking at community groups—our school systems, for example, offer an excellent opportunity to deal positively with teenagers and children at every level.

We have demonstrated the cost effectiveness of school– based education, and yet, there is too little of it taking place in this country. The school system is a very important ally. Churches and business communities are also very important. For example, The Rotary Clubs of this country have contributed almost $250 million to our polio eradication program. They have also been very active in our AIDS prevention program. More than ever before, new partnerships are going to be critical for the future.

Community involvement must include the local , state and national community, but the also the world community, in order for us to solve these problems.

For many of the world's health crises, such as AIDS, knowledge and information can be a most important injury prevention tool. We will test and duplicate what works best. We have a lot of knowledge about what works and will have a great impact, such as immunization and bicycle helmets in terms of injuries—we know how effective they have been. The effectiveness of seat belts is probably the best example.

We must continue to evaluate what works. Good data are critical. I want to emphasize the importance of data. The publication Injury in America highlights the role of data in injury research. A prerequisite for the scientific study of injury is the acquisition of data, on which we base priorities and research. Despite the obvious importance of injury as a public health problem, information to permit the study of the epidemiology of most injuries is still not available. We still don't have the information base.

No data is available on time, place and persons for some injuries and deaths, and even basic information is often lacking, such as the numbers and characteristics of people injured in nonfatal incidents. We must improve our databases.

Data are needed for planning, research, prevention, intervention, evaluation, setting priorities and measuring progress. Data help us to identify causes, risk factors, and groups at greater risk. Data are also used to develop consensus, to motivate citizens, to empower communities, and to provide policy. Data are a powerful force.

In the United States, statistics documenting the epidemics of firearm violence are an example of how data have been used to inform the debate. If you have been reading our papers this week—USA TODAY, NEW YORK TIMES—you have seen these articles on violence, substantiated by current scientific data.

Statistics showing that firearms are the second leading cause of death to Americans from the age of 15 to 34 have quantified a problem that people experience personally in their neighborhoods or in nearby communities. Data are what give meaning to these experiences. These numbers have moved people and policy makers to an array of decisions, from limiting access to weapons—the numbers helped pass the Brady bill and the bill against assault weapons. Numbers helped to prove the point in developing programs for conflict resolution among teenagers.

Many of you from other parts of the world are faced with a different set of challenges, but we share mutual need for data to help us understand the magnitude of the problem, to assess risk factors, and to guide us in developing strategies to lessen the burden of injury.

We must improve injury statistics. For example, in the United States, there are very sophisticated and highly technological processes for coding cause of death from a death certificate. Yet, more specific information about circumstances leading up to the fatality is needed to ultimately prevent the deaths. That is what we don't have.

In terms of morbidity, our national knowledge level is even more basic. We know how many people are hospitalized as a result of fractures, but, from the records, we can't tell what caused those fractures—whether it was a fall, or a motor vehicle crash.

We need community level data, as well as national data. Injury statistics need to be complete, comparable, timely, and appropriate for analysis and interpretation. We must be able to link data from various systems, in order to expand the knowledge and the analytical capacity of the data.

We have a lot of data systems at CDC. You wouldn't believe how many we have! The problem is that the systems don't communicate with each other very well. So, the real challenge we face today is figuring out a way to link and integrate these data systems, as we move ahead. It is going to be critical for our health care and public health reform.

We must be able to improve the ability of data systems to relate and communicate with each other, not just at CDC. For example, The Substance Abuse and Mental Health Services Administration (SAMHSA) is the agency that deals with drug abuse in this country. Just think about the relationship of drug abuse and injury, and how important it is to be able to link data from SAMHSA and other programs to CDC data bases. Improvements are being made, however. Hospitals are being encouraged to use the E codes in the International Classification of Diseases, to capture information about the cause of injuries. And so, it is beginning.

Just two months ago, NCHS published the first national estimates of the causes of injury based on a national sample of emergency department visits.

To improve data on non- fatal workplace injury, NIOSH is now using the Consumer Products Safety Commission's electronic surveillance system to monitor occupational injuries among young and mature workers.

NIOSH would like to expand this system to track workplace injuries treated in emergency rooms, among workers of all ages.

One of my favorite stories concerns an experience I had in Morocco. Teenagers from throughout Africa were invited to attended the Eighth International Symposium. This was the first time they had been invited, and they were there because of the obvious role that teenagers play in the spread of this epidemic. The teenagers discovered that the new director of CDC was there, so they asked if I would participate in a roundtable discussion. I did and it was an interesting experience. They asked me about CDC, its history and its commitment to solving the AIDS problem. They asked me a lot of questions. As I sat there with these teenagers from throughout Africa, I realized they reminded me very much of teenagers in this country.

So, I decided to ask them a question. I said, "I am curious. Why is it that teenagers today—I have a couple at home, too, by the way—why is it that teenagers today engage in so many high risk behaviors? I mean, if it is not violence or drug abuse, it's early school drop-out or tobacco use. Teenagers today seem to be attracted to high risk behaviors, at least from an adult's point of view." One young man from Southern Africa responded, "Dr. Satcher, are you familiar with the expression that in Africa it takes a whole village to raise a child? I responded that I had heard that before. He said, "Then, I'd like to ask you another question—Where is our village? Where is our community? Where are people who care about children; not just their own children but all children? Where are people who care about the environment?" I thought about that a lot. So, I say to you today that teenagers in this country are probably asking the same question—Where is their community when they need it?

We need a world community involved in solving these problems. And in order to achieve that, we have to begin with conferences like this, where we look to the future and say, "How are we going to cooperate and collaborate in solving some serious world problems?"

Thank you for your attention.

Welcome

Duane Alexander, M.D.

It is a pleasure to be here on behalf of the National Institute of Child Health and Human Development, and join in welcoming you to this landmark event, and to state how pleased we are to be a part of this effort.

We have been a part, from the start, of the international cooperative effort on infant mortality, and have seen the successes of that program, how it has contributed to our knowledge through the development of standard definitions, of standard data collection efforts, and understanding in infant mortality rates across countries by our joint activities in this area.

We hope that this international cooperative effort on injury statistics will be similarly fruitful and productive.

I want to start by talking a little bit behind Dr. Satcher's back, and point out to you the special role he has played, not only in getting this started, but in assuring that we have inclusion of violence and intentional injury statistics in this whole effort.

This has been something that has required his leadership, and not only in this particular effort, but in bringing activities of research and prevention activities within states and state health departments, to bear on the whole problem of violence and intentional injury in our society.

You heard him speak a little bit about this in his opening remarks here, but I think that you should be aware of the fact that this is a very sensitive topic and it took a person not only with the broad public health perspective of the importance of this as an issue, but with the personal courage and commitment to make it a priority item for the CDC and the Public Health Service.

I want to salute Dr. Satcher particularly for that activity and that effort.

The NICHD, over the past eight to ten years, has developed a major research program in injury research and injury prevention in children, with the encouragement of the American Academy of Pediatrics, and the Congress. During this time, that program has grown from one lonely research grant to a multi–million dollar program in grants and contracts in epidemiology and statistics activities, as well as in the epidemiology and prevention research program.

This has been done under the guidance and direction initially of Dr. Pete Scheidt, later joined by Mary Overpeck, by Bruce Simons Morton, by Yossi Harel, and by Jordan Finkelstein. And you will be hearing from some of them later in this program, about some of those activities and efforts.

The interests of the Institute, however, extends beyond just that part of the program in injury prevention. It also has a component of intervention studies in violence reduction among adolescents, that is part of this activity. And also, we extend our interests to the role of injury in causing disability, and approaches to rehabilitation of persons injured by either violence, or unintentional injuries.

So, we have a program that really spans the scope of injury related activity. Thus, we are pleased to be part of this new international cooperative effort. We think that we have something to contribute. We certainly have much to learn from this effort, on a broad scale. We look forward not only to this symposium, but to the continuing interaction with our colleagues at the Centers for Disease Control, specifically in the National Center for Health Statistics, and colleagues throughout the world, as represented here.

So, enjoy your conference, and we look forward to continuing to work with you. Thank you.

Charge to Participants

Manning Feinleib, M.D., Dr.P.H.

I am glad Dr. Satcher was able to be here to address us this morning. He spoke on many critical and important issues and I think he did a fine job outlining the importance of this symposium, this ICE effort, and the overall efforts of CDC. And Duane Alexander, I would like to thank you for your generous support for this conference, and, if we are halfway as successful as we have been with the ICE on infant and perinatal mortality, it will be a real accomplishment also. I would like to thank all of those who have been involved in the planning of this meeting, particularly, in addition to the NCHS staff, the staff of NCIPC, who had a major role in the development of the program and the selection of the topics. And welcome to all of you, especially our guests from abroad.

This international collaborative effort is made up of researchers from NCHS, other units in CDC, other public health services agencies, and researchers from selected foreign governments and research organizations. We all share a mutual concern for the quality of data. All of you have made, and continue to make, valuable contributions, providing data of high quality related to injury control.

This ICE on injury statistics has two main purposes. First, to learn more about ourselves through comparisons with others. And secondly, to improve international comparability and quality of injury data. During the three days of this meeting, we will begin to achieve an in-depth understanding of different national practices for defining and measuring injury, morbidity, and mortality. This understanding will provide a sound context for analyzing differences in injury rates, as a developing strategy to improve the quality, reliability, and comparability of international statistics on injuries. The ultimate goal is to provide the data needed to better understand the causes of injury and the most effective means of prevention.

The ICE program at NCHS consists of multinational collaborative activities, usually of several years duration. Our meeting today is the beginning of an ongoing process that will continue through other meetings, consultations, further research and analysis, and many collaborative projects. As you have heard, this ICE is the third in a series. And it will follow the patterns developed and successfully utilized through the earlier international collaborative efforts. The first ICE was on perinatal and infant mortality; the second, on issues related to aging. The ICE on injury statistics is, in part, a natural extension of the previous efforts. The ICE on aging, for example, has a project on significant morbidity related to osteoporosis and hip fractures caused by falls. In the ICE on infant and perinatal mortality, injuries have been identified as an oftentimes overlooked source of mortality and morbidity among infants.

In selecting participants for the ICE, we are particularly interested in countries and programs that have successfully tackled some of the data issues that we are concerned about, and who are willing to explore the establishment of comparable methods and definitions so that international comparisons can be valid.

NCHS, as the principal health statistic agency in the federal government, plays an important role in the coordination of data activities. Like charity, coordination begins at home. As in many countries, NCHS obtains injury data from such diverse sources as health interviews, hospital records, emergency and outpatient department visits, physician office visits and death certificates. You will hear about the findings from these diverse activities later in this meeting. But let me give you just a few examples of the relevance of this information to some of our current and evolving priorities.

First, the year 2000 objectives include reducing both unintentional injury and violence. Practically all of the data that are required for the monitoring of these objectives come from NCHS and CDC's data systems.

Another example, work is proceeding on a contract to evaluate the E-code systems for morbidity reports. Many of those involved in that contract are here with us at this symposium. A basic challenge to implementation of these codes to ICD-10 is that it will require the recording and coding of information that is not universally collected at the present time.

A third example, as Dr. Satcher referred to earlier, are the new data collection instruments in the National Hospital Ambulatory Medical Care Survey and the National Health Interview Survey, which are collecting and coding cause-specific injury data for the first time.

We hope, through this ICE on injury statistics, to build on these data efforts and get a clear understanding of remaining issues facing us in this country, as well as those facing those of you from other countries. We hope to begin to identify topics of mutual concern for cross-national investigations, and to identify data bases that can serve as research tools for further collaborative research. Through collaboration with our colleagues in other countries; with federal, state and local agencies in this country; and with researchers in academia and the private sector, we expect that in the long run—and we hope it is not too long—the process of refining data will lead to greater public awareness and stronger public policy on the prevention of injuries. Therefore, I am very pleased to be a part of this effort, to welcome all of you, and to wish you all a very successful meeting.

Levels and Trends in Injury Mortality and Morbidity in Selected Participating Countries

Australian Injury Morbidity and Mortality Data:
Issues for Comparability

by James E. Harrison, M.B., B.S., M.P.H.

Thank you for the opportunity to participate in this ground–breaking international meeting. The goal of the International Collaborative Effort on Injury Statistics is to improve "the quality, reliability, and comparability of international statistics on injuries." Achievement of this goal will have both direct and indirect value for Australia.

Attempts are made quite frequently to compare Australian experience of injury occurrence and control with experience elsewhere. More often than not, comparisons are difficult to make. Sometimes this is because data are not available. Often, however, the difficulty is that data are available for Australia and another country, but their trustworthiness and comparability are uncertain. A direct benefit of the ICE to Australia is that it should assist us in making valid international comparisons, just as it will assist others.

Achievement of the goal will bring other, more important benefits. Many of the problems which must be confronted when using and comparing injury data internationally are the same as those which arise in the course of national or regional injury surveillance and control. This is, I suspect, particularly true in the case of countries (such as Australia), which have a federal structure. Federal agencies confront problems of "the quality, reliability, and comparability of inter*state* statistics on injuries", and lessons learned at the international level are likely to have application at national level.

I have two aims in presenting this paper: to provide a brief picture of injury in Australia, and to relate this illustration of injury in a particular country to the objectives of the symposium.

I shall begin by presenting a definition of injury: "Disruption of the structure or function of the human organism, resulting from exposure to excessive or deficient energy." Typically, both the exposure to energy, and the onset of disruption, are acute. Often the energy is kinetic, but it may be another type (thermal, chemical, etc.).

I do not present this definition (which is based on definitions presented by others) to suggest that it is the last word on the matter but, rather, to underscore the need for clear definitions as the basis for our work in injury statistics. Something close to this definition is, I think, widely accepted in public health circles in Australia, and the following statistical sketch of injury in Australia is based on it. It should be noted that this definition includes injuries irrespective of the role of human intent.

The injury experience of a population is often presented as a pyramid. The apex represents the relatively small number of fatal injury cases, and the broader, lower parts of the pyramid represent the more numerous injuries of lesser severity. Figure 1 is an injury pyramid based on recent Australian data. I introduce the injury pyramid here to make two points about injury data in Australia (and, I think, elsewhere) which are pertinent to international comparability.

First, injury data availability is in direct proportion to case *severity*, and in inverse proportion to case *frequency*. We know quite a lot about the relatively small number of injury deaths, less about hospital inpatient cases, and still less about cases resulting in neither death nor hospital admission. The priorities implied by this hierarchy of information availability may be correct, though the present situation certainly did not result from careful planning of injury data systems. We should be careful not to under–rate the importance, in human and economic terms, of 'less severe' injuries.

Second, constructing the pyramid reminds me of the rough–and–ready nature of many injury case categories used in Australia and elsewhere. For want of more direct measures, we tend to use hospital admission, or attendance at a hospital emergency department, as a proxy for case severity. We do this despite knowing that clinical criteria for admission may vary considerably, that economic and other factors do much to determine which cases will go to which service, and that these factors vary with time and place. Improving our ability to measure the severity of injury (particularly injury that is not life threatening) rigorously and practicably is a challenge for injury researchers, and is important for international comparability of injury data.

Figure 2 shows incidence rates for injury deaths registered in Australia in 1992, by 5–year age groups, and sex. I would like to draw your attention to three points revealed by these data. First, male rates were higher than female – this is so for nearly all classes of injury for which data are available. Second, rates were highest in old age. Third, rates were relatively high for young adult males.

This figure can also be used as a reminder of several technical aspects of injury data that should be specified when reporting data, and kept in mind when comparing them.

The *event being reported* Note that I have reported cases by year of registration, not year of death. At present, about 12% of injury deaths in Australia are registered during a year later than the year of occurrence – nearly all in the following year. Improved death data collection is likely to facilitate early reporting of injury mortality by year of occurrence. This is a worthwhile improvement, particularly for classes of deaths whose rates vary substantially over short periods of time, and enables close monitoring of high priority types of injury.

Denominators In calculating rates, I have used age and sex specific estimates of the Australian population at the mid–point of the period covered by the figure. These estimates, published by the Australian Bureau of Statistics, are based on a national census each five years (most recently in 1991), with estimates for intercensal years being adjusted using birth, death, immigration, and emigration data. Usually (as in this figure) the population estimates used are on the basis of 'place of usual residence'.

Figure 3 is the same as Figure 2, except that the vertical axis shows numbers of injury deaths rather than incidence rates. The salient point is that most injury deaths involve young adult males. Note, also, the small peak in cases in young childhood (this has diminished in recent years).

The prominence of injury mortality in early adult life is still more evident in terms of the age–specific proportions of all deaths which are injury deaths (Figure 4). For males, injury accounted for more than half of all deaths from early childhood until the end of the fourth decade of life. The proportions of female deaths were smaller but were, nonetheless, substantial.

While mortality rates show injury to be an important cause of death, particularly in the first half of life, it is even more prominent in terms of some other measures of ill health. Years of Potential Life Lost ('YPLL'; here measured to age 65 years) due to injury is high because of the early ages at which most injury deaths occur. (Aspects of the method used to calculate YPLL, such as the choice of age thresholds, may warrant consideration by the ICE).

Injury is a frequent reason for admission to hospital, accounting for about one in ten cases in Australia. Surveys of reasons for visiting a doctor, and of self–reported recent illness also reveal the prominence of injury as a source of morbidity.

Surveillance of injury experience in Australia is, as elsewhere, restricted by data limitations (some attempts to overcome the limitations are mentioned at the end of this paper). At present, long term injury data are available, at national level, only for deaths. Figure 6 shows injury death rates since 1921. The main point to note is that both male and female injury rates have tended to decline since the late 1960s, and are now at historically low levels. Since 1968, male rates have declined by about 2.4% per year, and female rates have declined by about 3.1% per year. Note the continuing male excess.

On a technical note again, the rates in this figure have been standardised, by the direct method, to the Australian population in 1988. The use of standardisation as an aid to comparison of injury data is another matter which the ICE may care to consider.

While the recent decline in injury mortality has been considerable, and welcome, it should not be overstated. Other causes of death have declined at about the same rate, and so the proportion of all deaths which are injury deaths has changed less than the rate of injury deaths (Figure 7). Indeed, injury has accounted for a relatively high proportion of male deaths in Australia in recent years.

"Injury" is, of course, a mixed bag of conditions, occurring in diverse circumstances, and involving a wide range of causal factors. Figure 8 shows male rates since 1968 for three major categories of injury deaths, distinguished according to 'external cause': motor vehicle crashes; suicides; and falls. Motor vehicle crash death rates have dropped by more than half during this period – a dramatic decline, which accounts for much of the total decline in injury mortality during the period. Overall, suicide rates changed little during the period (as we shall see, some age–specific rates have risen). Suicide is now more common as a cause of male death than road crashes. Mortality attributed to falls declined gradually.

Figure 9 presents equivalent data for females, which tell a somewhat different story. Female rates were lower than male rates for road deaths and suicides, but similar for falls (falls death *case counts* are higher for females than males, reflecting the sex–distribution of the elderly population at risk). Rates for all three categories showed noticeable decline during the period.

Australian injury mortality data are coded according to the 'External Causes' classification of the 9th revision of the International Classification of Diseases (ICD9). Only one 'E–code' is provided per case, and 'injury and poisoning' codes (from Chapter 17 of ICD9) are not provided. A single E–code is useful, but provides limited insight into the circumstances of injury occurrence, and no direct information on the nature of the trauma sustained.

The data items and classifications used in injury statistics do much to determine what is – and can be – revealed. For example, alcohol is known to be an important factor in the occurrence of many types of injury, yet routine injury data collections generally do not record information on alcohol involvement (greater efforts have been made for road injury). Many significant categories of injury cannot be distinguished easily in Australian mortality and hospital admission data – occupational injuries and sports–related injuries for example. To a large extent, these defects reflect national reliance on ICD9. The National Injury Surveillance Unit (NISU) and others involved on injury surveillance and prevention are seeking to extend the information available about injury deaths in Australia, by co–operating with coroners to develop a national coroner case data system.

Geographic, social, economic and demographic factors contribute to injury risk. Groups attracting particular interest and concern differ between countries and with time. I have chosen to present the injury mortality experience of Aboriginal Australians as an example of the impact of these types of factors. The health disadvantage of Aboriginal Australians is becoming well known. Figure 10 shows a comparison of the injury mortality of Aborigines with that of all other Australians, during the three year period 1990 to 1992. The Aboriginal rates were much higher than those for the rest of the population.

This figure provides a good opportunity to mention another technical aspect of comparison of injury data, which might well be considered by the ICE: assessment of the significance of apparent differences between rates, particularly when case numbers (or populations) are small. For example, the rate shown in Figure 10 for Aboriginal Australians aged 75 years and above is derived from 12 deaths over three years, in a population whose mid–point size was 1583 persons.

The data source on which case counts in this figure are based – routine mortality data – is supposed to contain a record for every death registered. As such, it can be seen as a census of deaths, and case counts derived from this data collection are not subject to sampling error. The population estimate is also from a census. Where a rate is calculated on the basis of a large numbers of cases, it can be regarded, more or less, as an absolute value. If the number of cases is small, however, it should be recognised that the rate estimate is subject to chance variation in the precise number of cases that occurred in the period under consideration (e.g., two cases rather than one in a category would double the rate estimate).

A method used to take chance variation into account assumes that the number of injuries occurring in any time period is an independent variable which tends to follow a Poisson probability distribution (the National Center for Health Statistics presents formulae for calculating approximate confidence intervals based on this assumption in a technical appendix to many of its publications). Application of this approach to the data in Figure 10 confirms that the Aboriginal rates are significantly higher than non–Aboriginal rates overall, and for most of the age groups shown. For the age groups 10–14 years, and 75 years and over, however, the Aboriginal rate excess was not significant at the p=0.05 level.

Note that one Australian state (Queensland) did not supply information on Aboriginality for deaths registered during this period. This can serve as a reminder of the many situations in which data on a subject of interest are incomplete. The incomplete data on Aboriginal mortality are a lot better than no data – the situation that prevailed until a few years ago.

Routine injury data can be used in a number of ways. Analysis of historical data reveals events which may be important for the future control of injury. For example, the change from coal gas to petroleum gas for domestic purposes appears to have been associated in Australia (as it was in Britain and elsewhere) with a decline in suicide by this means (Figure 11). A more dramatic example is the rise and fall in suicide using pharmaceutical substances that coincided with the widespread use, then restriction, of barbiturates in Australia (Figure 12). The significance of such examples for the present is that awareness of historical trends is helping to ensure that environmental factors are taken into account in current attempts to develop strategies for suicide control in Australia.

Injury data can also lead to new recognition of problems, and may prompt causal hypotheses. For example, initial analysis of the Aboriginal injury mortality data mentioned a moment ago reveals striking differences between Aboriginal and non–Aboriginal suicide patterns (Figure 13). Is the peak in Aboriginal rates in early adulthood seen here a data artifact, or a stable pattern, or is this a breaking wave of suicide beginning with recent birth cohorts? While these data alone don't provide an answer, they can prompt us to ask the questions.

Increasingly, the available data are being used for priority setting in injury control, and for setting quantitative injury control targets. Figure 14 concerns one of a set of draft national targets which is presently out for public comment prior to refinement and anticipated adoption by Australia's governments. The aim is to achieve a year 2000 'All injury' mortality rate 20 percent lower than the rate in 1992.

An issue for the ICE raised by this Figure is the definition of 'all injury'. In the proposed Australian target, injury is defined as all deaths receiving an ICD 'External Cause' code except those attributed to medical and surgical complications and misadventures (i.e. E870–879), or to adverse effects of medications in therapeutic use (i.e. E930–949). These groups, account for only a small proportion of E–coded deaths, but about one–quarter of injury hospital admissions receive an E–code in these ranges. They have been excluded on the basis of a view that these cases are part of a rather different issue from that represented by other 'E–codes', and require different responses.

Another proposed injury control target is for drowning at ages 0 to 4 years (Figure 15). Drowning accounted for more than one–third of all 'External Causes' deaths in this age group in Australia in 1992. More than half of the drowning deaths occurred when a child fell or wandered into a private swimming pool.

We know this latter point because a special classification is being applied to drowning deaths in Australia. The International Classification of Diseases (9th revision), used to classify 'causes of death', treats drowning in a way that is not sufficient for current circumstances in Australia. Responding to the lack of necessary detail on circumstances of drownings, special supplementary classifications were developed in several states. Beginning with 1992 death registrations, one of these classifications is being applied nation–wide. This provides an example of a general challenge to classification of injury: information requirements change over time, and differ between settings, suggesting a need to try to design systems that can accommodate changes, and to allow for special local or regional requirements.

Rates of non–intentional drowning, and of most other categories of non–intentional injury in Australia, are declining or steady. The same cannot be said for intentional injury. While still low by world standards, homicide rates are tending to rise (Figure 16 shows rates for males and females aged 20 to 39 years).

More dramatic is the thirty–year rise in suicide rates amongst young adult males (Figure 17). Male suicide rates at older ages declined a little during the same period. A proposed year 2000 target appears optimistic, in the light of the historic trends. Reversals in Australian suicide rates almost as dramatic as the one implied by the target have occurred (see Figure 12), when a specific environmental factor changed. While a number of suicide control measures are being proposed now, I know of none for which there is substantial evidence that would warrant prediction of a turnaround of the magnitude implied by this target, and I suspect that these trend data were not taken into account in framing the draft target.

Proposed Australian injury control goals and targets address a number of other topics which have also been identified as warranting special attention. A problem for target–setting is the lack of adequate baseline data for many topics on which we might wish to set targets. Data are imperfect for mortality, scantier for injury morbidity than mortality, and very limited for exposure to risk factors.

The need to improve injury data is recognised, and the National Injury Surveillance Unit has a key role in bringing about the necessary changes. Here is a list of my priorities for improving injury data in Australia. In the light of these priorities, my interest in the ICE should come as no surprise.

Issue	Developments	Expected Benefits
• Data standards	• National Health Data Dictionary • National Minimum Dataset for Injury Surveillance	• better comparability • efficiency
• Injury mortality	• coroner data system	• timeliness • detailed information
• In–patient injury morbidity	• national morbidity collection	• comparability • accessibility
• Ambulatory injury morbidity	• integrated special purpose emergency department collection	• quantitative rigour • efficient collection
• Special purpose injury surveillance	• trauma service information systems • rare injury registers (e.g., spinal injury) • sector–specific information system (e.g., sports injury; farm injury	• various benefits

At national level, a key task is the first—standard setting. In collaboration with several injury surveillance and control groups, NISU has developed a National Minimum Data Set for Injury Surveillance (NMDS–IS). The principles which have guided its design are public health usefulness; ease of data collection; capacity for integration in general purpose data systems; and compatibility, with the ICD, and with the Australian National Health Data

Dictionary (a developing standard for national reporting of hospital admission data). An outline of the core data items in the NMDS–IS is shown in Figure 18.

Apart from the narrative injury description item (which is of crucial importance), the NMDS–IS maps very closely onto both the 9th and 10th revisions of the International Classification of Diseases. The minimum data set is in use in a number of emergency departments, and is being assessed for inclusion in the National Health Data Dictionary, and by groups developing ambulatory services data systems at state and regional level. We expect that further development of data standards, together with projects to improve national aggregation of data on injury admissions, and the collection of enhanced injury mortality data by coroners, will result in further improvement of injury surveillance and control in Australia over the next few years. These developments will improve "the quality, reliability, and comparability" of Australian statistics on injuries. In undertaking this work, we will try to learn from experience gained in other countries, and will be pleased if others find worthwhile lessons in the Australian experience.

Thank you for your attention. I hope I have achieved my twin aims of introducing Australian injury data to you, while also raising some of the issues which we'll be considering during the rest of this Symposium, and afterwards, during the very welcome International Collaborative Effort on Injury Statistics. I trust that some fruit of the Effort will be on display at the 3rd International Conference on Injury Prevention and Control, in Melbourne, Australia in February 1996.

Note on data: Unless stated otherwise, data in this paper were analysed by NISU using mortality and population data supplied by the Australian Bureau of Statistics.

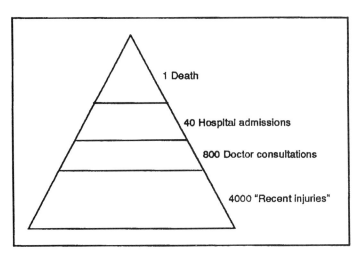

Figure 1. Australian "Injury Pyramid" (approximate values)

Figure 2: Injury deaths Australia, 1992: Incidence rates by age group and sex.

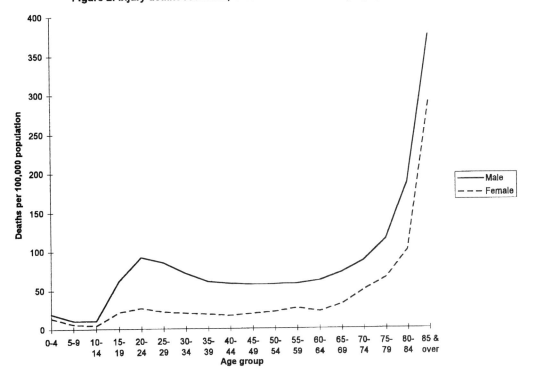

Figure 3: Injury deaths Australia, 1992: case counts by age group and sex.

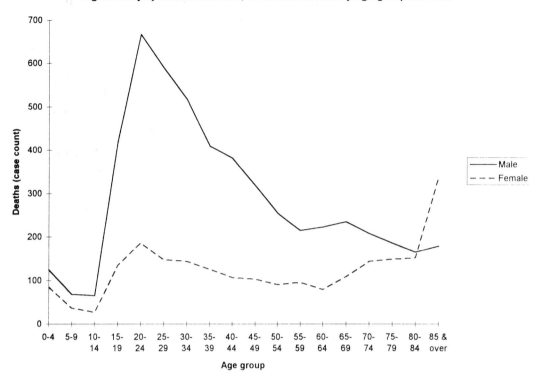

Figure 4: Injury as a proportion of all deaths, Australia 1992: by age and sex.

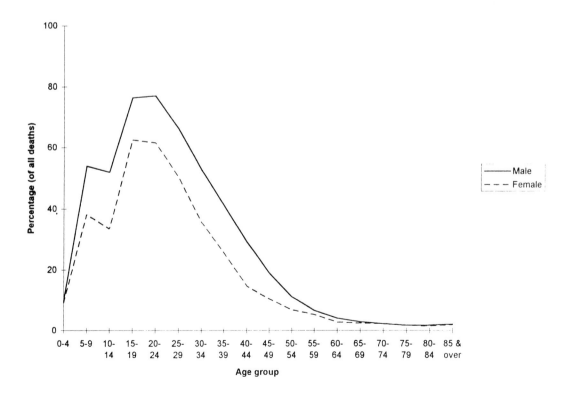

Figure 5: Rank of injury and other causes of ill-health, Australia 1990/91 (or closest available year)

Rank	Mortality	YPLL (<65)	Admissions	Bed-days	Doctor visits	Recent illness
1	circulatory	other	other	other	other	other
2	neoplasm	**INJURY**	**INJURY**	circulatory	respiratory	respiratory
3	other	neoplasm	circulatory	**INJURY**	circulatory	circulatory
4	respiratory	circulatory	respiratory	neoplasm	**INJURY**	**INJURY**
5	**INJURY**		neoplasm	respiratory	infectious	infectious
6	infectious		infectious	infectious	neoplasm	neoplasm

YPLL(<65)=Years of Potential Life Lost before age 65 years.   Recent Illness=episodes reported at interview.

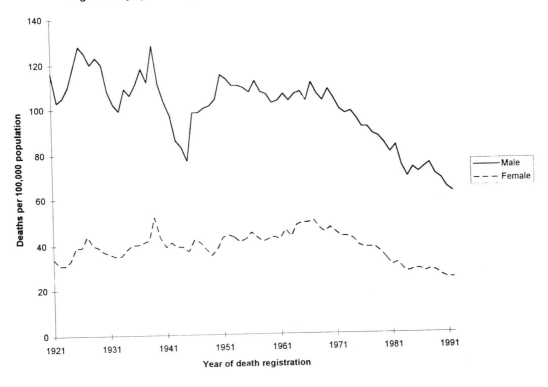

Figure 6: Injury mortality, Australia 1921-1992: age standardised rates, by sex.

Figure 7: Injury deaths as a proportion of all deaths, Australia 1921-1992: by sex.

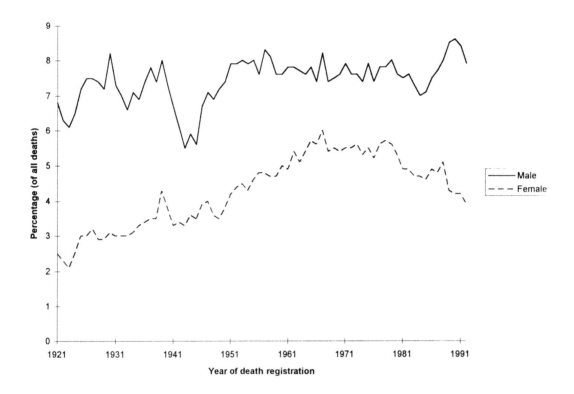

Figure 8: Mortality from three major types of injury, Australia 1964-92: males, age standardised rates.

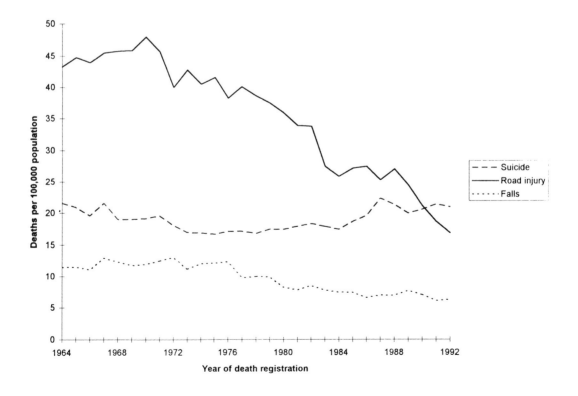

Figure 9: Mortality from three major types of injury, Australia 1964-92: females, age standardised rates.

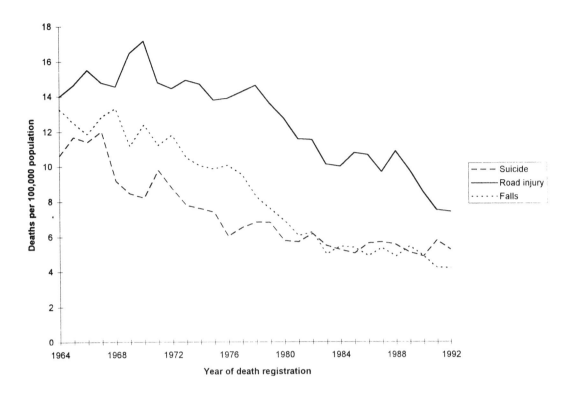

Figure 10: Aboriginal and non-Aboriginal injury mortality, 1990-92: Australia (except Queensland)

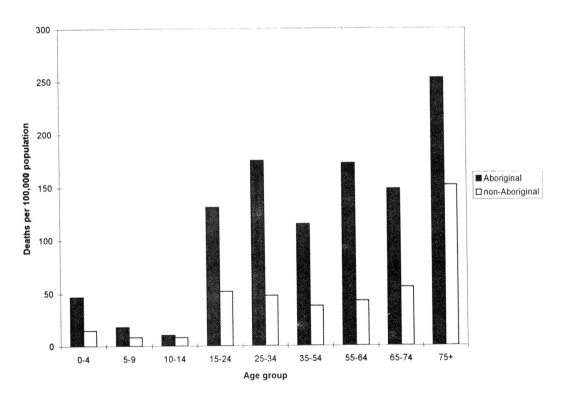

Figure 11: Suicide by gas, Australia 1922-92: females.

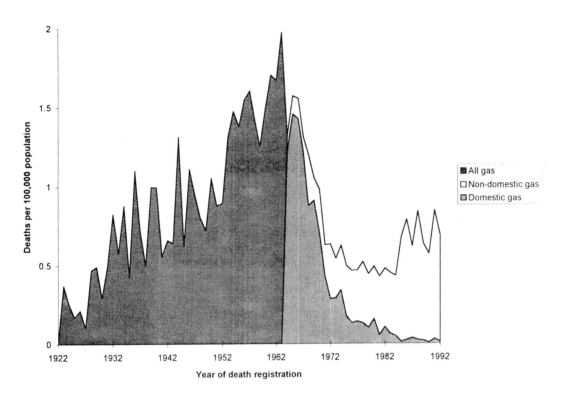

Figure 12: Common methods of suicide Australia 1922-92: female, age standardised rates.

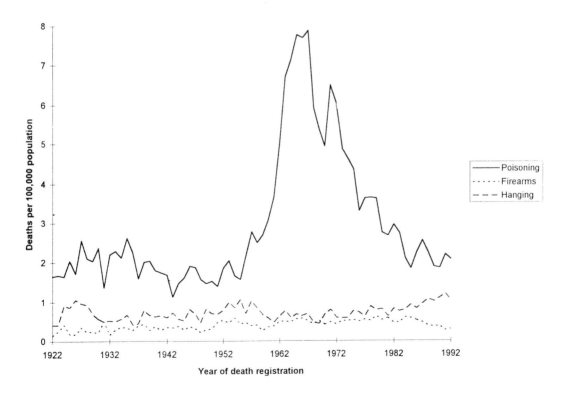

Figure 13: Suicide mortality, Aboriginal and other persons, Australia (except Queensland) 1990-92

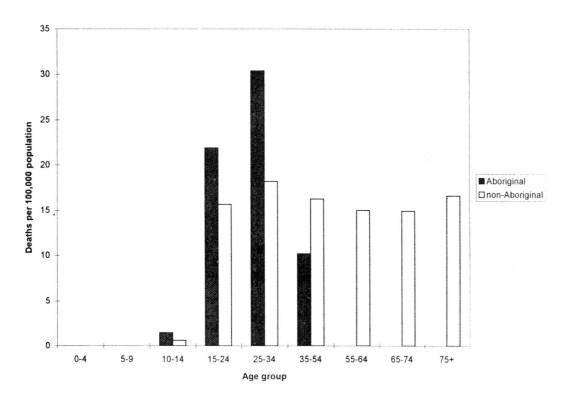

Figure 14: Injury mortality Australia, 1968-92: age standardised rates, by sex

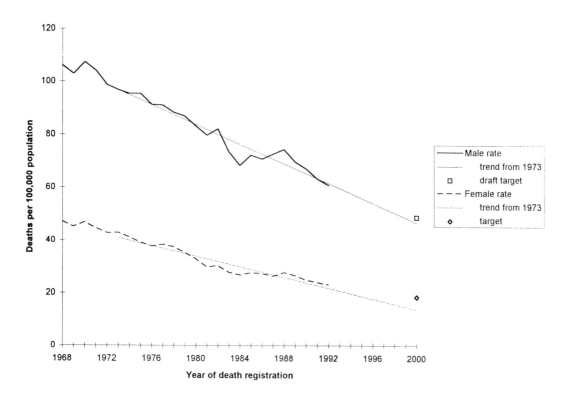

Figure 15: Australian injury trends and targets: drowning, 0-4 years, 1964-92.

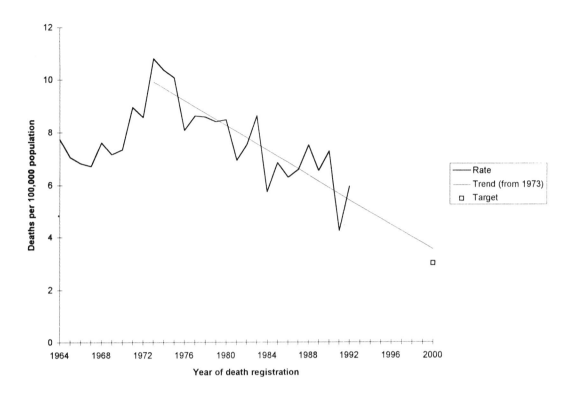

Figure 16: Australian injury trends and targets: homicide, 20-39 years, 1964-92

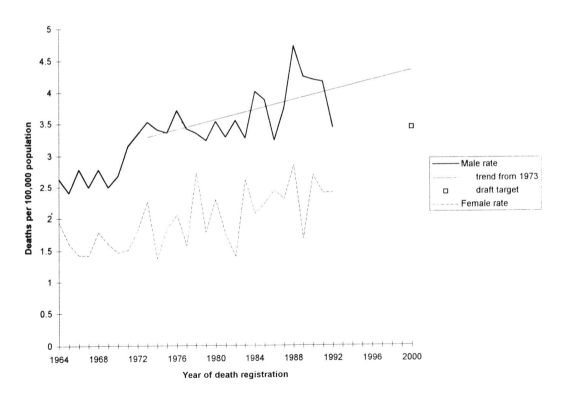

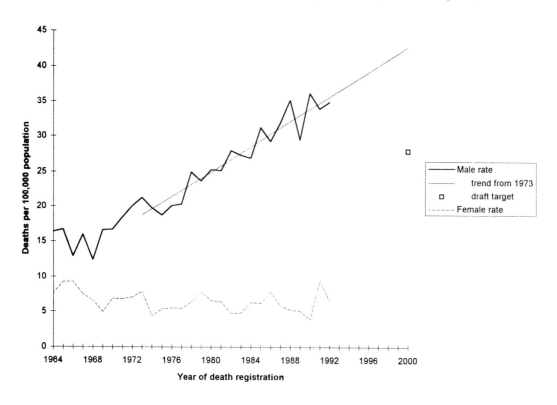

Figure 17: Australian injury trends and targets: suicide, males 20-24 years, 1964-92

Figure 18: National Minimum Data Set for Injury Surveillance

	Minimum	Extended
Narrative description of injury event	<=100 characters	unlimited
Main 'external cause'	29 'cause' groups	full ICD9 E-codes
	11 'intent' groups	
Type of place of occurrence	13 categories	
Type of activity	9 categories	
Trauma	30 'nature' groups	full ICD9 Chapter 17 codes
	22 'body part' groups	

Levels and Trends in Injury Mortality and Morbidity in Sweden Since 1978

by Leif Svanström, Ph.D., Lars Berg, M.D., Anders Åberg, and Lothar Schelp

Abstract

Sweden has after the Second World War established itself as a Welfare State, with a high life expectancy. However the reputation of a leading statistical system goes even further back. All citizens are covered in the national population register, since 1749. Death diagnoses are known since 1911, but there are reports on mortality pattern as early as in the late 18th century. The population is now 8,700,000, with 18 percent above 65 years of age.

Overall mortality has decreased substantially after the second world war. Injuries are the leading cause of death up to 45 years of age. However the rate of fatal injuries has decreased from above 100 per 100,000 mean population for men 1977 to 75 the year 1991. The corresponding figures for women are from 70 to 40. All types of injuries, intentional as well as non- intentional, have decreased about the same, for both genders.

Forty people per 100,000 cars in traffic (14 per 100,000 population) were killed in traffic injuries the year 1975. Corresponding figures 1992 were 19 (9 per 100,000 population). The number of work related fatal injuries were around 400 in 1955, and in 1992 it was less than 80.

About 10 percent of hospital care is due to injuries. About 1/3 of care days for males and more than 1/2 for females are caused by femoral fractures.

This means that there are new priorities above the traditional in injury prevention. A National Injury Prevention Programme has been established since 7-8 years ago.

Background

Sweden has after the Second World War established itself as a Welfare State, with a high life expectancy. However the reputation of a leading statistical system goes even further back. All citizens are covered in the national population register, since 1749.

Life expectancy at current rates in Western Europe, the United States, Canada, Australia, New Zealand and Japan exceeds 75 years; in Japan and the Scandinavian countries (and in some states of the United States such as Hawaii and Minnesota) life expectancy for women is around 80 years . The most reliable data on mortality rates up to the most advanced ages over a long period of time pertain to Sweden. Excellent data exists for Sweden since 1750; "superlative" data have been achieved since 1895 (Vaupel and Lundström 1993). Death diagnoses are known since 1911, but there are reports on mortality pattern as early as in the late 18th century.

The Swedish population is now 8,700,000. Twenty-four and six-tenths percent (1990) are below 20 years of age, 17.8 percent 65 and above. The projection for the year 2025 is 23.2 percent and 21 percent respectively.

Injury Mortality Trends

After heart disease and cancer injury is the most common cause of mortality, while in the age groups -45 years injury is the number one cause of death. Looking at *a long term* perspective nonintentional injuries have been increasing as a cause of death since the beginning of this century but has constantly decreased since 1971 (figure 1). However that development is basically due to the traffic mortality, while drownings has constantly decreased and falls increased during this century.

Looking at *a short term* perspective there has been a decrease in the overall fatal injury rate from around 100 per 100,000 of mean population for males 1976 to 75 per 100,000 in 1991 (figure 2). Corresponding rates for females are 70 per 100,000 and 40 per 100,000. Looking at causes for males all show a decrease during this period with the exception of homicide, which however stays on a very low level (figure 3).

Suicide, falls and motor vehicle dominate as causes. For females there is a corresponding decrease of all causes, however falls are by far the dominating cause of mortality (figure 4).

In general the current picture of mortality is for intentional injuries dominated by suicide. The non-intentional injuries as a cause of death are dominated by falls, about 40 percent, motor vehicles and other traffic, about 30 percent, drownings, another 10 percent, while fire only causes 3 percent (figure 5).

Looking into some *specific* causes *traffic* injuries has decreased substantially both per population and per vehicles (table 1). In 1975 40 persons per 100,000 vehicles were killed, 1992 the rate had decreased to 19. The corresponding rates per 100,000 mean population were 14 and 9 respectively.

These rates places Sweden among the leading countries in the world together with Norway and Great Britain (table 2). There is a more intermediate group with Denmark, Italy and Finland, while countries like USA and France shows the double rate. The bicycle injury rate is high but is now slowly decreasing (figure 6).

There is a remarkable decrease of *work* related fatal injuries (figure 7).

Fatal *drownings* are to 1/3 related to boats activities, 29 out of 167 are related to activities on ice or with snowmobiles and only 18 of 167 are related to bathing (table 3). The figures have varied during the last decade from 145 to 203, with an average of 172.

In general there has been a remarkable decrease of *childhood* injuries in Sweden. A comparison made by Bergman and Rivara shows that USA and Sweden had the same injury mortality in the age group 5-14 years 1957-59 and Sweden had a higher rate for age 1-4 years, while 30 years later Sweden showed a rate of 1/4 to 1/3 of that of USA (figure 8).

Falls account to a major part of the mortal nonintentional injuries. Looking at trends (figure 9) for females as well as for males (figure 10) there is a remarkable decrease from 1980 to 1986. This is explained by changes in coding routines. However there seems to be a decrease for females from 1988 onwards, but an increase for males during the same period.

Injury "Morbidity" Trends

Hospital discharge registers is the main source of information on injuries besides the mortality register. By far the most dominating cause of hospital in-patient care due to *non-intentional injuries* is falls, 57 percent in 1988, thereafter transport, 13 percent (figure 11). Actually about 1/3 of the hospital care days for males and more than 1/2 for females in Sweden were caused by femoral fractures (table 4).

There has since long been an increase in the rate of non-intentional injuries leading to hospital care for females, dominated by falls (figure 12). However there is now a levelling of, even a decrease. There is also a corresponding development for males (figure 13).

Looking at hospital care due to *intentional injuries* shows that almost 60 percent are caused by suicide attempts and 20 percent by assaults (figure 14).

During the last 15-20 years there is a growing source of information on injuries through local surveillance systems based on all kinds of doctor's and hospital visits. In table 5 are reported percent distribution of registered injuries in two counties and one municipality. About 1/3 of injuries occur at home, 1/6 at transport, production/commerce and sports environment respectively.

Looking at a similar surveillance in Falköping 1978 (Schelp and Svanström 1986) indicates an injury incidence in total of 113 per 1,000 inhabitants and year out of which 27 per 1,000 are home injuries, 22 per 1,000 are work related injuries and 9 per 1,000 are transport injuries. The surveillance system from Motala municipality shows for 1983‑84 that 38 percent of *traffic‑related injuries* are caused by cyclists and another 29 percent by pedestrians (figure 15). A similar study from Lidköping municipality 1984 shows that the dominating age group is 15‑24 followed by 0‑14 (table 6).

The study from the Motala surveillance system also shows that 40 percent of *sports injuries* are caused by soccer, 10 percent by basket/volleyball/handball and 10 percent by bandy and ice‑hockey.

Summary and Conclusion

The rate of fatal injuries has decreased from above 100 per 100,000 mean population for men 1977 to 75 the year 1991. The corresponding figures for women are from 70 to 40. All types of injuries, intentional as well as non-intentional, have decreased about the same, for both genders.

Forty people per 100,000 cars in traffic (14 per 100,000 population) were killed in traffic injuries the year 1975. Corresponding figures 1992 were 19 (9 per 100,000 population). The number of work related fatal injuries were around 400 in 1955, in 1992 it was less than 80. Actually more people are now killed in bicycle injuries yearly than at work!

About 10 percent of hospital care is due to injuries. About 1/3 of care days for males and more than 1/2 for females are caused by femoral fractures.

This means that there are new priorities than the traditional in injury prevention. A National Injury Prevention Programme has been established since 7‑8 years ago in order to formulate national targets and strategies as well as to support regional and local preventive activities. There is also a priority to improve the quality of national, regional and local registers and surveillance systems.

References

1.   Bergman AB and Rivara FP. Sweden's Experience in Reducing Childhood Injuries. Pediatrics 1991:88(1).

2.   Causes of Death 1987. Stockholm: Statistics Sweden, 1989.

3.   Causes of Death 1988. Stockholm: Statistics Sweden, 1991.

4.   Causes of Death 1991. Stockholm: Statistics Sweden, 1993.

5.   Drowning statistics 1993. Stockholm: Press Information, Swedish Life Saving Society, 1994.

6.   Hospital Discharge Registry. Stockholm: National Board of Health and Welfare, Centre for Epidemiology, 1994.

7.   Lindqvist K. Towards Community‑Based Injury Prevention. The Motala Model. Linköping: Linköping University, Dept. of Community Medicine, 1993. Thesis.

8.   Schelp L and Svanström L. One-Year Incidence of Home Accidents in a Rural Swedish Municipality. Scand J Soc Med 1986;14:75-82.

9.   Strategies for a Safe Sweden. Stockholm: National Board of Health and Welfare, 1991.

10.   Traffic Injuries 1991. Stockholm: Statistics Sweden, 1992.

11.   Vaupel J W and Lundström H. Longer Life Expectancy?: Evidence from Sweden of Reductions in Mortality Rates at Advanced Ages. Odense University, Denmark and Duke University, USA and Statistics Sweden. Manuscript. 1993.

12.   Work- related Injuries. Stockholm: Statistics Sweden, 1992.

Table 1. Fatal traffic injuries in Sweden 1975-1992, by 100 000 vehicles in traffic, 100 000 mean population and year. Source: Traffic Injuries 1991. Stockholm: Statistics Sweden 1992.

	Year				
	1975	1980	1985	1990	1992
Killed/100 000 veh		40	28	24	20	19
Killed/100 000 pop		14	10	10	9	9

Table 2. No. of killed in traffic injuries per 100 000 inhabitants in some selected countries, by year. Source: Traffic Injuries 1991. Stockholm: Statistics Sweden 1992.

	Year			
	1975	1980	1985	1990
Norway	13	9	10	8
Sweden	14	10	10	9
GB	12	11	9	9
Denmark	16	13	15	12
Italy	18	16	13	12
Finland	19	12	11	13
USA	21	22	18	18
France	27	25	21	20

Table 3. Number of fatal drownings in Sweden 1992, by cause and age. Source: Drowning statistics 1993. Stockholm: Press Information, Swedish Life Saving Society, 1994.

Cause	Children			Adults	Total
	0-4	5-9	10-14		
Ice/ snowmobile	1	2	1	25	29
Bathing	0	2	0	16	18
Sport boats	0	0	2	52	54
Vessels	0	0	0	2	2
Other	6	0	1	57	64
Total	7	4	4	152	167

Table 4. Number of hospital discharges and care days caused by injuries in Sweden 1989, by diagnosis and gender. Source: Hospital Discharge Registry. Stockholm: National Board of Health and Well, Centre for Epidemiology, 1994.

Diagnosis	Gender	No. discharges	No. care days	%
Scull fractures	M	2 846	19 558	
	F	1 080	8 400	
Femoral fractures	M	6 599	196 069	31
	F	18 117	693 081	54
Other fractures	M	18 234	181 319	
	F	21 292	366 627	
All other injuries	M	38 796	243 653	
	F	28 850	209 285	
Total	M	66 475	640 599	100
	F	69 339	1 277 393	100

Table 5. Injuries by environment in two Swedish counties and one municipality. %- distribution. Source: Strategies for a Safe Sweden. Stockholm: National Board of Health and Welfare, 1991.

Environment	Geographical area Bohus county	Lidköping municip	Västmanland county
Transport	12	16	15
Home	37	33	29
Production/ Commerce	14	20	16
School	7	7	11
Sport	15	16	18
Entertainment	3	2	4
Nature	6	3	3
Sea,lake etc	3	1	1
Other	2	1	3
Total	100	100	100

Table 6. Traffic injuries in Lidköping, Sweden, 1984, by age group and gender. In numbers, % and per 1 000 mean population/ year. Source: Lindqvist K. Towards Community- Based Injury Prevention. The Motala Model. Linköping: Linköping University, Dept. of Community Medicine, 1993. Thesis.

Age	Gender M	F	Total	%	Per 1 000 pop/year
0-14	25	27	52	29	8
15-24	34	23	57	31	11
25-34	8	3	11	6	2
35-44	5	9	14	8	3
45-54	8	7	15	8	4
55-64	3	10	13	7	3
65-74	6	9	15	8	4
75-	3	2	5	3	2
Total	92	90	182	100	5

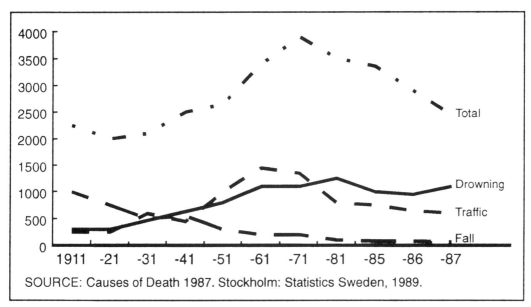

Figure 1. Number of non-intentional injuries in Sweden 1911-87, by cause and year

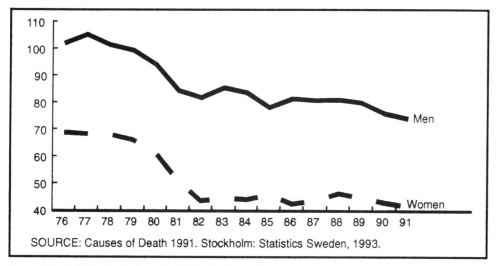

Figure 2. Fatal injuries in Sweden 1976-91, by gender and year. Rate year 100,000 of mean population.

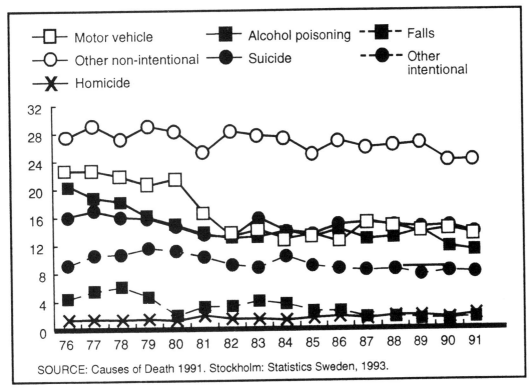

Figure 3. Fatal injuries in Sweden 1976-91, by cause and year. Rates per 100,000 of mean population. Males.

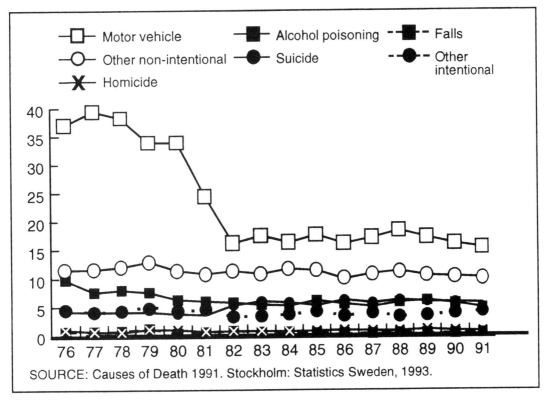

Figure 4. Fatal injuries in Sweden 1976-91, by cause and year. Rates per 100,000 of mean population. Females.

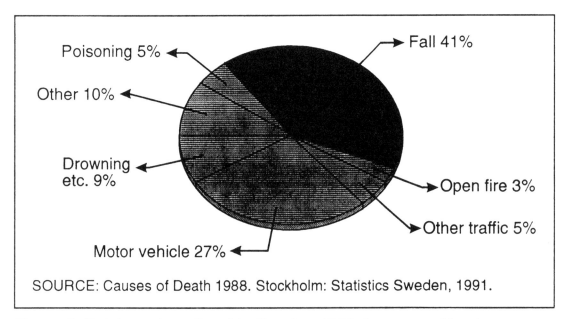

SOURCE: Causes of Death 1988. Stockholm: Statistics Sweden, 1991.

Figure 5. Fatal non-intentional in Sweden 1988, by cause. Number (n=1804) and percent.

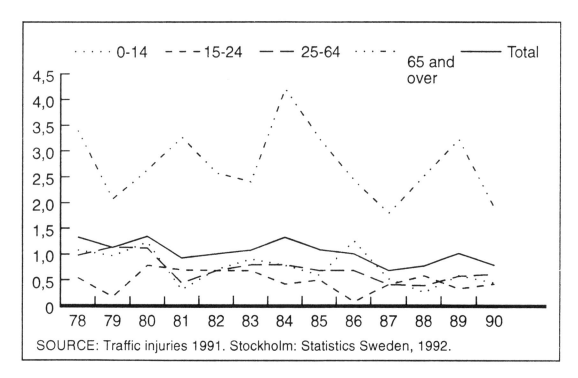

SOURCE: Traffic injuries 1991. Stockholm: Statistics Sweden, 1992.

Figure 6. Fatal bicycle injuries in Sweden 1978-90, by age group and year. Rates per 100,000 of mean population

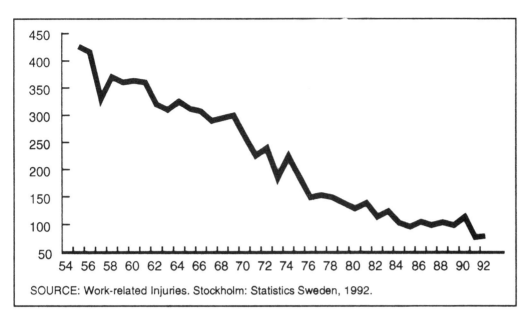

Figure 7. Number of work related fatal injuries in Sweden 1955-92, by year

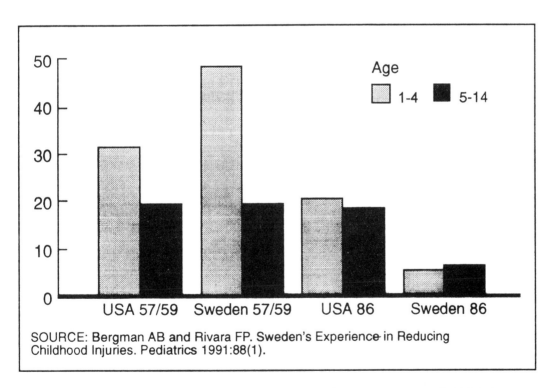

Figure 8. Fatal child injuries in USA and Sweden 1957-59 and 1986, by age group and year. Rates per 100,000 of mean population

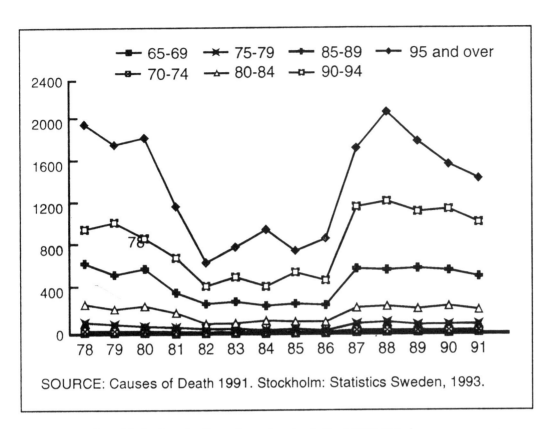

Figure 9. Fatal injuries in Sweden due to falls 1978-91, by age group and year. Rates per 100,000 of mean population

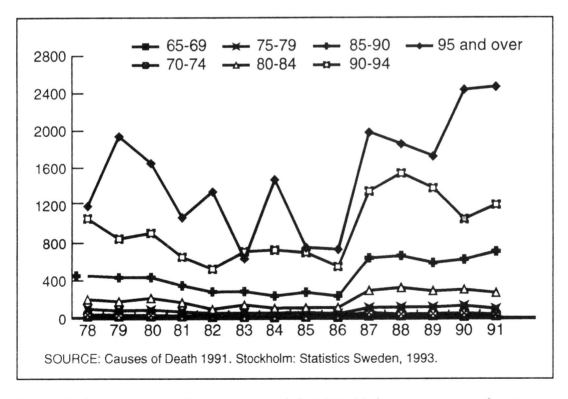

Figure 10. Fatal injuries in Sweden due to falls 1978-91, by age group and year. Rates per 100,000 of mean population

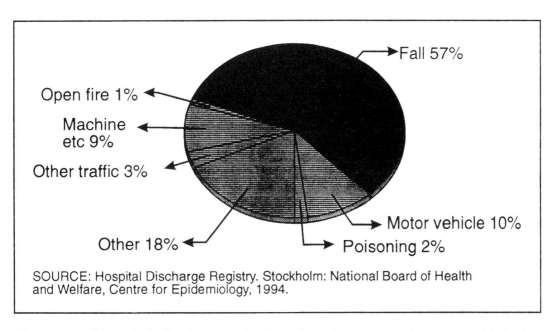

Figure 11. Hospital discharges in Sweden due to non-intentional injuries 1988, by cause, number (n=143,589) and percent

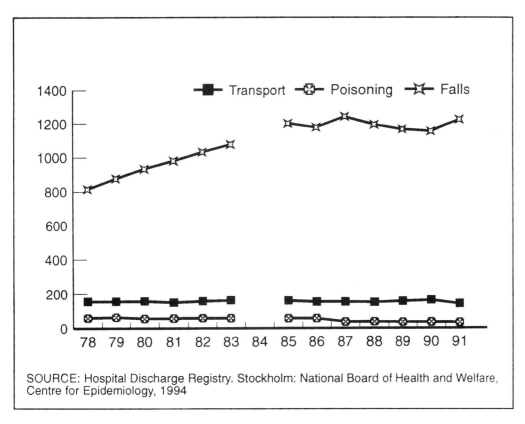

Figure 12. Hospital discharges in Sweden due to non-intentional injuries 1978-91, by cause and year. Rates per 100,000 of mean population

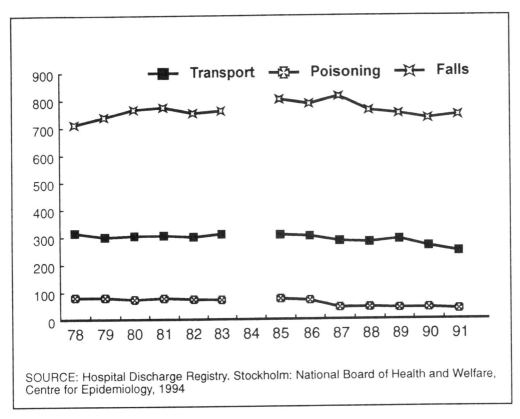

SOURCE: Hospital Discharge Registry. Stockholm: National Board of Health and Welfare, Centre for Epidemiology, 1994

Figure 13. Hospital discharges in Sweden due to non-intentional injuries 1978-91, by cause and year. Rates per 100,000 of mean population

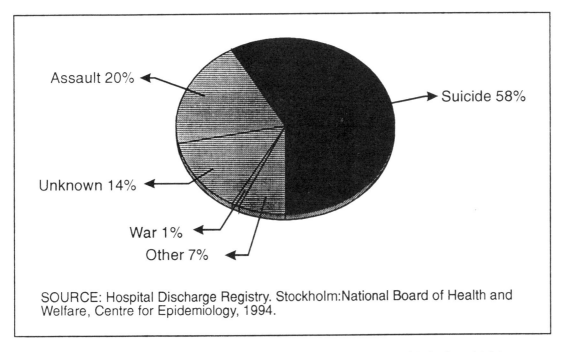

SOURCE: Hospital Discharge Registry. Stockholm:National Board of Health and Welfare, Centre for Epidemiology, 1994.

Figure 14. Hospital discharges in Sweden due to intentional injuries 1991, by cause, number (n=14,069 and percent)

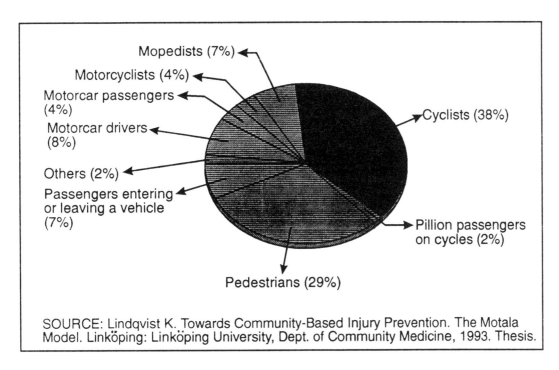

Figure 15. Traffic injuries in Motala, Sweden 1983-84, by category and percent (n=632)

Injury Among Persons 1–24 Years of Age In the United States: Data From The National Center for Health Statistics

by Lois A. Fingerhut, M.A. and Brenda S. Gillum, M.A.

Introduction

Data systems of the National Center for Health Statistics (NCHS) are the source of national estimates of injury morbidity and injury mortality in the United States. Each of the data systems collects, defines and disseminates injury data differently. Briefly, mortality data are from the National Vital Statistics System and are based on information recorded by physicians or coroners on the death certificate for **all** deaths from the 50 States and the District of Columbia. National estimates of injury morbidity are derived from several different NCHS **survey**–based data systems. Two are hospital–based medical abstract surveys: the National Hospital Discharge Survey (NHDS) and the National Hospital Ambulatory Medical Care Survey (NHAMCS)–Emergency Department component. A third is a household–based door–to–door survey: the National Health Interview Survey (NHIS). The technical details for each of these data systems can be found in published documents of the NCHS (1,2,3,4).

Definitions of injury

Rules for defining injury as an underlying cause of death are set forth in the International Classification of Diseases (ICD) published by the World Health Organization. Methods and rules for classifying injury morbidity are less clear and are often developed by individual users (5). The ICD provides codes that are specific to the nature and the cause of injury. In the United States, it is common practice to code nonfatal injuries using codes defined in the ICD's Chapter 17 (Injury and Poisoning) for nature of injury and in the Supplementary Classification of External Causes of Injury and Poisoning for cause of injury. The completeness of external cause (E) coding for morbidity data varies with the data collection site (e.g., hospital inpatient versus hospital emergency department). Beginning in 1979, the Ninth Revision of the ICD was adopted for in use in the United States.

Mortality

Cause of death statistics are based on the *underlying cause* of death which is defined as "(a) the disease or injury which initiated the train of events leading directly to death, or (b) the circumstances of the accident or violence which produced the fatal injury." (5) Thus, it is the cause of the injury (i.e., the motor vehicle crash) rather than the nature of the injury (i.e., intracranial injury) that is selected as the underlying cause of death. These "external" or E–codes are E800–E999 from the ICD–Ninth revision.

Contributing causes of death: Data on the nature of the injury, that is for example, a fracture, burn, poisoning or head injury are found in the multiple cause of death files (6). These are not routinely published by NCHS, but are available on public use tapes.

Morbidity

Cause–specific morbidity data from the NHDS are based on the ICD, 9th revision, Clinical Modification (CM) and are coded and published by the nature of the injury, based on codes 800–999. Because only about 40 percent of hospital injury discharge records have E–codes, they are not considered valid for making national estimates of cause–specific hospitalizations. Cause–specific injury data from the NHAMCS–ED are coded by both E–code and N–code. Annual household interview data on acute injury conditions are based on self–reports and are usually categorized by nature of the injury. In addition, NHIS data on episodes of injury differentiate between injuries involving motor vehicles. (2,3,4)

Cross–system comparisons

Injury rates are often published on different bases making the potential for confusing cross system comparisons quite likely. For example, death rates are generally published per 100,000 population, hospitalization discharge rates are per 10,000 population, and emergency department visit rates and reported conditions are per 100 persons. Injury pyramids can be useful for simplifying this. Based on NCHS data systems, for every 1000 injury conditions reported for persons 1–24 years of age in the NHIS, there are approximately 510 visits to emergency department; 25 hospitalizations; and 1 injury death (fig.1). Looked at another way, for every injury death at ages 1–24 years, there are 17.4 injury related hospitalizations, 356 injury visits to emergency departments and 700 self– reported injuries.

Mortality (figures 2 through 9)

Approximately 1 in a thousand or one tenth of one percent of reported injuries in this age group result in death. Despite this, most national analyses of injury data in this country are based on mortality. One can offer several reasons: 1) the data are coded as to the external cause of the injury which is crucial for prevention, 2) the data are for all persons and not based on a sample, 3) the level of geographic detail is far more extensive than for morbidity data, and 4) the high quality of mortality data (due, in part, to State laws which mandate the completion of a standard death certificate for every death occurring in the State). Information on the death certificate is also subject to local, and national quality control measures concerning the completion, filing and later amendments to the certificate.

In 1991, 36,140 persons 1–24 years in the United States died as a result of an injury compared with 16,005 who died as a result of a natural cause of death. Overall, 70 percent of deaths among persons 1–24 were the result of an external cause of death– varying from 43 percent for those aged 1–4 years to 81 percent for teenagers 15–19 years. Approximately 40 percent of deaths at ages 1–24 (with very minimal variation by age) were the result of an unintentional injury. Intentional injury (which includes homicide and suicide) varies significantly by age, from 3.5 percent for those 5–9 years, to 36 percent of all deaths among persons 20–24 years of age.

The single leading cause of death for persons 1–24 years is motor vehicle crashes. Among young children 1–4, drowning and fires are also among the top ranked causes of unintentional injury death. At 20–24 years, homicide and suicide together cause more deaths than do motor vehicle crash related injuries.

Differences by sex in injury mortality increase with age. Among young children 1–4 years, the death rate from drowning among young boys is twice that for young females. At 5–9 years, the sex difference in drowning is about 3:1, and the motor vehicle death rate for boys is 1.6 times that for females. At 10–14 years, the sex ratio from drowning is 4:1; the motor vehicle death rate for boys is twice that for females; for suicide it is 3:1 and for homicide it is 2:1. Injury death rates for males 15–19 and 20–24 are 3–4 times those for females, with the larger differences in homicide and suicide rates, than in unintentional injury mortality.

At ages 10–14, 15–19 and 20–24 years, firearms are associated with more deaths than any cause with the exception of motor vehicles. More than half of these firearm deaths are associated with homicide. Death rates associated with firearms for persons 10–24 years have been increasing, while motor vehicle death rates have been falling. Even among children as young as 10–14 years, the firearm death rate has been increasing. From ages 25–34 on, both firearm and motor vehicle crash death rates have been stable or have been declining.

Mortality data also have the benefit of geographic detail. County level data are often beneficial in helping to target prevention activities. As an example, one can look at county level firearm death rates among males 15–24 years of age. In 1990–91, the death rate in Orleans, Louisiana and Washington, DC were similarly high, more than three times the rate in Duval, Florida.

Hospital discharge data (figures 2, 10 and 11):

In 1991, there were approximately 629,000 injury related discharges from short–stay hospitals among persons 1–24 years. These national estimates are based on a sample of discharges from short–stay hospitals. Demographic, diagnostic, and procedure data are collected using both manual and automated abstracting. The NHDS has been conducted annually since 1965. In 1991, there were approximately 25 discharges for every 1,000 reported injury conditions, with the ratio being slightly higher for those 15–24 years than for those 1–14 years.

Discharge rates for persons 1–24 follow an age pattern similar to that for mortality, with discharge rates for children 1–4 years higher than for children 5–14 years, but considerably lower than at 15–24 years. Also, at each age, the discharge rate for males exceeds that for girls.

Among children 1–4 and 5–14 years, hospitalization rates for males with head injuries and burns are about 3 times the rates for girls. At 15–24 years, laceration and open wound rates are about 3 times higher for males than for females. Discharge rates associated with poisoning, on the other hand, are higher for females than for males.

Emergency department visits: (figures 2, 12 and 13)

The first national estimates of cause–specific visits for injury are from the 1992 NHAMCS–ED component which is based on a sample of visits to emergency rooms. The cause–specific data were manually abstracted and coded according to the ICD–9–CM.

In 1992, there were an estimated 13 million injury related visits to ED's among persons 1–24 years of age. ED visit rates for injury show less variation by age than do mortality or hospitalization rates for injury. Unlike mortality, visits to EDs are often related to falls. For children 1–14 years, one third of injury visits that were E–coded were fall–related. Among those 15–24 years, 16 percent were falls, 21 percent were motor vehicle and 8 percent were assault related.

Household Interview Survey (figures 2 and 14)

In the NHIS, injuries are defined by whether or not medical attention was received or if there were any days of restricted activity associated with the injury. In 1992, there were about 26 million injuries reported for persons 1–24 years of age, with the incidence of reported injuries higher for males than for females at ages 5–14 and 15–24 years and similar at 1–4 years.

Childhood injury incidence data have been the subject of several of the rotating NHIS supplements, but are not reported in detail on an annual basis.

One reason for the lack of annual detail has been that the sample size is too small as a result of only using a two week recall period. Plans are currently underway to revise the injury questions in the NHIS (in addition to other parts of the core questionnaire) so as to enable a more detailed and comprehensive understanding of injury morbidity in the US.

In 1961, Drs. Kerr White, Franklin Williams and Bernard Greenberg described an illness pyramid very similar to the injury pyramid that has been referred to. (7) To paraphrase from their summary: "in a population of 1,000 adults, in an average month 750 will experience an episode of illness; 250 will consult a physician; 9 will be hospitalized; 5 will be referred to another physician and 1 will be referred to a university medical center. The latter sees biased samples of one tenth of one percent of the sick adults from which students of the health professions must get an unrealistic concept of medicine's task ..."

So too, must injury researchers be cautious in not relying solely on injury mortality statistics for the characterization of injury. We must always be cognizant of the very important differences between the epidemiology of fatal and of nonfatal injuries.

References

1.   National Center for Health Statistics. Advance report of final mortality statistics, 1991. Monthly vital statistics report; vol 42 no 2, suppl. Hyattsville, Maryland: Public Health Service. 1993.

2.   Graves EJ. 1992 Summary: National Hospital Discharge Survey. Advance data from vital and health statistics; no 249. Hyattsville, Maryland: National Center for Health Statistics. 1994.

3.   McCaig LF. National Hospital Ambulatory Medical Care Survey: 1992 emergency department summary. Advance data from vital and health statistics; no 245. Hyattsville, Maryland: National Center for Health Statistics. 1994.

4.   Benson V and Marano MA. Current estimates from the National Health Interview Survey, 1992. National Center for Health Statistics. Vital Health Stat 10(189). 1994.

5.   World Health Organization. Manual of the International Statistical Classification of Diseases, Injuries, and Causes of Death, based on the recommendations of the Ninth Revision Conference, 1975. Geneva: World Health Organization, 1977.

6.   National Center for Health Statistics. Vital statistics, instructions for classifying multiple causes of death. NCHS instruction manual; part 2b. Hyattsville, Maryland: Public Health Service. Published annually.

7.   White KL, Williams F, and Greenberg BG. The ecology of medical care. The New England Journal of Medicine. vol 265, no 18, pp.885–92. Nov 2, 1961.

	Defined by:	Number of events	Published per	For every 1,000 conditions
Death	E800-E999	36,140	100,000	1
Hospitalization	N800-N999	629,000	10,000	25
Emergency department visit (1992)	E800-E999	12,883,000	100	510
Reported condition	Self report	25,267,000	100	

Figure 1. Injury in the population 1-24 years of age: United States, 1991

Injury resulting in:	All, 1-24 years	1-24 years	1-14 years	15-24 years
	Number	For every 1,000 reported conditions:		
Death	36,140	1	0.6	3
Hospital discharge	629,000	25	19	32
Emergency department visit 1992	12,883,000	510	513	506
Reported conditions	25,267,000			

Figure 2. Injury in the population 1-24 years of age: United States, 1991

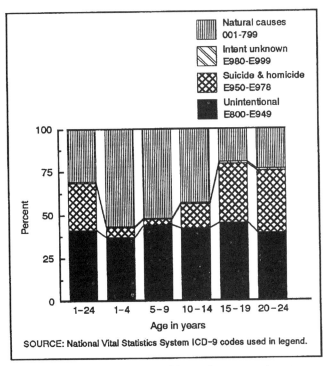

Figure 3. Deaths among persons 1-24 years by cause and age: United States, 1991

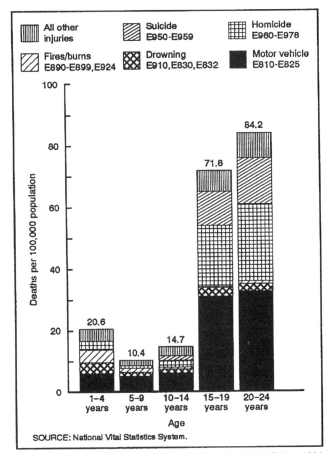

Figure 4. Injury mortality among persons 1-24 years: United States, 1991

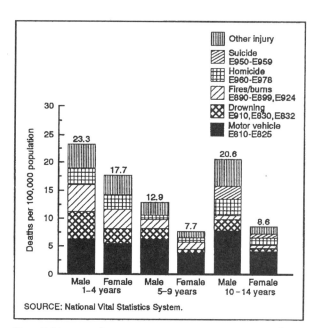

Figure 5. Injury mortality among males and females 1–14 years: United States, 1991

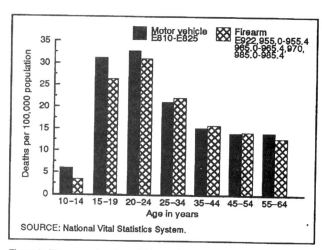

Figure 7. Firearm and motor vehicle crash death rates for persons 10–64 years by age: United States, 1991

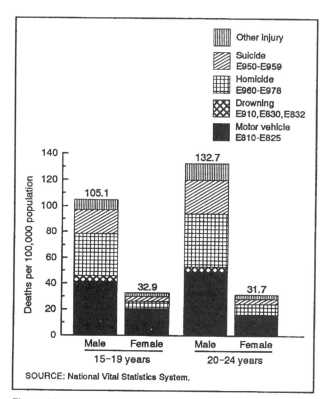

Figure 6. Injury mortality among males and females 15–24 years: United States, 1991

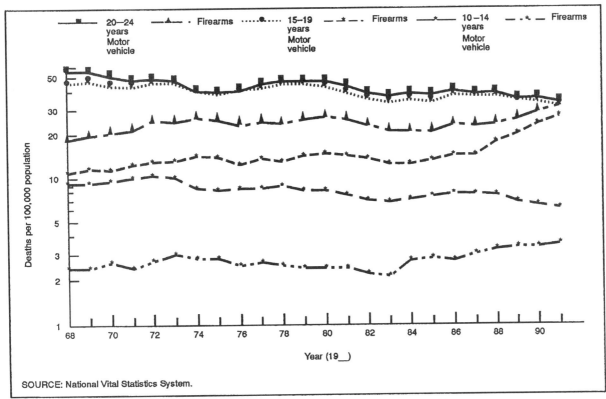

Figure 8. Firearm and motor vehicle mortality among persons 10–24 years by age: United States, 1968–1991

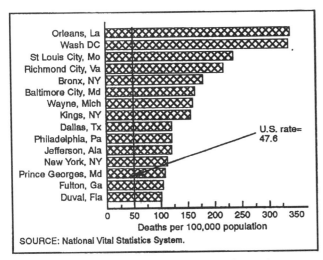

Figure 9. Firearm death rates for males 15–24 years by county: United States, 1990–91

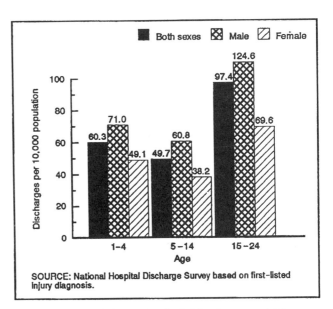

Figure 10. Hospital discharge rates due to injury for persons 1–24 years, by age and sex: United States, 1992

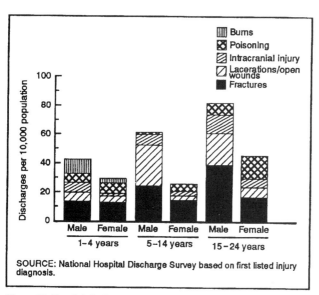

SOURCE: National Hospital Discharge Survey based on first listed injury diagnosis.

Figure 11. Hospital discharge rates for selected injuries for persons 1–24 years: United States 1992

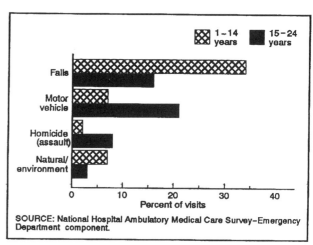

SOURCE: National Hospital Ambulatory Medical Care Survey–Emergency Department component.

Figure 13. Selected leading causes of injury visits to emergency departments by age: United States, 1992

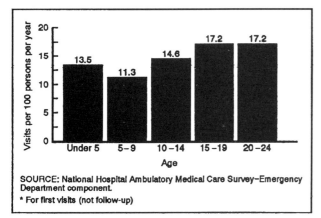

SOURCE: National Hospital Ambulatory Medical Care Survey–Emergency Department component.

* For first visits (not follow-up)

Figure 12. Emergency department visit rates for injuries* among persons under 25 years: United States, 1992

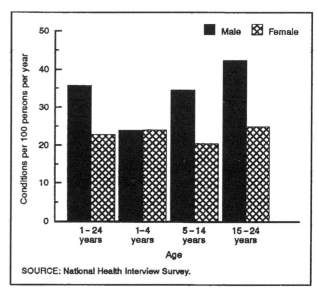

SOURCE: National Health Interview Survey.

Figure 14. Injuries reported in household interviews among persons 1–24 years by sex: United States, 1991

Levels and Trends in Injury Mortality and Morbidity Israel

by Pnina Zadka, Batja Halperin, Suzana Zaritzky, Sharon Goldman, and Vita Barell

Introduction

Injuries are often looked upon as preventible. Thus the main targets for prevention are the circumstances of the event, rather than the outcome—nature of injury. These circumstances are studied, qualified, quantified and classified. The medical care delivery approach deals with the nature and severity of injury and the most appropriate and efficient route of delivering medical care after an injury has occurred. An information system for collection and analysis is needed for all of these aspects in order to improve prevention programs and services for acute and rehabilitative treatment of injuries.

Accordingly, there are two major approaches to injury statistics classification of mortality and morbidity;

A.   The external cause (circumstances).

B.   Nature of injury (type and severity).

A.   The external cause may be categorized as:

     I.   Accidental (non–intentional)

     II.   Intentional

          1.   Self inflicted (suicide)

          2.   Inflicted by others (homicide, war etc.)

B.   The nature of injury falls into three main groups:

     I.   Type of force

          1.   Injuries caused by mechanical forces.

          2.   Injuries caused by heat.

          3.   Injuries caused by chemical agents.

     II.   Site or organ affected

          1.   Head & neck

          2.   Chest

          3.   Back

          4.   Abdomen

          5.   Upper limb

          6.   Lower limb

III.   Type of wound

    1.   Fracture

    2.   Superficial

    3.   Open wound

    4.   Crushing injury

Classification of injuries and external causes is primarily based on the International Classification of Diseases (ICD). In some cases, the data do not enable precise classification, but in most cases maintain the principles of the ICD.

Data sources

Injury statistics in Israel may be obtained from different sources, none of which has been designed for data collection purposes. Thus, each of the sources has limitations.

Traditionally data on the "external cause" of the injury, which is usually tailored for the prevention approach, are more available than data on type of injury (nature of injury) and severity of injury.

The main sources for national data regarding injury are the following:

1.   Mortality Data: Data on fatal injuries have been available since 1950 for each year and up to 1992 from the mortality files. The advantage of this source is its completeness, reliability and continuity. Mortality data are classified according to the ICD external causes (E–code). The main limitation is that this is the only code, since only one cause is coded on mortality files, reflecting mainly the circumstances of the event and the type of force. Details on the forces involved are not always listed on the death notification. Another drawback is that up to 1965 the data for non–Jews in Israel were incomplete.

2.   Hospitalization Data: Hospitalization data in Israel have been available since 1952. The latest available year is 1987 (1990 being in process). The data on injuries are mostly limited to the "nature of injury" and information on the external cause is poor. Attempts to improve the reporting and coding of the external cause on hospitalization records have not been successful. Hospitalizations are classified by ICD injury code as well as E–code, whenever available.

3.   Suicides: Information on suicides is available through two sources: death notification, and a special Health Monitoring system for reporting suicides and suicide attempts. Suicide and suicide attempts were a criminal felony up to 1967, and all cases were police obligatory reports. This law was abolished in 1967 and a special reporting system was established by the Ministry of Health for cases of suicides and suicide attempts. Suicides statistics are based on these notifications.

Agencies reporting suicide attempts are: general (short stay) hospitals, psychiatric hospitals and District Health Bureaus. The reporting agent for suicides is the Coroner's Office. Reporting of suicide and suicide attempts is incomplete, with an estimated coverage of 75 percent for suicides and no estimate for suicide attempts. There is under–reporting by certain hospitals, and non–reporting by others. Since 1985 the reports on suicides are checked against death notifications and missing cases are added. Statistics on suicides and suicide attempts are categorized by background factors and the means used by the victim as well as some demographic characteristics.

4.   Health Interview Survey: The 1993 Health Interview Survey contained a battery of questions on injuries: type, circumstances of the event, and agent of first medical contact. The recall period was two weeks and the questions were limited to injuries that caused any limitation in daily activity. As the sample was 6000 households (20,000 persons), the number of injury cases was small and cross–classification of injuries was limited.

Nevertheless, the data obtained in the survey enable combination of information on type of injury with the external cause.

5. Road Accidents: Data are based on reports of road accidents with casualties compiled by the police. Since 1990, the data are based on computerized files created by the police at the initial report. Accidents and casualty files are matched against other data sources to correct and complete the information obtained at the time of the initial report. These data sources are: the Vehicle Registration file and the Driver License files held by the Ministry of Transportation, as well as the Population Register. The data on road accident casualties are limited to the severity of injury and the "type" of person injured (pedestrian, passenger, driver, motorcyclist, bicycle rider, etc.). Severe injuries are those for whom there were at least 24 hours of hospitalization; a fatality is a death within one month of the accident. Other information available on road accidents are details of the place, time, and environmental conditions at the scene of the accident.

6. Emergency Room Admissions: A National Injury Surveillance System using emergency room data bases and associated hospitalization records, is currently under development. The first stage, a pilot study, was carried out in 1993.

Levels and Trends

Mortality:

Fatal injuries are coded as external causes in mortality statistics. Deaths due to external causes have decreased by over 45 percent in the last two decades (1970–1991). Deaths due to external causes decreased more rapidly than total mortality (table 1) and comprised about 5 percent and 8 percent of total deaths among females and males respectively in Israel in 1991. The proportion of external causes of death ranged from a high of 10.6 percent among males in 1970 to a low of 3.4 percent among females in 1982 (table 1). In general, deaths due to external causes are 35 percent more frequent among males than among females.

The main cause of fatal injuries are transportation accidents (tables 2a, 2b), followed by suicides for males and accidental falls for females. While deaths due to transportation accidents (TA) and accidental falls have decreased in the last decade among both genders, the suicide rate increased in both genders to the extent that suicide rates are almost equal to TA (and to accidental falls in females) in the latest period (1990–1992). The proportion of external deaths assigned to undetermined external causes has increased two fold in the last period. This increase is mainly due to an increase in deaths assigned to undetermined causes over the last two years (In 1991 one of the sources for editing the recorded causes on the death notification, the Coroner's Office, was cut off).

The decrease in deaths due to injuries can be seen in almost all sub–categories, (tables 2a, 2b) except for suicides and undetermined causes. In all sub–categories except for accidental falls, the rate for males is higher (almost double) than that for females. Special note should be made of deaths due to firearm accidents and military and terror casualties, almost all of these are males, there are 1:100,000 cases in each of the two subcategories (table 2a). Despite the "Intifada" there was no noticeable increase in these cases.

The differences between the two population groups in Israel, Jews and non–Jews reflect a major cultural difference. The death rate due to external causes among non– Jewish males is higher by about 20 percent than that among Jewish males in most of the sub–categories, with major exception, deaths due to suicides (tables 4a, 4b). The rate of suicides among Jewish males is triple the rate for non–Jewish males, about 12:100,000 and 4:100,000 respectively. Another minor exception are homicide deaths, which is two–fold higher among non–Jewish males.

Contrary to the pattern among males, among females the rates for external causes are 20 percent higher for Jewish females than for non–Jewish females (tables 3a, 3b). The suicide rate pattern for females is similar to that of males. There are almost no cases of suicides among non–Jewish females, 1:100,000 on the average (4–5 cases per year). The differences in suicide rates seen among men are even more extreme among females; the rate for Jewish women is four times higher than the rate for non–Jewish women. Another minor exception are deaths due to accidental falls; the rate for Jewish women is almost double the rate for non–Jewish females. The only two sub–categories in which non–Jewish females have a higher injury rate are burns and drowning.

Even though the proportion of injuries among all deaths does not exceed 10 percent, in some age groups the proportion is much more significant. About one–third to one–fourth of total deaths are related to injuries among school boys and girls (aged 5–14 years) respectively. The two main causes responsible for these deaths are TA and drowning. Among youngsters aged 15–24 years, about two–thirds of the deaths are caused by external causes, the two principal causes being TA and suicides. Among the elderly men aged 65–74 years, the two major causes of injuries are also TA and suicides, but in women in that age group, TA is the major cause followed by suicides and accidental falls. While accidental falls among elderly women declined, from 13:100,000 in 1984–1986 to 6.5:100,000 in 1990–1992, suicides rates in this group increased.

Trends of transportation accidents over the last decade will be dealt with more detail in the chapter on road accidents.

Hospitalizations:

In 1987, 38,172 (6 percent) of hospitalizations in short stay hospitals were due to injuries; a rate of 87:10,000. There were 223,870 hospitalization days for care of injuries, 502 days per 10,000 (table 5). The hospitalization rate due to injuries for Jews and non–Jews are similar at most age groups except for infants and toddlers (under 5 years) among whom non–Jews have significantly higher rates for both boys and girls, and for the elderly, among whom, Jewish women have significantly higher rates than men (Jews and non–Jews) and non–Jewish women (2). Females have, in general, lower hospitalization rates due to injuries at all age groups (except for elderly Jewish women as mentioned before). The same pattern is seen in hospitalization days rate and for average length of stay. Average length of stay for injury patients is directly associated with age in both genders and both population groups.

The main type of injury among inpatients with injuries were fractures (30 percent), regardless of gender and age (table 5).

Information concerning hospital inpatients is classified by nature of injury, the external cause is seldom available. In general, the rate for injury hospitalizations is decreasing. Between 1979 and 1987, the injury hospitalization rates decreased by 20 percent for all age groups except for elderly women (age 75+), for whom it increased by almost 25 percent (from 242:10,000 to 309:10,000). That increase is mainly attributed to the increase in hospitalizations due to fractures among women aged 75 years and over. Elderly men experienced a decrease in hospitalizations due to fractures at that period, from 139:10,000 to 96:10,000.

Although the total rate of fracture hospitalizations among elderly increased from 1979 to 1987, the hospitalization days rate decreased from 0.04 days per person to 0.02 per person (table 6). The total hospitalization days rate spent on injuries decreased by almost 40 percent (0.09 per person in 1979 to 0.05 per person in 1987).

Among infants, hospitalization rates due to injuries, increased by almost 40 percent over the eight years under consideration. The increase is evident in almost all sub–categories presented (table 5). Despite the increase in the rate of hospitalization among infants, hospitalization days rates for infants decreased by 40 percent. The same pattern is reflected in each injury sub–category for infants, an increase in hospitalization rate combined with a decrease in hospitalization days rate.

Internal injuries, including intra–cranial injuries, are the second leading cause in hospital injury patients.

The total internal injury hospitalization rate decreased by half over the eight years, for both genders. The hospitalization days rate decreased by 75 percent for almost all age groups.

The most severe injuries among infants and toddlers (under 5 years) were burns. About 7–10:10,000 infants were burned, each of these cases needed about 20 hospitalization days on the average. Even though hospitalizations days rate due to burns among infants and toddlers decreased from 2 days per 100 infants in 1979 to 1:100 in 1987, it is often a traumatic and costly event.

The main cause for admission for injury patients are fractures (30 percent). Intracranial and internal injuries comprise another 13 percent and poisonings 8 percent. In children under 15, internal and intracranial injuries are more frequent than fractures in hospital admissions; also burns are a significant cause for hospital admissions in children.

Road accidents:

Since 1949, the number of road accident casualties has increased continuously with a higher growth rate than in the total population. The number of fatal casualties has continuously increased up to 1973, but since the mid 70's the number has fluctuated in a decreasing trend. The number of bicycle–rider casualties has decreased continuously and so has the number of pedestrian casualties. At the same time, the number of drivers and car passengers injured in road accidents has increased continuously.

The rate of fatal injuries in road accidents (RA) has not changed in the last decade for the total population (table 8). Nevertheless there are different trends in some of the age groups. The rate of RA fatalities dropped by 40 percent among children (age 0–14) and by 20 percent among elderly (age 65 and over). For those aged 15–24 and those aged 45–64, the rate of RA fatalities has increased slightly.

The rate of severely injured persons from RA (hospitalized for more than 24 hours) has fluctuated over the years. The fluctuation may be accounted for by changes in legislation with regard to use of seat belts in cars and helmets for motorcycles and moped riders; 1. Compulsory wearing of seat belts in front seats on non–urban roads and wearing of helmets on non–urban roads (1983). 2. Compulsory wearing of seat belts in front seats and helmets also in urban roads (1988). 3. Compulsory wearing of seat belts also in rear seats (1993).

The rate of total casualties in RA has increased as a result of a continuous increase in the rate of those slightly injured in RA in all age groups. Special attention should be drawn to the high growth rate of those slightly injured among the 15–24 and the 25–44 years age groups, a 100 percent and 80 percent increase respectively in the rate, over the last decade.

Self–reported injuries:

A question on limitations in daily activities caused by injury was asked in the last Use of Health Services Survey, conducted in Israel in 1993. The question referred to injuries which occurred during the past two weeks. There were about 200 cases of injuries reported in the sample (among 21,000 respondents). The rate of injuries causing limitation in daily activity was 53:1,000, 60:1000 in males and 45:1,000 in females. As seen in data available from other sources, males have a higher rate of injuries than females at all age groups up to age 45; the difference peaks for children (ages 0–14). At age 45 and over, the gender differences are not statistically significant.

The main type of injury is cuts, bruises, and blows—about 52:1,000 for all ages, and 77:1,000 for children aged 0–14 (table 10). The reported burns rate was 12:1,000 for all ages, and among elderly (65+) 17:1,000.

One–third of all reported injuries occurred at home, another fifth occurred in outdoors About half of the injuries of children (0–14) occurred at school or other day care institutions.

One third of all persons injured to an extent that their daily living activities were limited, did not seek any formal medical care. Among those who did get formal medical care, more than half were treated in clinics and about 45 percent were treated in hospitals (ER and inpatients). The percent who did not get any formal medical care peaks among elderly (65+), at 50 percent, and is lowest at 17 percent among youngsters age 15–24 years. Among the latter 52 percent got their first medical care in a hospital. That phenomenon probably reflects that, for the elderly, minor injuries often caused limitation in daily activities, while among young persons more severe injuries caused limitations in daily activities and needed professional medical care.

Suicides:

The information presented here for 1990, is based on the reports received by the Ministry of Health, while there is an estimated coverage of 75 percent (compared to cause of death reports). No estimate exist on the coverage of suicide attempts reported to the Ministry of Health.

Suicides are more frequent among men while suicide attempts are more frequent among women. The ratio of suicides to suicide attempts is 1:22 among women and 1:4 in men (table 13). The suicide rate peaks among elderly regardless of gender. Suicides among youth is still a rare event in Israel. Nevertheless, suicide attempts were reported in 4:100,000 teenage boys and 29:100,000 teenage girls.

The main incentive for suicides are depressive disorders. The main incentive for suicide attempts are familial difficulties, whereas depressive disorders rank second (table 14). Mental diseases are the incentive in 10 percent and 24 percent in men and women respectively, and 13 percent and 8 percent respectively in suicide attempts. The main form of suicide among men is hanging or other form of strangulation, 48 percent. Among women the most common method is jumping from a height, 49 percent. More drastic means such as gun shots are responsible for 23 percent and 11 percent of the suicides for men and women respectively, but for less than 1 percent of suicide attempts in both men and women. Sixty-four percent of men and 83 percent of women tried to commit suicide by an over dose of medications, with a very low "success rate", 6 cases out of 300 attempts.

Discussion

Injuries are a health problem that should be attacked from different angles. The preventive measures can be achieved from different actions: 1. Health education, especially geared to more susceptible population groups, such as youth and elderly. 2. Legislation and setting of obligatory commercial standards for equipment. 3. Developing an information system which can identify population at risk.

Since injuries often relate to different behavioral and environmental conditions, there is a need to identify high risk groups and then determine the most appropriate course of action for these targets. For example, if burns are a hazard among infants, than a prevention program should be targeted towards educating parents and developing safety standards.

One of the major health problems associated with injuries are long lasting and permanent disabilities resulting from severe injuries, as well the emergency medical service for life threatening injuries. The delivery of medical care for injuries should be organized in a comprehensive approach for the three main stages of medical care: evacuation, medical treatment and rehabilitation.

The information currently available in Israel does not enable efficient target–oriented strategies either for prevention or for medical care. There is an urgent need for a more comprehensive information systems as well as appropriate classification system specific to injury statistics.

Internationally agreed minimum data sets, including uniform classification systems, will advance data collection and classification in developed countries. Such uniform minimum data sets will enable comparative studies to the advantage off all countries.

References

1. Central Bureau of Statistics, Causes of Death 1987–1989, Special Publication Ser. 923, Jerusalem, 1993.

2. Central Bureau of Statistics, Diagnostic Statistics on Hospitalizations, Special Publication Ser. 941, Jerusalem 1993.

3. Central Bureau of Statistics, Road Accidents With Casualties 1992(A), Part I: General Summary, Special Publication Ser. 942, Jerusalem 1993.

4.   Stein, N and T Kline, <u>Ministry of Health</u>, Suicides and Suicide Attempts 1990, Statistical Publication, No.4, Jerusalem 1991.

Table 1: Standardized(*) Mortality Rates

	External causes		Percent of total deaths	
Year	Males	Females	Males	Females
1970	83	37	10.6	5.8
1971	68	42	8.9	6.9
1972	65	36	8.5	5.6
1973	56	34	7.2	5.4
1974	67	36	8.6	5.6
1975	65	35	8.6	5.8
1976	57	31	7.8	5.5
1977	56	32	7.7	5.6
1978	55	28	7.7	5.1
1979	53	31	7.6	5.8
1980	46	22	6.6	4.2
1981	43	19	6.5	3.7
1982	42	18	6.2	3.4
1983	53	25	7.8	4.7
1984	53	25	8.1	5.0
1985	56	31	8.8	6.4
1986	56	30	8.6	6.1
1987	58	28	9.1	5.9
1988	55	26	8.8	5.6
1989	53	27	9.0	6.1
1990	49	24	8.6	5.6
1991	44	21	7.7	4.8

Source: 1.   Central Bureau of Statistics, Causes of Death 1 special publication Ser. 923, Jerusalem
          2.   Data in process of publication.
          (*) the standard population is the world population given Doll R., Muir C. and Waterhouse J.
          in Cancer Incuden in Five continents.

Table 2a: Causes of Death - Males

Rates per 100,000

Cause	Total	0	1-4	5-14	15-24	25-34	35-44	45-54	55-64	65-74	75+
					1984-1986						
Transportation accident	14.1	2.0	4.6	4.6	18.8	15.3	12.6	14.7	19.4	26.9	46.2
Suicide	7.7	0.0	0.0	0.1	5.8	9.3	9.1	11.9	14.3	24.7	29.5
Accidental Falls	4.0	0.0	2.2	0.8	1.1	1.2	1.6	2.0	4.2	8.8	55.4
Homicide	2.5	0.0	0.2	0.1	3.4	4.8	4.9	3.2	2.6	2.5	2.4
Drowning	2.2	1.3	1.2	1.7	3.2	2.4	1.9	1.6	1.9	3.1	4.4
Suffocation	1.5	14.5	2.6	0.1	0.4	0.1	0.6	0.6	1.9	2.2	13.1
Firearms	1.3	0.0	0.0	0.1	5.2	1.7	0.9	0.8	0.0	0.0	0.0
Military and Terror	1.2	0.0	0.0	0.1	4.3	1.3	1.3	0.6	0.0	0.0	0.0
Burns	1.1	0.7	1.4	0.2	1.1	0.7	0.1	1.6	2.3	3.8	4.0
Electric & Explosi	1.0	0.0	0.2	0.4	2.0	1.8	0.9	1.2	0.0	0.6	0.8
Undetermined	2.6	0.7	0.7	0.2	3.6	2.4	2.4	3.4	3.7	6.6	10.8
Other accident	3.6	7.2	2.7	0.9	2.8	2.5	3.0	4.2	5.4	7.8	16.7
Other non-injury	665.6	1253.0	45.6	17.4	27.7	45.3	114.1	457.7	1372.0	3409.0	7857.8
All causes	708.4	1279.3	61.3	26.9	79.3	88.7	153.3	503.7	1427.7	3496.1	8041.0

1987-1989

Transportation accident	14.4	3.3	4.8	5.7	20.0	16.1	12.4	16.9	16.7	20.2	56.0
Suicide	10.2	0.0	0.0	0.3	7.7	12.3	11.6	15.9	23.3	25.8	45.7
Accidental Falls	3.9	1.3	0.5	0.5	0.8	1.0	1.0	1.2	1.9	7.8	79.9
Homicide	2.2	1.3	0.8	0.6	3.3	3.8	2.2	3.6	2.8	1.2	2.2
Drowning	2.5	0.7	1.6	1.9	4.0	2.4	2.1	1.8	2.8	2.5	5.8
Suffocation	1.8	9.8	0.7	0.1	0.3	0.5	0.6	1.4	2.8	4.4	24.4
Firearms	1.1	0.0	0.2	0.1	4.5	0.7	0.7	0.4	0.0	0.0	0.0
Military & Terror	0.9	0.0	0.0	0.1	3.1	1.5	0.6	0.2	0.0	0.0	0.4
Burns	0.6	0.7	1.2	0.2	0.0	0.3	0.2	1.0	0.5	0.9	5.3
Electric & Explosi	0.7	0.0	0.2	0.4	2.1	0.8	0.4	0.2	0.2	0.6	0.4
Undetermined	4.9	3.3	0.3	0.9	4.1	5.5	5.0	6.8	5.9	12.8	26.6
Other accident	2.4	1.3	2.1	0.8	1.9	2.2	2.5	3.6	4.7	3.1	8.9
Other non-injury	647.1	1093.6	41.5	14.1	24.0	50.9	111.9	405.7	1271.1	3176.2	9564.8
All causes	692.7	1115.3	53.8	25.6	75.8	98.2	151.2	458.6	1332.7	3255.5	9820.6

1990-1992

Transportation accident	9.8	1.2	3.3	2.3	17.2	11.4	7.6	7.2	13.3	16.3	31.1
Suicide	10.4	0.0	0.0	0.7	9.9	12.4	12.3	15.5	19.3	27.8	36.7
Accidental Falls	2.4	0.0	0.2	0.0	0.5	1.2	1.0	1.0	2.4	5.9	44.4
Homicide	1.8	0.6	0.2	0.1	2.0	3.2	2.5	3.1	3.0	2.0	2.4
Drowning	1.6	0.0	0.6	1.4	2.8	0.9	1.7	1.2	1.5	1.7	4.0
Suffocation	1.7	11.8	1.1	0.1	0.1	0.2	0.3	0.7	2.6	3.9	24.2
Firearms	0.3	0.0	0.0	0.0	1.6	0.2	0.2	0.0	0.0	0.0	0.0
Military & Terror	0.9	0.0	0.0	0.1	2.9	1.1	1.0	0.2	0.0	0.6	0.4
Burns	0.3	0.0	0.5	0.1	0.5	0.2	0.1	0.3	0.2	0.6	1.6
Electric & Explosi	0.6	0.0	0.6	0.1	0.9	1.2	0.6	0.2	0.4	0.6	0.0
Undetermined	7.4	1.9	1.4	0.9	7.3	6.6	7.5	8.9	12.0	16.3	44.4
Other accident	1.6	3.7	0.6	0.6	2.1	1.5	1.6	2.1	1.7	1.1	6.1
Other non-injury	626.2	1000.0	37.3	13.7	24.7	44.3	105.0	352.2	1162.9	3032.3	9576.0
All causes	665.1	1019.2	45.7	20.1	72.4	84.5	141.5	392.6	1219.4	3109.1	9771.3

Source: Central Bureau of Statistics, Causes of Deaths 1987-1989 Special Publication ser. 923, 1993 data, in press

Table 2b: Causes of Death - Females

Rates per 100,000

Cause	Total	0	1-4	5-14	15-24	25-34	35-44	45-54	55-64	65-74	75+
					1984-1986						
Transportation accident	6.1	0.0	4.5	2.8	5.7	3.7	4.3	5.9	8.0	23.8	19.3
Suicide	3.9	0.0	0.0	0.1	2.9	3.6	5.2	4.4	9.1	13.3	12.6
Accidental Falls	5.2	0.7	0.9	0.3	0.1	0.3	0.3	1.1	2.7	13.0	87.4
Homocide	1.1	0.7	0.0	0.3	1.8	1.0	1.5	0.8	2.3	1.5	1.4
Drowing	0.6	0.0	1.6	0.3	0.4	0.0	0.8	0.4	0.2	2.2	2.1
Suffocation	1.3	9.8	1.1	0.1	0.1	0.2	0.3	0.6	0.9	4.6	11.2
Firearms	0.1	0.0	0.0	0.0	0.6	0.0	0.0	0.0	0.0	0.0	0.0
Military & Terror	0.0	0.0	0.0	0.0	0.1	0.0	0.0	0.0	0.0	0.0	0.0
Burns	0.6	0.0	0.7	0.2	0.2	0.6	0.6	0.4	0.5	2.2	3.2
Electric & Explosi	0.2	0.0	0.0	0.1	0.1	0.2	0.3	0.2	0.0	1.2	0.0
Undetermined	1.6	0.0	0.4	0.1	1.6	1.2	1.0	2.1	2.5	4.9	7.7
Other accidents	2.0	8.4	2.2	0.7	0.1	0.3	0.1	1.1	1.6	4.0	21.1
Other non-injury	610.1	1124.1	48.9	14.7	19.9	34.6	88.5	277.7	957.5	2927.4	7030.5
All causes	632.7	1143.7	60.3	19.6	33.6	46.0	102.9	294.6	985.2	2998.1	7196.6

1987-1989

Cause											
Transportation accident	6.2	1.4	4.5	3.3	5.9	4.3	3.8	6.2	8.4	15.1	26.9
Suicide	4.2	0.0	0.0	0.1	2.6	4.1	4.5	4.5	8.6	11.6	22.0
Accidental Falls	4.9	0.0	0.7	0.3	0.4	0.1	0.2	0.8	1.2	9.2	102.2
Homocide	1.2	0.7	0.2	0.2	1.9	2.0	1.2	1.7	0.8	1.6	1.9
Drowning	0.6	0.7	0.5	0.7	0.7	0.3	0.5	0.0	0.6	1.3	2.6
Suffocation	1.5	13.7	0.5	0.1	0.1	0.4	0.4	0.2	2.2	3.2	15.5
Firearms	0.0	0.0	0.0	0.0	0.2	0.0	0.0	0.0	0.0	0.0	0.0
Military & Terror	0.1	0.0	0.0	0.0	0.1	0.1	0.1	0.2	0.0	0.0	0.0
Burns	0.6	3.4	0.2	0.1	0.2	0.2	0.2	0.4	0.6	2.1	4.5
Electric & Explosi	0.1	0.0	0.0	0.1	0.1	0.0	0.4	0.2	0.2	0.0	0.4
Undetermined	2.4	0.7	1.2	0.7	0.7	1.5	0.6	2.3	4.0	5.5	23.5
Other accidents	1.0	4.1	1.2	0.4	0.2	0.4	0.2	0.4	0.4	1.8	11.7
Other non-injury	590.1	952.6	38.3	12.8	18.3	32.5	82.6	257.7	808.5	2327.3	8404.2
All causes	612.9	977.3	47.4	18.7	31.2	46.0	94.7	274.5	835.4	2378.9	8615.4

1990-1992

Cause											
Transportation accidents	4.5	3.4	4.7	1.8	4.7	3.1	3.1	4.4	6.0	8.7	17.8
Suicide	4.3	0.0	0.0	0.1	2.9	4.1	4.2	7.2	8.2	13.2	17.4
Accidental Falls	4.0	0.7	0.3	0.1	0.1	0.2	0.2	0.6	0.6	6.3	86.3
Homocide	1.0	0.0	0.2	0.1	1.0	2.0	1.4	1.5	1.0	1.1	2.3
Drowning	0.5	0.0	1.4	0.3	0.5	0.2	0.1	0.6	0.4	0.8	2.6
Suffocation	1.7	14.4	0.7	0.3	0.1	0.0	0.2	0.8	1.4	3.7	20.8
Firearms	0.0	0.0	0.0	0.0	0.0	0.0	0.0	0.0	0.0	0.0	0.0
Military & Terror	0.1	0.0	0.0	0.1	0.2	0.0	0.1	0.0	0.2	0.5	0.0
Burns	0.2	0.7	0.3	0.1	0.0	0.1	0.0	0.6	0.0	0.5	1.5
Electric & Explosi	0.0	0.0	0.2	0.0	0.1	0.0	0.0	0.0	0.0	0.0	0.0
Undetermined	4.1	4.1	2.8	0.7	2.4	2.2	1.9	3.2	5.0	10.3	37.1
Other accidents	0.5	3.4	0.9	0.2	0.1	0.0	0.2	0.0	0.6	0.5	3.8
Other non-injury	647.0	928.6	37.5	15.3	19.8	33.3	104.2	278.1	808.8	2458.7	9536.7
All causes	667.9	955.4	48.9	19.2	31.9	45.2	115.7	296.8	832.2	2504.4	9726.3

Source: Central Bureau of Statistics, Causes of Deaths 1987-1989 Special Publication ser. 923, 1 1990-1992 data, in press

Table 3a: Deaths Due to External Causes - Jewish - Females

Rates per 100,000

1984-1986

Cause	Total	0	1-4	5-1	15-24	25-34	35-4	45-5	55-64	65-74	75+
Transportation accident	6.3	0.0	2.1	2.8	6.2	3.8	4.3	6.2	7.8	23.6	20.0
Accidental Falls	5.8	0.0	0.7	0.3	0.1	0.4	0.3	1.3	2.5	13.6	86.5
Suicide	4.5	0.0	0.0	0.1	3.2	4.0	5.9	5.0	9.8	13.9	13.3
Other accidents	1.8	2.8	1.2	0.3	0.1	0.4	0.2	1.3	1.8	3.3	20.0
Suffocation	1.4	8.3	1.2	0.1	0.0	0.2	0.3	0.6	1.0	4.6	11.5
Homicide	1.1	0.9	0.0	0.4	1.7	1.1	1.4	0.9	2.3	1.3	1.5
Burns	0.4	0.0	0.2	0.0	0.0	0.0	0.5	0.4	0.5	2.0	2.6
Drowning	0.5	0.0	0.5	0.1	0.4	0.0	0.8	0.2	0.0	2.3	2.2
Electric & Explos	0.2	0.0	0.0	0.0	0.1	0.2	0.3	0.2	0.0	1.3	0.0
Firearms	0.1	0.0	0.0	0.0	0.7	0.0	0.0	0.0	0.0	0.0	0.0
Military & Terror	0.0	0.0	0.0	0.0	0.1	0.0	0.0	0.0	0.0	0.0	0.0
Undetermined	1.5	0.0	0.0	0.0	0.9	1.1	0.8	2.2	2.5	5.0	8.1
Other non-injury	666.7	893.6	34.1	11.1	17.6	33.3	85.0	272.0	952.8	2935.3	6909.4
All causes	690.3	905.5	40.0	15.2	31.2	44.5	99.9	290.3	980.9	3006.3	7075.1

7–13

Cause											
Transportation accidents	6.5	0.0	3.0	2.4	6.9	4.7	3.5	6.8	8.3	15.8	27.4
Accidental falls	5.6	0.0	0.5	0.3	0.3	0.1	0.3	0.9	0.9	9.3	103.0
Suicide	4.9	0.0	0.0	0.1	3.1	4.8	4.9	5.0	9.2	12.4	22.9
Other accidents	1.0	1.9	0.9	0.4	0.1	0.4	0.3	0.2	0.4	2.0	12.5
Suffocation	1.5	9.3	0.2	0.0	0.1	0.5	0.4	0.2	2.2	3.4	16.1
Homocide	1.2	0.0	0.2	0.3	1.5	2.1	1.1	1.7	0.9	1.7	2.0
Burns	0.5	2.8	0.2	0.1	0.2	0.1	0.3	0.4	0.0	2.0	4.0
Drowning	0.5	0.9	0.2	0.3	0.5	0.1	0.1	0.0	0.7	1.4	2.8
Electric & Explos	0.1	0.0	0.0	0.0	0.1	0.0	0.3	0.0	0.0	0.0	0.4
Firearms	0.0	0.0	0.0	0.0	0.2	0.0	0.0	0.0	0.0	0.0	0.0
Military & Terror	0.1	0.0	0.0	0.0	0.1	0.1	0.1	0.2	0.0	0.0	0.0
Undetermined	2.4	0.9	0.7	0.5	0.5	1.5	0.5	1.7	3.7	5.6	24.1
Other non-injury	647.9	730.5	25.2	8.8	15.5	29.9	81.3	254.1	789.9	2293.9	8322.2
All causes	672.2	746.3	31.1	13.1	29.2	44.4	93.1	271.3	816.2	2347.4	8537.4

Cause											
Transportation accident	3.9	1.8	2.2	1.3	4.6	2.6	2.7	3.4	5.0	7.8	15.1
Accidental falls	4.1	0.0	0.2	0.1	0.1	0.2	0.1	0.6	0.4	5.6	73.1
Suicide	4.4	0.0	0.0	0.1	3.1	4.2	3.6	7.0	8.3	11.4	15.4
Other accidents	0.4	1.8	0.7	0.2	0.1	0.0	0.1	0.0	0.4	0.5	3.4
Suffocation	1.4	2.7	0.4	0.3	0.1	0.0	0.2	0.8	1.2	3.1	17.4
Homocide	0.9	0.0	0.0	0.1	0.9	1.9	1.3	1.3	1.0	0.5	2.0
Burns	0.1	0.0	0.2	0.0	0.0	0.0	0.0	0.6	0.0	0.2	1.3
Drowning	0.4	0.0	0.2	0.2	0.4	0.0	0.0	0.6	0.4	0.7	2.3
Electric & Explos	0.0	0.0	0.2	0.0	0.1	0.0	0.0	0.0	0.0	0.0	0.0
Firearms	0.0	0.0	0.0	0.0	0.0	0.0	0.0	0.0	0.0	0.0	0.0
Military & Terror	0.1	0.0	0.0	0.1	0.2	0.0	0.1	0.0	0.2	0.5	0.0
Undetermined	3.7	3.6	1.8	0.4	2.1	2.0	1.5	2.8	4.8	7.8	30.2
Other non-injury	642.7	658.2	24.2	10.2	14.8	30.1	88.4	231.6	730.8	2066.8	7933.6
All causes	662.2	668.2	30.2	12.8	26.5	41.0	97.9	248.6	752.5	2104.9	8093.9

Source: Central Bureau of Statistics, Causes of Death 1987-1989, Sp 1990-1992 data, in press.

Table 3b: Deaths Due to External Causes - non Jewish - Females

Rates per 100,000

Cause	Total	0	1-4	5-14	15-24	25-34	35-44	45-54	55-64	65-74	75+
					1984-1986						
Transportation accident	5.2	0.0	12.1	2.9	3.9	3.6	4.4	3.2	9.8	27.0	6.9
Accidental falls	2.0	2.9	1.5	0.3	0.0	0.0	0.0	0.0	4.9	4.5	103.4
Suicide	0.7	0.0	0.0	0.0	1.7	1.4	0.0	0.0	2.5	4.5	0.0
Other accident	2.9	26.2	5.3	1.9	0.0	0.0	0.0	0.0	0.0	13.5	41.4
Suffocation	0.8	14.5	0.8	0.0	0.4	0.0	0.0	0.0	0.0	4.5	6.9
Homicide	0.9	0.0	0.0	0.0	2.1	0.7	2.2	0.0	2.5	4.5	0.0
Burns	1.6	0.0	2.3	0.6	0.9	4.3	1.1	0.0	0.0	4.5	13.8
Drowning	1.3	0.0	5.3	1.0	0.4	0.0	1.1	1.6	2.5	0.0	0.0
Electric & Explos	0.1	0.0	0.0	0.3	0.0	0.0	0.0	0.0	0.0	0.0	0.0
Firearms	0.0	0.0	0.0	0.0	0.0	0.0	0.0	0.0	0.0	0.0	0.0
Military & Terror	0.0	0.0	0.0	0.0	0.0	0.0	0.0	0.0	0.0	0.0	0.0
Undetermined	1.9	0.0	1.5	0.3	4.3	2.2	2.2	1.6	2.5	4.5	0.0
Other non-injury	337.6	1854.7	96.3	26.2	27.8	42.4	112.7	320.1	1002.5	2819.8	9289.7
All causes	355.1	1898.3	125.1	33.6	41.6	54.6	123.6	326.4	1027.0	2887.4	9462.1

7-15

1987-1989

Transportation accident	5.1	5.3	9.3	5.9	2.3	2.9	5.7	2.9	8.6	4.2	19.2
Accidental Falls	1.8	0.0	1.4	0.3	0.4	0.0	0.0	0.0	4.3	8.4	89.7
Suicide	0.8	0.0	0.0	0.3	0.8	1.1	1.9	1.4	2.2	0.0	6.4
Other accident	0.9	10.5	2.1	0.3	0.4	0.6	0.0	1.4	0.0	0.0	0.0
Suffocation	1.3	26.3	1.4	0.3	0.0	0.0	0.0	0.0	2.2	0.0	6.4
Homicide	1.2	2.6	0.0	0.0	3.1	1.1	1.9	1.4	0.0	0.0	0.0
Burns	0.8	5.3	0.0	0.0	0.0	0.6	0.0	0.0	6.5	4.2	12.8
Drowning	1.4	0.0	1.4	1.9	1.6	1.1	2.9	0.0	0.0	0.0	0.0
Electric & Explos	0.3	0.0	0.0	0.3	0.0	0.0	1.0	1.4	2.2	0.0	0.0
Firearms	0.0	0.0	0.0	0.0	0.0	0.0	0.0	0.0	0.0	0.0	0.0
Military & Terror	0.0	0.0	0.0	0.0	0.0	0.0	0.0	0.0	0.0	0.0	0.0
Undetermined	2.3	0.0	2.9	1.5	1.6	1.7	1.0	5.7	6.5	4.2	12.8
Other non-injury	325.1	1581.6	79.3	25.6	27.5	44.1	91.7	281.2	991.4	2824.3	9711.5
All causes	341.0	1631.6	97.9	36.4	37.6	53.2	106.0	295.6	1023.8	2845.2	9859.0

1990-1992

Transportation accident	4.9	6.9	10.8	3.3	2.8	3.9	2.4	6.2	14.0	4.4	12.7
Accidental Falls	1.2	2.3	0.6	0.3	0.0	0.0	0.8	0.0	2.3	4.4	63.3
Suicide	1.3	0.0	0.0	0.0	1.0	2.4	3.3	1.2	2.3	13.2	0.0
Other accidents	0.6	6.9	1.3	0.3	0.0	0.0	0.8	0.0	2.3	0.0	0.0
Suffocation	2.0	41.4	1.3	0.3	0.0	0.0	0.0	0.0	2.3	4.4	19.0
Homicide	0.8	0.0	0.6	0.0	0.7	1.4	0.8	1.2	0.0	8.8	0.0
Burns	0.5	2.3	0.6	0.6	0.0	0.5	0.0	0.0	0.0	4.4	0.0
Drowning	1.1	0.0	4.4	0.6	0.7	1.0	0.8	0.0	0.0	0.0	0.0
Electric & Explos	0.0	0.0	0.0	0.0	0.0	0.0	0.0	0.0	0.0	0.0	0.0
Firearms	0.0	0.0	0.0	0.0	0.0	0.0	0.0	0.0	0.0	0.0	0.0
Military & Terror	0.0	0.0	0.0	0.0	0.0	0.0	0.0	0.0	0.0	0.0	0.0
Undetermined	3.6	4.6	5.1	1.5	2.1	1.9	2.4	2.5	4.7	30.7	50.6
Other non-injury	316.1	1443.7	67.8	27.9	26.4	34.3	90.5	306.4	1222.0	3386.0	9734.2
All causes	331.9	1508.0	92.5	34.7	33.7	45.4	102.0	317.6	1250.0	3456.1	9879.7

Source: Central Bureau of Statistics, Causes of Death 1987-1989, Special publication Ser 1990-1992 data, in press.

7-16

Table 4a: Deaths Due to External Causes - Jewish - Males

Rates per 100,000

Cause	Total	0	1-4	5-14	15-24	25-34	35-44	45-54	55-64	65-74	75+
					1984-1986						
Transportation accident	14.2	1.7	2.9	3.7	20.5	14.3	11.8	13.6	18.0	28.1	48.0
Accidental Falls	4.2	0.0	2.0	0.4	1.2	1.0	1.5	2.1	3.8	9.0	55.3
Suicide	8.9	0.0	0.0	0.1	6.4	10.0	10.3	13.2	15.4	26.1	31.3
Other accident	3.1	4.3	1.1	0.5	1.7	2.0	2.2	3.7	5.3	8.4	18.0
Suffocation	1.4	7.8	1.8	0.0	0.5	0.1	0.5	0.7	1.8	2.3	14.2
Homicide	2.4	0.0	0.0	0.2	2.9	4.6	5.1	2.3	2.5	1.7	2.1
Burns	1.1	0.9	0.7	0.1	1.3	0.7	0.2	1.4	2.0	3.7	3.4
Drowning	1.9	0.9	0.2	1.0	2.6	2.3	1.8	1.6	2.0	3.3	4.7
Electric & Explos	0.9	0.0	0.0	0.0	2.2	1.7	0.8	1.4	0.0	0.7	0.9
Firearms	1.5	0.0	0.0	0.1	6.3	1.8	1.0	0.9	0.0	0.0	0.0
Military & Terror	1.3	0.0	0.0	0.0	5.3	1.6	1.5	0.5	0.0	0.0	0.0
Undetermined	2.8	0.9	0.0	0.2	3.7	2.6	1.8	3.7	3.8	7.0	11.2
Other non-injury	733.4	1053.6	33.7	13.4	24.3	43.4	107.3	442.3	1344.2	3430.9	7870.0
All causes	777.1	1070.0	42.4	19.7	78.8	86.2	145.8	487.3	1398.9	3521.0	8059.2

7–17

Transportation accident	14.1	3.5	3.0	4.9	20.5	14.7	11.5	16.4	15.8	18.2	56.3
Accidental Falls	4.2	1.8	0.4	0.4	0.8	1.1	1.1	1.4	2.1	7.9	75.4
Suicide	11.6	0.0	0.0	0.0	8.2	13.3	12.5	17.8	24.6	27.1	48.7
Other accident	2.2	0.0	0.9	0.9	1.4	1.8	2.6	3.0	4.9	2.6	8.1
Suffocation	1.9	6.2	0.7	0.1	0.2	0.4	0.7	1.6	3.1	4.3	24.8
Homicide	1.9	0.9	1.1	0.4	2.4	3.3	1.9	3.0	2.6	0.7	2.4
Burns	0.5	0.0	0.9	0.2	0.0	0.3	0.1	1.2	0.5	0.7	4.8
Drowning	2.1	0.0	1.3	1.3	2.5	1.9	1.9	1.8	3.1	2.6	6.2
Electric & Explos	0.6	0.0	0.0	0.3	1.7	0.6	0.3	0.2	0.3	0.7	0.5
Firearms	1.3	0.0	0.2	0.0	5.7	0.9	0.8	0.5	0.0	0.0	0.0
Military & Terror	1.1	0.0	0.0	0.0	4.0	1.6	0.7	0.2	0.0	0.0	0.5
Undetermined	4.9	1.8	0.0	0.5	3.8	5.9	5.3	6.7	6.0	12.9	23.9
Other non-injury	714.5	891.5	30.8	10.3	21.5	52.8	107.1	385.4	1248.1	3158.9	9583.8
All causes	760.7	905.6	39.2	19.2	72.7	98.4	146.7	439.3	1311.0	3236.7	9835.3

1990-1992

Transportation accident	9.4	0.9	1.9	1.9	16.7	11.7	6.5	6.4	11.5	15.5	29.8
Accidental Falls	2.7	0.0	0.2	0.0	0.6	1.3	0.9	1.2	2.1	6.3	44.1
Suicide	12.0	0.0	0.0	0.7	11.2	14.1	13.4	17.6	20.8	29.0	38.1
Other accident	1.4	1.7	0.6	0.7	2.0	1.3	1.3	1.6	1.0	0.6	6.5
Suffocation	1.7	8.7	0.6	0.1	0.1	0.1	0.2	0.6	2.4	3.9	25.1
Homicide	1.4	0.0	0.0	0.0	1.7	2.4	1.4	2.6	1.9	1.8	2.6
Burns	0.3	0.0	0.4	0.2	0.4	0.2	0.1	0.4	0.2	0.3	1.7
Drowning	1.2	0.0	0.2	1.0	1.4	0.7	1.4	1.2	1.7	1.8	4.3
Electric & Explos	0.5	0.0	0.4	0.1	0.8	1.1	0.7	0.2	0.2	0.3	0.0
Firearms	0.4	0.0	0.0	0.0	1.8	0.1	0.2	0.0	0.0	0.0	0.0
Military & Terror	1.0	0.0	0.0	0.1	3.4	1.1	1.1	0.2	0.0	0.6	0.4
Undetermined	6.8	0.9	0.8	0.5	6.0	5.3	6.7	8.6	9.1	15.5	43.3
Other non-injury	694.0	833.9	26.2	10.0	22.7	44.8	102.4	334.9	1120.7	3014.9	9625.4
All causes	732.8	846.0	31.4	15.2	68.8	84.2	136.5	375.4	1171.6	3090.5	9821.4

Source: Central Bureau of Statistics, Causes of Death 1987-1989, Special publication Ser 1990-1992 data, in press.

7–18

Table 4b: Deaths Due to External Causes - Non Jewish - Males

Rates per 100,000

Cause	Total	0	1-4	5-14	15-24	25-34	35-44	45-54	55-64	65-74	75+
					1984-1986						
Transportation accident	13.6	2.8	10.0	7.6	13.3	20.7	18.2	22.6	36.6	10.1	22.3
Accidental Falls	2.9	0.0	2.9	2.1	0.7	2.7	2.1	1.6	9.1	5.0	55.9
Suicide	2.2	0.0	0.0	0.3	4.0	5.3	1.1	3.2	0.0	5.0	5.6
Other Accident	5.6	16.6	7.9	2.4	6.1	5.3	8.5	8.1	6.1	0.0	0.0
Suffocation	2.1	36.0	5.0	0.6	0.0	0.0	1.1	0.0	3.0	0.0	0.0
Homicide	3.2	0.0	0.7	0.0	5.0	5.3	3.2	9.7	3.0	15.1	5.6
Burns	1.4	0.0	3.6	0.6	0.4	0.7	0.0	3.2	6.1	5.0	11.2
Drowning	3.5	2.8	4.3	3.7	5.4	2.7	2.1	1.6	0.0	0.0	0.0
Electric & Explos	1.3	0.0	0.7	1.8	1.4	2.0	1.1	0.0	0.0	0.0	0.0
Firearms	0.5	0.0	0.0	0.0	1.8	0.7	0.0	0.0	0.0	0.0	0.0
Military & Terror	0.4	0.0	0.0	0.3	1.1	0.0	0.0	1.6	0.0	0.0	0.0
Undetermined	2.2	0.0	2.9	0.3	3.2	1.3	6.4	1.6	3.0	0.0	5.6
Other non-injury	357.4	1892.0	83.8	30.1	38.2	56.0	158.1	565.4	1707.3	3080.4	7698.3
All causes	396.3	1950.1	121.8	49.9	80.7	102.7	201.9	618.7	1774.4	3120.6	7804.5

1987-1989

	1	2	3	4	5	6	7	8	9	10	11
Transportation accident	15.9	2.5	10.2	8.2	18.2	22.8	18.0	19.8	25.6	52.1	51.0
Accidental Falls	2.5	0.0	0.7	0.9	0.7	0.6	0.0	0.0	0.0	5.2	140.1
Suicide	4.1	0.0	0.0	1.2	6.3	8.0	5.7	4.2	10.2	5.2	6.4
Other Accident	3.5	5.1	6.1	0.6	3.7	4.0	1.9	7.1	2.6	10.4	19.1
Suffocation	1.4	20.4	0.7	0.3	0.4	1.1	0.0	0.0	0.0	5.2	19.1
Homicide	3.8	2.5	0.0	1.2	6.3	6.3	3.8	7.1	5.1	10.4	0.0
Burns	0.8	2.5	2.0	0.3	0.0	0.6	0.9	0.0	0.0	5.2	12.7
Drowning	4.4	2.5	2.7	3.8	8.9	4.6	2.8	1.4	0.0	0.0	0.0
Electric & Explos	1.3	0.0	0.7	0.6	3.3	1.7	0.9	0.0	0.0	0.0	0.0
Firearms	0.2	0.0	0.0	0.3	0.7	0.0	0.0	0.0	0.0	0.0	0.0
Military & Terror	0.2	0.0	0.0	0.3	0.0	1.1	0.0	0.0	0.0	0.0	0.0
Undetermined	4.6	7.6	1.4	2.3	5.2	4.0	2.8	7.1	5.1	10.4	63.7
Other non-injury	348.3	1676.8	75.1	26.1	32.6	42.2	144.9	529.7	1498.7	3447.9	9312.1
All causes	391.0	1720.1	99.7	46.0	86.4	96.9	181.8	576.3	1547.3	3552.1	9624.2

1990-1992

	1	2	3	4	5	6	7	8	9	10	11
Transportation accident	11.9	2.2	7.3	3.7	18.9	10.6	15.5	12.2	30.3	29.0	47.9
Accidental Falls	1.1	0.0	0.0	0.0	0.3	1.0	1.6	0.0	4.3	0.0	47.9
Suicide	3.3	0.0	0.0	0.6	5.4	5.3	4.9	2.4	6.5	9.7	18.0
Other Accident	2.4	8.7	0.6	0.3	2.4	2.4	3.3	4.9	8.7	9.7	0.0
Suffocation	1.6	19.7	2.4	0.3	0.0	0.5	0.8	1.2	4.3	4.8	12.0
Homicide	3.8	2.2	0.6	0.6	3.0	6.7	9.8	6.1	13.0	4.8	0.0
Burns	0.3	0.0	0.6	0.0	0.7	0.0	0.0	0.0	0.0	4.8	0.0
Drowning	3.2	0.0	1.8	2.8	7.8	1.4	3.3	1.2	0.0	0.0	0.0
Electric & Explos	0.9	0.0	1.2	0.0	1.4	1.9	0.0	0.0	2.2	4.8	0.0
Firearms	0.2	0.0	0.0	0.0	0.7	0.5	0.0	0.0	0.0	0.0	0.0
Military & Terror	0.5	0.0	0.0	0.0	1.0	1.4	0.8	0.0	0.0	0.0	0.0
Undetermined	9.8	4.4	3.0	2.0	11.8	12.0	13.0	11.0	39.0	29.0	59.9
Other non-injury	328.2	1419.2	69.4	26.0	31.8	42.3	123.0	458.0	1545.5	3314.0	8892.2
All causes	367.3	1456.3	87.0	36.2	85.3	86.1	175.9	497.0	1653.7	3410.6	9077.8

Source: Central Bureau of Statistics, Causes of Death 1987-1989, Special publication Ser 1990-1992 data, in press.

Table 5: Hospitalizations by Type of Injury (First Listed Diagnosis)

Age	Total injuries	Fracture	Internal injuries	Burns	Poisonings	Other
			Rates per 10,000			
			1979			
			Males			
0	57	23	8	7	6	14
1-4	121	44	21	23	18	14
5-14	103	53	27	8	4	11
15-24	155	68	42	10	10	26
25-44	102	44	27	6	5	19
45-54	92	43	19	5	4	21
55-64	91	39	17	4	4	27
65-74	109	56	14	4	2	33
75+	238	139	44	8	7	38
All ages	117	53	27	9	7	20
			Females			
0	38	14	7	7	4	6
1-4	82	33	12	16	12	9
5-14	49	26	10	6	3	5
15-24	56	21	16	4	4	11
25-44	50	16	16	3	2	13
45-54	58	27	8	3	2	18
55-64	75	45	8	2	2	18
65-74	135	94	10	3	3	26
75+	242	186	21	6	2	28
All ages	69	35	13	5	4	13

		Males				
0	76	10	15	10	9	32
1-4	121	17	24	12	16	52
5-14	97	26	21	3	4	43
15-24	126	27	18	5	7	69
25-34	90	20	11	4	6	49
35-44	72	18	8	3	5	38
45-54	69	18	8	3	5	35
55-64	69	23	6	3	6	31
65-74	94	38	12	2	7	35
75+	160	96	15	3	8	38
All ages	96	26	15	4	7	44

		Females				
0	61	10	14	8	5	24
1-4	80	11	18	8	11	32
5-14	45	10	10	2	3	20
15-24	49	8	6	3	9	23
25-34	34	6	4	1	6	17
35-44	34	10	3	2	5	14
45-54	44	16	4	2	5	17
55-64	63	31	5	1	6	20
65-74	119	72	4	2	10	31
75+	309	219	19	1	15	55
All ages	62	23	7	3	7	22

Source: 1.   **Central Bureau Of Statistics**, Diagnostic Statistics of h___ special series No. 803, 1987.
          2.   **Central Bureau Of Statistics**, Diagnostic Statistics of h___ special series No. 941, 1993.

Table 6: Hospitalization Days Due to Injuries First Listed Diagnosis

Age	Total injuries	Fracture	Internal injuries	Burns	Poisonings	Other
			Rates per 10,000			
			1979			
0-4	591	212	59	213	32	75
5-14	455	198	118	87	10	42
15-24	828	379	211	85	15	139
25-34	601	281	135	63	12	111
25-44	646	300	135	48	10	152
45-54	862	445	125	50	9	232
55-64	1249	733	115	39	11	351
65-74	1729	1241	108	53	10	318
75+	4830	3668	392	158	24	588
All ages	860	466	138	88	14	153
			1987			
0	287	33	43	101	14	96
1-4	359	69	46	82	27	135
5-14	263	77	39	21	7	119
15-24	464	127	40	39	15	243
25-34	348	97	30	29	15	177
25-44	319	105	24	28	9	153
45-54	381	152	28	32	14	155
55-64	539	292	30	23	22	172
65-74	1104	727	40	33	45	259
75+	2882	2283	113	29	68	389
All ages	502	228	39	36	18	181

Source: 1. Central Bureau Of Statistics, Diagnostic Statistics of hospital special series No. 803, 1987.
2. Central Bureau Of Statistics, Diagnostic Statistics of hospital special series No. 941, 1993.

Table 7: Road Accident Casualties by Type of Road and Severity

Year	All roads				Thereof: urban road			
	All casual	Fatality	Severely injured	Slightly injured	All casual	Fatality	Severely injured	Slightly injured
1983	19867	436	3437	15994	14305	213	2086	12006
1984	19116	399	3274	13604	13604	184	1910	11510
1985	18709	387	3064	15258	13192	169	1828	11195
1986	21206	415	3277	17514	14942	212	1968	12762
1987	22173	493	3641	18038	15232	225	2173	12834
1988	23088	511	3797	18780	15744	241	2178	13325
1989	24062	475	3536	20051	16299	223	2039	14037
1990	27668	427	3965	23276	18790	195	2282	16313
1991	31541	444	4147	26950	21425	204	2421	18800
1992	37838	507	4676	32655	25350	205	2634	22511

				Percentages				
1983	100	2	17	81	100	1	15	84
1984	100	2	17	71	100	1	14	85
1985	100	2	16	82	100	1	14	85
1986	100	2	15	83	100	1	13	85
1987	100	2	16	81	100	1	14	84
1988	100	2	16	81	100	2	14	85
1989	100	2	15	83	100	1	13	86
1990	100	2	14	84	100	1	12	87
1991	100	1	13	85	100	1	11	88
1992	100	1	12	86	100	1	10	89

Source: Central Bureau of Statistics, Road accidents with Casual special Publication Series no. 842, Jerusalem 1993

Table 8: Road Accidents Casualties by Age and Severity

			Rates per 10,000				
Year	Severity of	TOTAL	0-1	15-24	25-	45-	65+
1983	Fatal	1.1	0.5	1.1	0.8	0.9	2.5
	Severe	8.3	4.4	12.0	8.0	6.7	8.6
	Slight	38.8	14.4	52.5	48.0	39.4	29.2
1984	Fatal	1.0	0.4	0.9	0.9	0.9	2.2
	Severe	7.8	4.3	11.2	7.2	7.2	8.3
	Slight	36.8	14.0	49.3	45.8	38.0	28.9
1985	Fatal	0.9	0.4	0.9	0.7	0.9	2.4
	Severe	7.2	4.2	9.7	6.7	6.0	7.2
	Slight	35.8	12.8	47.9	44.3	36.6	27.7
1986	Fatal	1.0	0.3	1.1	0.5	1.2	2.2
	Severe	7.6	4.2	10.6	7.1	6.1	7.7
	Slight	40.4	14.1	53.4	47.9	41.2	30.8
1987	Fatal	1.1	0.5	1.0	1.0	1.2	2.5
	Severe	8.3	4.4	11.4	7.7	6.4	7.8
	Slight	43.2	14.3	56.2	50.0	38.3	28.2
1988	Fatal	1.1	0.4	1.2	1.0	1.3	2.7
	Severe	8.8	4.6	12.3	7.4	7.3	8.0
	Slight	41.9	13.6	58.7	50.6	26.1	28.0
1989	Fatal	1.0	0.4	1.3	0.9	1.1	2.4
	Severe	7.8	4.3	11.7	6.9	7.3	7.6
	Slight	44.0	14.5	65.4	53.4	41.2	28.9
1990	Fatal	0.9	0.3	1.2	0.8	0.9	2.2
	Severe	8.2	4.5	14.0	8.0	7.9	9.5
	Slight	48.3	17.1	81.6	64.1	49.5	32.2
1991	Fatal	0.9	0.3	1.2	0.8	0.9	2.3
	Severe	8.2	4.8	14.0	8.2	7.8	8.8
	Slight	53.3	19.5	92.5	71.2	54.5	33.3
1992	Fatal	1.0	0.3	1.3	0.9	1.3	2.0
	Severe	9.0	4.7	14.6	97.5	8.9	10.2
	Slight	62.9	22.9	*****	86.9	60.4	32.8

Source: Central Bureau of Statistics, Road accidents special Publication Series no. 842, Jerus

Table 9: Injured(*) Persons I-III/1993

	Rates per 1000		
Age	Both sexes	Males	Females
0-14	45	57	33
15-24	43	52	34
25-44	56	68	44
45-64	57	53	61
65+	77	77	77
All ages	53	60	45

Source: Use of Health Services survey, unpublished data
(*)   Injuries in two weeks, causing disability in daily activities.

Table 10: Injuries(*) Persons by Type of Injury I-III/1993

	Rates per 1000				
Age	Total(*)	Cut & Bruises	Burns	Other	Unknown
0-14	89.1	76.9	9.6	0.8	1.8
15-24	71.8	56.9	8.7	0.9	5.3
25-44	77.8	56.1	12.2	1.5	8.0
45-64	58.2	43.1	14.0	1.1	0.0
65+	64.1	44.9	17.4	1.8	0.0
All ages	68.9	52.5	11.6	1.2	3.6

Source: Use of Health Services survey, unpublished data
(*)   Injuries in two weeks, causing disability in daily activities
(**)   Total number of injuries, a person could be counted more th___ _____ _____

Table 11: Injured(*) Persons by Place of Occurrence I-III/1993

		Percent			
Age	Total	Home	Institute	Open field	Other & un
0-14	100.0	29.7	53.4	10.1	7.0
15-24	100.0	31.6	16.2	29.0	22.9
25-44	100.0	18.9	33.6	31.0	15.9
45-64	100.0	40.7	27.1	25.9	6.5
65+	100.0	54.3	2.7	21.2	21.8
All ages	100.0	32.0	31.0	23.1	13.9

Source: Use of Health Services Survey, unpublished data
 (*) Injuries in two weeks, causing disability in daily activities.

Table 12: Injured(*) Persons by First Agent of Care I-III/1993

		Percent			
Age	Total	Clinic	Hospital & Emergency Room	Other	No medical care
0-14	100.0	44.7	23.8	3.6	27.9
15-24	100.0	28.7	51.9	2.1	17.3
25-44	100.0	32.1	38.2	0.0	29.7
45-64	100.0	40.4	28.0	3.7	27.9
65+	100.0	33.0	17.2	0.0	49.9
All ages	100.0	36.4	31.8	1.9	29.9

Source: Use of Health Services Survey, unpublished data
 (*) Injuries in two weeks, causing disability in daily activities.

Sources of Injury Related Data and Special Methodological Problems

The Death Certificate as a Source of Injury Data

by Harry M. Rosenberg, Ph.D. and Kenneth D. Kochanek

Introduction

The death certificate is one of our oldest sources of data on injuries, representing a system that has evolved over hundreds of years and one that has achieved a modicum of international comparability. In lieu of well established, comprehensive, and comparable data sets for morbidity, heavy reliance continues to be placed on death certificate information for both national and international injury surveillance and research. The mortality data system based on the death certificate may provide a model for other data systems in terms of its legal basis, statistical content, processing, and international standards to promote comparability. While the death certificate as a source of injury data is described in terms of the U.S. experience, it is believed that many of the examples and observations are applicable more generally.

Examples are provided of the use of death certificate information for injury prevention and control. This is followed by a description of the structure and content of the death certificate with an emphasis on items of particular relevance to injury data, and by the way in which death certificate information is processed and processing changes that are likely in the foreseeable future as a result of automation increasingly applied to information and statistical systems. The paper concludes with a discussion of some issues in the use of death certification information for injury research and injury monitoring.

Importance of Death Certificate Information

As a cause of death, the average level of mortality from Accidents and adverse effects in the United States has decreased almost 50 percent since 1950 (Figure 1) (1). Yet while the level of age–adjusted death rates from this cause decreased, the relative importance of accident mortality increased, that is, its rank a leading cause of death increased because the mortality from other leading causes of death, principally heart disease and stroke, decreased even more sharply than accidents during this period. Thus, accidents was the 5th leading cause of death in the United States in 1991 for all age groups combined but the leading cause of death for each of the age groups 1–4 years, 5–14 years, 15–24 years, and 25–44 years (Table 1). At older ages, the relative importance of accidents decreases because the high age–specific mortality of chronic diseases enables them to compete successfully for a higher ranking as the leading cause (2). By ages 45–64, accidents dropped to a ranking of 4th, and by ages 65 and over, accidents further declined to a rank of 7th. Still in the older age groups, accidents are a significant cause of death accounting for a total of 26,444 deaths to persons 65 and older in 1991.

In terms of it impact on health, society, and family, the toll of accident mortality as usually measured is greatly understated because of its great impact among the young and therefore its much greater effect on life expectancy than chronic diseases whose mortality is concentrated at older ages. This effect is well known, of course, and is reflected in the use in injury presentations of alternative measures such as Potential Years of Life Lost rather than age–adjusted death rates when depicting the health impact of accident mortality.

The continuing importance of death certificate data from the national vital statistics system is underscored by the major undertaking to monitor the health status of the U.S. population described in Healthy People 2000: National Health Promotion and Disease Prevention Objectives (3). This comprehensive statistical effort involves monitoring the well–being of the U.S. population in terms of the 22 priority areas of which Unintentional injuries is priority area No. 9 (Figure 2). In Healthy People 2000, injury mortality and morbidity are measured using a variety of indicators (Figure 3), four of which are based on mortality data from the death certificate. These areas are deaths for all injuries combined, for falls, for drownings, and for residential fire deaths.

Death certificate data are also the foundation of major occupational injury information published by the National Institutes for Occupational Safety and Health through the National Traumatic Occupational Fatality Reporting System

(4), or NTOF, and by the U.S. Bureau of Labor Statistics through its Census of Fatal Occupational Injuries (5). A recent occupational mortality report of the National Center for Health Statistics (NCHS) based on information from death certificates shows that accidents are a major source of mortality in certain occupation groups (6). Examples from this report illustrate the use of death certificate information for identifying high risk occupations. Shown in Figure 4 are the ten highest statistically significant Proportionate Mortality Ratios (PMR's) for occupations and causes of death in 12 states in 1984. Thus, in the extractive occupations, for males 20 years and over, mortality from accidents was almost five times higher than that in all occupations combined, reflected in a PMR of 456. For men working in Forestry, fishing and hunting, the relative risk of death measured by the PMR was 361; for male farm workers the PMR was 248; and for electricians, 246. These were all statistically significant. For females, occupations with elevated risk of death from accidents include persons working in mail distributing occupation with a PMR of 203 (Figure 5); and protective service occupations, a PMR of 199. The report shows that there were many other occupations where accidents are a major risk, but these were the most prominent in terms of an elevated PMR. A report with more recent data and a much larger data base is now in preparation as a collaborative project of NCHS and NIOSH.

These illustrations underscore the continuing importance of information from the death certificate as an important source of data to define and to monitor the health burden of injuries both in the United States and in other countries.

The Death Certificate

The document that is the basis for mortality data in the U.S. and other countries in the death certificate. In the decentralized vital statistics of the U.S., death certificates are legal and statistical documents of the states, not of the Federal government. However, some degree of standardization in the structure and content of the various death certificates used by the states is achieved by their willingness, for the most part, to adhere to a "model" certificate promulgated by NCHS. Shown in Figure 6 is the U.S. Standard Certificate of Death that was promulgated by NCHS in 1989 (8) and adopted in a form very close to this by all of the states.

In the United States, two persons complete the information on the death certificate. The bottom half of the certificate is the medical certification of death which is completed by the attending physician, medical examiner, or coroner; and the top half, which contains the demographic information, is completed by the funeral director, who also has the ultimate responsibility for filing the certificate with the appropriate state registration officials, who are custodians of the original records. The state registration officials also have the authority and responsibility to conduct queries for questionable or incomplete information (such as followup for death whose cause is pending investigation), or where the particulars of an accident are not adequately described.

On the U.S. Standard Certificate of Death, the format of the medical certification of death is consistent with the International Form of Medical Certificate of Cause of Death required by the World Health Organization (9). To the extent that there are differences between the WHO standard and the certificate format recommended by NCHS to the states, it is the additional line in Part I of the U.S. Standard to allow for more medical conditions in the chain of events leading to death.

For injury–related deaths, the U.S. Standard Certificate of Death has a number of items including the date and time of the injury, whether the injury occurred at work, a description of how the injury occurred, the place of injury, and the actual street location of the injury. Clearly, the death certificate is a potentially rich source of statistical information on injuries. It is also instructive to note what the standard death certificate does not ask regarding injuries. It does not, for example, ask explicitly about drug or alcohol involvement; and it does not clearly specify the degree of detail that is acceptable when describing how the injury occurred. Moreover, it does not include prompts specific for accidents that would encourage the medical provider to provide useful information in an automobile accident whether the decedent was the driver or a passenger, or the location of the accident in terms of such categories as mine, farm, or residence. As the death certificate is now structured, the level of reporting detail for accidents is left entirely to the judgement, ingenuity, and energy of the certifier.

The reverse side of the U.S. Standard Certificate of Death contains instructions for completing the death certificate (Figure 7). At the bottom of the instructions are two examples of properly–completed medical certifications. One of these—the upper example—is a so–called "natural" cause of death; the lower example is an injury, in this case an automobile accident that resulted in death from a skull fracture. Inclusion of these examples in the death certificate instructions in the two dozen states that adopted them greatly assisted in proper completion of death certificates, according to the many appreciative calls received by NCHS staff. The impact of the revised certificates is also reflected in NCHS and state mortality statistics, where improvements were observed in the specificity of medical certifications and the reporting of some ill–defined certifications. In terms of the latter (Table 2), for example, the trend in deaths reported for Heart failure, which had been increasing annually from 1979 to 1988 declined by 10 percent between 1988 and 1989, a reduction presumably attributable to the introduction of the revised death certificates. Introduction of the revised death certificate resulted in a number of other trend discontinuities among the leading causes of death such as for diabetes and for atherosclerosis, as noted in the NCHS annual mortality report for 1989 (10).

The statistical consequences of the revision in the U.S. death certificates is instructive in the sense that it shows that almost any change in a vital statistics data collection instrument may have an effect on the resultant information that is collected. That should be borne in mind as the U.S. and other countries move toward electronic systems of data entry for vital records, as discussed below.

Processing Death Certificate Information

The nature and quantity of injury information on the death certificate has been substantially and positively affected by changes in the way in which information from the death certificate has been processed. Additional changes are underway that will further affect the types of data on injury available to researchers and others. These changes have implications for international studies of health and for the international comparability of mortality statistics. While these processing systems were developed in the United States, they are being increasingly adopted by other countries, and may eventually become a model or a standard for processing mortality data.

Multiple Cause Coding

The first major change occurred in 1968, when NCHS began to routinely code multiple causes of death rather than just the underlying cause of death. While multiple causes had been periodically coded before, as early as 1917 and for a major study in 1955, this type of coding had never been done routinely because of the expense involved. But beginning with mortality data for 1968, multiple cause coding was introduced on a routine basis on the grounds that the resultant data would be more uniform and much more informative than underlying cause of death data alone. The software and data entry system is called "ACME," a well–known by now acronym that stands for Automated Classification of Medical Entities (11). The practical significance of the system is (1) that a medical coder codes not one but all of the conditions reported on the medical certification of death, (2) the computer system, not a medical coder, selects the single underlying cause of death resulting in much more consistency in selecting the underlying cause, and (3) most important, that both underlying and multiple cause–of–death data tapes and tabulations are available on an annual basis. For injury research, ACME opened up new doors by making available on a routine basis for the first time the "nature of injury" or N–codes. These codes describe the impact of an external cause of death. Thus, in the earlier example of a motor vehicle accident resulting in a skull fracture, the only information captured in underlying cause–of–death tabulations is the motor vehicle accident or the external cause; the skull fracture, or nature of injury, ordinarily would not be captured. But in multiple cause–of–death statistics, it is routinely available. Mortality data shown in Table 3 from a paper by Israel, Rosenberg, and Curtin, (12) show a cross–tabulation of injuries, suicides, and homicides by their respective nature of injuries. Thus, in 1979, a total of 54,479 nature of injury entries were reported for motor vehicle accidents (second column of the table); almost half were intracranial injuries, excluding those associated with skull fractures. Nature–of–injury codes are useful also in providing more specificity than the traditional E–codes for, for example, the types of poisons that resulted in a poisoning death, or in adverse effects and complications.

Multiple cause data are useful for injury research not only for analysis, but also for understanding the nature of the medical certification itself. For example, shown in Table 4 is the distribution of conditions reported on the death certificate for the ten leading causes of death (13). In 1991, of the 89,347 deaths due to injuries, 16.1 percent had three conditions reported on the death certificate. This percent could be examined over time to see if information on injuries is growing more or less informative, and in relation to the trend for other causes of death. In another example of using multiple cause data to evaluate the medical certification of death, Table 5 shows the average number of causes per death for selected underlying causes that are infrequently reported with other causes of death. For motor vehicle accidents, the average number of conditions reported on the death certificate is 1.94. External causes are more likely than other causes to be the only condition reported on the death certificate. For almost half of motor vehicle accidents, no other condition was reported on the death certificate. In contrast, other underlying causes are frequently reported with other causes (Table 6). For diabetes, for example, on only 2.8 percent of the certificates in 1991, was this the only cause reported on the death certificate; the average number of causes reported for these certificates was 3.46.

TRANSAX

Other changes in processing death certificate information have important implications for injury research. In 1977–78, NCHS developed the actual system by which multiple cause–of–death data are processed; this is called the "TRANSAX" system, for translation of axes (14). Under this system, for each death record, two types of information are made available, one in which the statistical record contains a code, called the "entity" code, for every condition reported on the death certificate, and the other, a "record" code which combines information from several codes when appropriate using linkages that are reminiscent of those used for underlying cause–of–death data. For example, acute myocardial infarction and hypertension as entities on a death certificate would be combined into Acute myocardial infarction with hypertensive disease.

MICAR

Another important development in processing mortality data occurred in 1990 when NCHS began implementing the "MICAR" system (15). MICAR, which stands for Mortality Medical Indexing, Classification, and Retrieval, is a major step toward simplifying data entry for medical information from the death certificate. The ultimate goal of NCHS in developing the MICAR system is entry of the full text of the medical certification of death and with computer identification of appropriate multiple cause–of–death codes, both entity axis and record axis codes, and—through ACME—selection, as now, the underlying cause of death. In 1990, the first year of implementation of MICAR, about five percent (94,372) of the U.S. death records were coded using MICAR with subsequent processing through ACME for underlying cause and through TRANSAX for multiple cause–of–death data. In 1991, the percent increased to 26, with 573,416 records (16). With MICAR and its successor SUPERMICAR, which is still under development, each entry on the death certificate is classified to an index or reference number that is independent of the International Classification of Diseases, and that will eventually permit retrieval of the full text of the medical certification of death. Examples of SUPERMICAR listings shown in Figures 8 through 11 show the potential of this system for retrieving information of value for injury surveillance and research.

Electronic Death Certificate

The next major development in both collecting and processing data from the death certificate will be the electronic death certificate (EDC). The EDC concept, and it is that to a large extent, is that the funeral director and the medical certifier will enter the literal information at a computer terminal from which it will be transmitted, without a paper copy, to the state, and then to NCHS. At the point of data entry, instructions can be given interactively; queries can be made for incomplete or inconsistent information; and edits can be implemented. At the state office, the information can be processed through TRANSAX and ACME, and the information can be used on a current basis for creating continuous data stream in real time at both the state and national level. Such a system, when fully implemented, could have a dramatically positive effect for both the timeliness and the quality of death registration data.

The development of an electronic vital record began with the birth certificate in the 1980's, and has been widely implemented. For 1991, a total of 19 states either partly or entirely collected their birth certificate information in this way. It is estimated that about 25 percent of the almost 4 million births annually are reported on electronic birth certificates. The impetus for an electronic death certificate has not been as compelling as for an electronic birth certificate; but the process has begun, most notably with early implementation of such a system in New Hampshire and now with a number of pilot tests in a number of states. Creating such a system for the death certificate is more complicated than for the birth certificate. For the birth certificate only one person is responsible for completing the record; but for the death certificate, both a medical certifier and a funeral director are now involved in the process. How the information from these two sources will be integrated and cross-checked will present a challenge. In addition, for the death certificate, the editing and querying process is much more complicated than for births. One will have to question the certifier for, for example, a lack of specificity for cause of death, such as failing to report the primary site of a cancer, or failing to adequately describe the circumstances under which an injury occurred.

In the next few years, it is likely that development and initial implementation of an EDC will occur, resulting in much better and more timely death registration data.

Mortality Data Dissemination

Mortality data from the death certificate are made available in both published and electronic form. "Final" mortality data—representing the entire death file and processed largely by the states using the automated systems—are available 1.5–2.0 years after the close of a data year. Processing the final mortality data is largely automated. In contrast, provisional mortality data are based on a 10–percent sample and are processed manually by NCHS; they are available about 4–5 months after the principal month of occurrence. Another difference is that final mortality data are available on both a multiple and underlying cause basis, while provisional mortality data are available only on an underlying cause basis. The final data has been available in electronic form on data tapes beginning with the 1968 data year; but provisional data are not yet available electronically.

Issues in the Use of Death Certificate Information for Injury Surveillance and Research

Death certificate information from the national vital statistics system constitute a basic and important element in a statistical system for monitoring injuries, as noted in the use of these data for Healthy People 2000 and for occupational injury surveillance. Yet, there are a number of issues and limitations in the use of mortality data that should be noted. Some of these are related to the quality and completeness of the information reported on the death certificate.

Completeness

Among the issues are the completeness of the information. For example, for 48,574 motor vehicle accident deaths in the U.S. in 1989, a total of 8,553 or almost one of five did not specify who was injured, that is, a driver or a passenger or a cyclist or a pedestrian (17). In the case of the 12,151 falls in the U.S. in 1981, the largest specified number, 1,163, was on steps; but 5,694, or almost half of these deaths were from Other and unspecified falls. In the important area of firearm mortality, it is important to identify which deaths are from handguns. In 1989, of the 1,489 deaths attributed to firearms, a total of 231 were reported as due to handguns. Yet, almost five times as many were not firearms unspecified as to type, which constituted the largest category of accidental firearm deaths. Thus, the area of completeness of reporting is a critical element in the effective use of death certificate information for injury prevention and control.

How can this be addressed? For one thing, better education of medical certifiers is needed on how to complete the death certificate. NCHS has initiated a number of efforts directed at physicians to improve cause–of–death reporting beginning with two national workshops, one in 1989 (18) and the other in 1991 (19). These initiatives are continuing. A second approach to addressing this problem is querying at the state level. Death certificates with incomplete information on injuries should not be permitted to pass to the stage of processing without asking the medical certifier for sufficiently complete information to make it useful for injury surveillance (20). These initiatives need to be national in scope if they are to result in good information on which to base injury prevention programs.

Information Augmentation

It needs to be recognized that even if all the items on the death certificate were answered completely and accurately, there would still be need for additional information on injuries that is not routinely captured on the death certificate, or, if captured, not in a standard, uniform, and dependable way. Examples include whether drugs or alcohol may have been involved in the accident. Without a direct question to the certifier asking about substance abuse, one can expect as many studies have shown that the impact of substance abuse on injuries cannot be adequately measured using information on the standard death certificate. Additional information from another source is needed to augment the information routinely collected on the death certificate.

What kinds of augmentation are possible? One type is what NCHS calls "followback" surveys. These are surveys using death certificates as a sampling frame that can be used to get additional information on deaths for a special subset of the decedent population, based on demographic characteristics or on causes of death. Last conducted in 1986 (21); the National Mortality Followback Survey focussed on obtaining socio-economic information such as income, and information on health care in the last year of life. A new NCHS mortality followback survey is going into the field this year.

Another approach to augmenting information reported on the death certificate is by linking information reported on the death certificate with that from another source. For example, the 1993 national mortality followback survey includes a component to link with abstracts of coroner/medical examiner records. This will not only augment information on the death certificate but will also be a useful basis for checking the reliability of the cause of death reported by the same medical examiner or coroner who completed the death certificate.

The death certificate can be linked to a variety of other sources including hospital records, health examination survey records, health interview records, and administrative records—each of which can potentially enrich the mortality data base for injury research.

Validity and Reliability

The question of validity and reliability is one that suffuses information from the vital registration system. The death certificate, and in particular cause of death, is always a prime suspect in these investigations. Many studies have been published on the validity of cause of death reflected in the NCHS annotated bibliography of 128 such studies carried out over a period of 23 years (22), with an update published in 1991 (23).

Some of these studies raise troubling questions regarding the medical certification of death, but these have been largely in the area of natural causes, or deaths related to disease processes of relatively long duration. For injuries, the cause of death tends to be more clear-cut and immediate in its fatal action. Nevertheless, questions of validity do often arise regarding manner of death, that is, whether the injury was accidental, suicidal, or homicidal. Only in-depth studies can shed light on this, and, even in some cases, the basic records will not reveal what the medical certifier has chosen not to report.

Conclusion

In conclusion, the death certificate is likely to continue to serve as a basic source of injury data despite its known limitations, because it still represents the only data source with mandatory reporting, universal coverage, and international standards for data collection, classification, and reporting (24). These are formidable attributes—developed over several centuries—to which other data systems aspire in their relative youth, but have not yet realized. Until they do, mortality data will continue to be a key data source for injury surveillance and research on an national and international basis.

References

1.   National Center for Health Statistics. "Advance Report of Final Mortality Statistics, 1991" <u>Monthly Vital Statistics Report</u>; Vol. 42, No. 2, Supplement. Hyattsville, Maryland: Public Health Service. 1993a.

2.   <u>ibid</u>.

3.   U.S. Department of Health and Human Services. <u>Healthy People 2000: National Health Promotion and Disease Prevention Objectives</u>. Washington: Public Health Service. 1991.

4.   National Institute for Occupational Safety and Health. <u>National Traumatic Occupational Fatalities: 1980–86</u>. September 1989.

5.   U.S. Department of Labor, Bureau of Labor Statistics, <u>Fatal Workplace Injuries in 1992: A Collection of Data and Analysis</u>, Report 870, April 1994.

6.   Rosenberg, HM, Burnett C, Maurer J, Spirtas R. "Mortality by Occupation, Industry, and Cause of Death: 12 Reporting States, 1984." <u>Monthly Vital Statistics Report</u>; Vol. 2, No. 4, Supplement. Hyattsville, Maryland. 1993b.

7.   National Center for Health Statistics. "Annual Summary of Births, Marriages, Divorces, and Death: United States, 1992. <u>Monthly Vital Statistics Report</u>; Vol. 41, No. 13. Hyattsville, Maryland: Public Health Service. 1993c.

8.   Tolson GC, Barnes JM, Gay GA, Kowaleski JL. "The 1989 Revision of the U.S. Standard Certificates and Reports." National Center for Health Statistics. <u>Vital and Health Statistics</u>. Series 4, No. 29. June 1991.

9.   World Health Organization. <u>International Classification of Diseases: Manual of the International Statistical Classification of Diseases, Injuries, and Causes of Death (ICD–9)</u>. Geneva, 1977.

10.   National Center for Health Statistics. "Advance Report of Final Mortality Statistics, 1989" <u>Monthly Vital Statistics Report</u>; Vol. 40, No. 2, Supplement. Hyattsville, Maryland: Public Health Service. 1991.

11.   National Center for Health Statistics. <u>Vital Statistics of the United States, 1989</u>, Vol. II, Mortality, part A. Washington: Public Health Service. 1993d. DHHS Pub. No. (PHS) 93–1101. U.S. Government Printing Office.

12.   Israel RA, Rosenberg HM, Curtin LR. "Analytical Potential for Multiple Cause–of–Death Data," <u>American Journal of Epidemiology</u>, Vol. 124, No. 2, pp. 161–179. August 1986.

13.   Kochanek K, Rosenberg HM. "Issues, Considerations, and Examples in the Use of Multiple Causes of Death in U.S. Government Statistics," paper presented at the Meeting on Multiple Causes of Morbidity and Mortality, World Health Organization. London, April 26–28, 1994.

14.   Chamblee RF and Evans MC. "TRANSAX, the NCHS System for Producing Multiple Cause–of–Death Statistics, 1968–78. National Center for Health Statistics. <u>Vital and Health Statistics</u>. Series 1, No. 20. June 1986.

15.   National Center for Health Statistics. "Vital Statistics, Data Entry Instructions for the Mortality Medical Indexing, Classification, and Retrieval System (MICAR). <u>NCHS Instruction Manual; Part 2g</u>. Hyattsville, Maryland: Public Health Service. Published annually.

16.   National Center for Health Statistics, op.cit., 1993a.

17.   National Center for Health Statistics, op.cit., 1993d.

18.   National Center for Health Statistics and The National Committee on Vital and Health Statistics, Report of the Workshop on Improving Cause-of-Death Statistics, Virginia Beach, Virginia, October 15–17, 1989.

19.   National Center for Health Statistics and The National Committee on Vital and Health Statistics, Report of the Second Workshop on Improving Cause-of-Death Statistics, Virginia Beach, Virginia, April 21–23, 1991.

20.   Rosenberg HM. "The Impact of Cause-of-Death Querying." Technical Papers, No. 45. International Institute for Vital Registration and Statistics. June 1991.

21.   Poe GS, Powell-Griner E, McLaughlin JK, et al. "Comparability of the Death certificate and the 1986 National Mortality Followback Survey. National Center for Health Statistics. Vital and Health Statistics. Vol. 2, No. 118. November 1993.

22.   Gittelsohn A, Royston PN, "Annotated Bibliography of Cause-of-Death Validation Studies, 1958–80." National Center for Health Statistics. Vital and Health Statistics. Vol. 2, No. 89. 1982.

23.   National Center for Health Statistics, op.cit., 1989.

24.   Rosenberg HM, "Improving Cause-of-Death Statistics," American Journal of Public Health, Vol. 79, No. 5, May 1989, pp. 563–564.

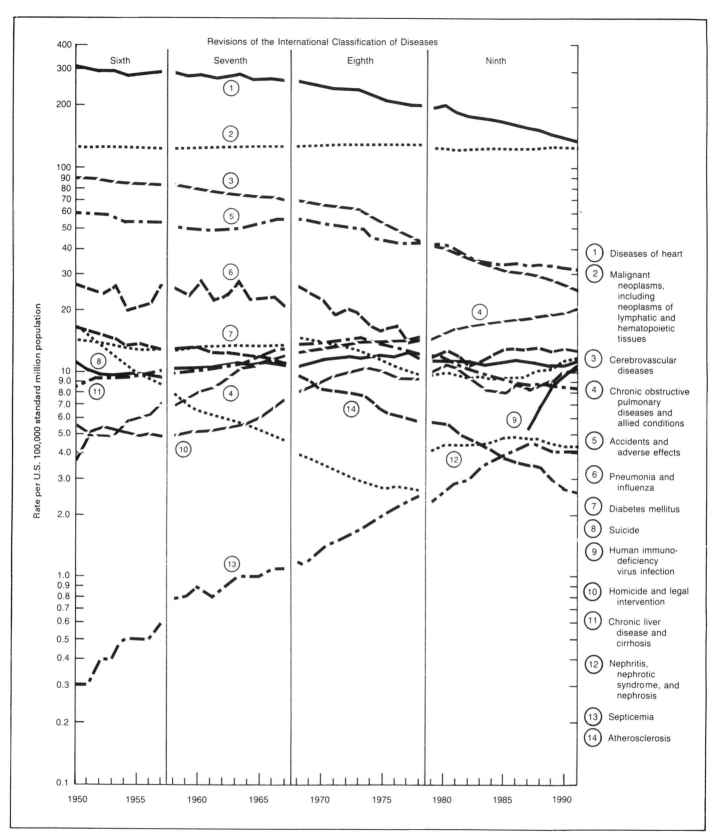

Figure 1. Age-adjusted rates for 14 of the 15 leading causes of death: United States, 1950–91

Figure 2. Priority areas for Healthy People 2000

1. Physical activity and fitness objective status
2. Nutrition objective status
3. Tobacco objuective status
4. Alcohol and other drugs bojective status
5. Family planning objective status
6. Mental health and mental disorders objective status
7. Violent and abusive behavior objective status
8. Educational and community based programs objective status
9. Unintentional injuries objective status
10. Occupational safety and health objective status
11. Environmental health objective status
12. Food and drug safety objective status
13. Oral health objective status
14. Maternal and infant health objective status
15. Heart disease and stroke objective status
16. Cancer objective status
17. Diabetes and chronic disabling conditions objective status
18. HIV objective status
19. Sexually transmitted diseases objective status
20. Immunization and infectious diseases objective status
21. Clinical preventive services objective status
22. Surveillance and data systems objective status

Figure 3. Unintentional injuries objective status, Healthy People 2000

Objective	Original	Revised
9.1 Unintentional injury deaths (age-adjusted per 100,000)...	34.5	34.7
a. American Indians/Alaska Natives (age-adjusted per 100,000).	82.6	66.0
b. Black males (age-adjusted per 100,000).....................	64.9	68.0
b. White males (age-adjusted per 100,000).....................	53.6	49.8
9.2 Unintentional injury hospitalizations (per 100,000)......	887	832
9.3 Motor vehicle crash-related deaths		
Per 100 million vehicle miles traveled (VMT).................	2.4	...
Age-adjusted per 100,000 people..............................	18.8	19.2
a. Children 14 years and under (per 100,000).................	6.2	...
b. People 15-24 years (per 100,000).........................	36.9	...
c. People 70 years and over (per 100,000)...................	22.6	...
d. American Indians/Alaska Natives (age-adjusted per 100,000).	46.8	37.7
e. Motorcyclist (per 100 million VMT).......................	40.9	...
(per 100,000)..	1.7	...
f. Pedestrians (per 100,000)................................	3.1	2.8
9.4 Fall-related deaths (age-adjusted per 100,000)...........	2.7	No change
a. People 65-84 years (per 100,000).........................	18.0	18.1
b. People 85 years and over (per 100,000)...................	131.2	133.0
c. Black males 30-69 years (per 100,000)....................	8.0	8.1
9.5 Drowning deaths (age-adjusted per 100,000)..............	2.1	No change
a. Children aged 4 and under (per 100,000)..................	4.2	4.3
b. Males 15-34 years (per 100,000).........................	4.5	No change
c. Black males (age-adjusted per 100,000)...................	6.6	No change
9.6 Residential fire deaths (age-adjusted per 100,000).......	1.5	1.7
a. Children 4 years and under (per 100,000).................	4.4	4.5
b. People 65 years and over (per 100,000)..................	4.4	4.9
c. Black males (age-adjusted per 100,000)...................	5.7	6.4
d. Black females (age-adjusted per 100,000).................	3.4	3.3
e. Residential fire deaths caused by smoking................	17%	26%
9.7 Hip fractures among older adults (per 100,000)...........	714	...
a. White females 85 years and over..........................	2,721	...
9.8 Nonfatal poisoning (per 100,000)........................	103	108
a. Among children 4 years and under.........................	650	648
9.9 Nonfatal head injuries (per 100,000)....................	125	118
9.10 Nonfatal spinal cord injuries (per 100,000).............	5.9	5.3
a. Males..	8.9	9.6
9.11 Secondary disabilities associated with head and spinal cord injuries		
Head injuries (per 100,000).................................	20.0	...
Spinal cord injuries (per 100,000)..........................	3.2	...
9.12 Motor vehicle occupant protection systems...............	42%	...
a. Children 4 years and under...............................	84%	...
9.13 Helmet use by motorcyclists and bicyclists		
Motorcyclists...	60%	...
Bicyclists..	8%	...
9.14 Safety belt and helmet use laws		
Number of States with safety belt laws......................	33	...
Number of States with Motorcycle Helmet Use Laws............	22	...
9.15 Number of States with handgun design to protect children.	0	...
9.16 Fire suppression sprinkler installation (number of localities)..	...	700
9.17 Residences with smoke detectors.........................	81%	...
9.18 Injury prevention instruction in schools................	---	...
9.19 Protective equipment in sporting and recreation events...	---	...
National Collegiate Athletic Association		
Football..	Required	...
Hockey..	Required	...
Lacrosse..	Required	...
High school football..	Required	...
Amateur boxing..	Required	...
Amateur ice hockey..	Required	...
9.20 Number of States with design standards for roadway safety	---	...
9.21 Injury prevention counseling by primary care providers...	---	...
9.22 Number of States with linked emergency medical services and trauma systems..................................	2	...

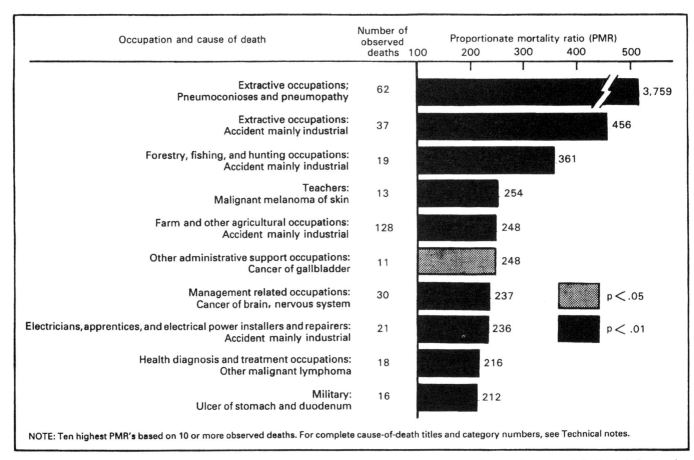

Figure 4. Ten highest statistically significant proportionate mortality ratios (PMR's) for occupations and causes of death and observed number of deaths for males 20 years of age and over: Total of 12 reporting States, 1984

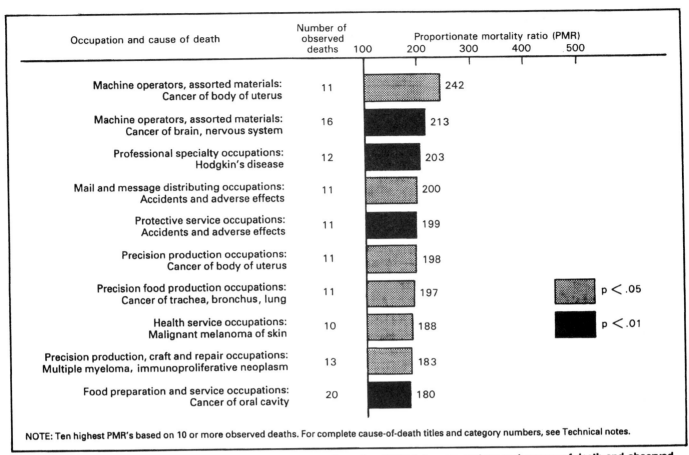

Occupation and cause of death	Number of observed deaths	Proportionate mortality ratio (PMR)
Machine operators, assorted materials: Cancer of body of uterus	11	242
Machine operators, assorted materials: Cancer of brain, nervous system	16	213
Professional specialty occupations: Hodgkin's disease	12	203
Mail and message distributing occupations: Accidents and adverse effects	11	200
Protective service occupations: Accidents and adverse effects	11	199
Precision production occupations: Cancer of body of uterus	11	198
Precision food production occupations: Cancer of trachea, bronchus, lung	11	197
Health service occupations: Malignant melanoma of skin	10	188
Precision production, craft and repair occupations: Multiple myeloma, immunoproliferative neoplasm	13	183
Food preparation and service occupations: Cancer of oral cavity	20	180

p < .05

p < .01

NOTE: Ten highest PMR's based on 10 or more observed deaths. For complete cause-of-death titles and category numbers, see Technical notes.

Figure 5. Ten highest statistically significant proportionate mortality ratios (PMR's) for occupations and causes of death and observed number of deaths for females 20 years of age and over: Total of 12 reporting States, 1984

FIGURE 6. U.S. STANDARD CERTIFICATE OF DEATH

TYPE/PRINT IN PERMANENT BLACK INK FOR INSTRUCTIONS SEE OTHER SIDE AND HANDBOOK

LOCAL FILE NUMBER

U.S. STANDARD
CERTIFICATE OF DEATH

STATE FILE NUMBER

DECEDENT

1. DECEDENT'S NAME *(First, Middle, Last)*		2. SEX	3. DATE OF DEATH *(Month, Day, Year)*

4. SOCIAL SECURITY NUMBER	5a. AGE—Last Birthday *(Years)*	5b. UNDER 1 YEAR		5c. UNDER 1 DAY		6. DATE OF BIRTH *(Month, Day, Year)*	7. BIRTHPLACE *(City and State or Foreign Country)*
		Months	Days	Hours	Minutes		

SEE INSTRUCTIONS ON OTHER SIDE

8. WAS DECEDENT EVER IN U.S. ARMED FORCES? *(Yes or no)*

9a. PLACE OF DEATH *(Check only one; see instructions on other side)*

HOSPITAL: ☐ Inpatient ☐ ER/Outpatient ☐ DOA   OTHER: ☐ Nursing Home ☐ Residence ☐ Other *(Specify)*

9b. FACILITY NAME *(If not institution, give street and number)*	9c. CITY, TOWN, OR LOCATION OF DEATH	9d. COUNTY OF DEATH

10. MARITAL STATUS—Married, Never Married, Widowed, Divorced *(Specify)*	11. SURVIVING SPOUSE *(If wife, give maiden name)*	12a. DECEDENT'S USUAL OCCUPATION *(Give kind of work done during most of working life. Do not use retired.)*	12b. KIND OF BUSINESS/INDUSTRY

13a. RESIDENCE—STATE	13b. COUNTY	13c. CITY, TOWN, OR LOCATION	13d. STREET AND NUMBER

13e. INSIDE CITY LIMITS? *(Yes or no)*	13f. ZIP CODE	14. WAS DECEDENT OF HISPANIC ORIGIN? *(Specify No or Yes—If yes, specify Cuban, Mexican, Puerto Rican, etc.)* ☐ No ☐ Yes Specify:	15. RACE—American Indian, Black, White, etc. *(Specify)*	16. DECEDENT'S EDUCATION *(Specify only highest grade completed)* Elementary/Secondary (0-12) | College (1-4 or 5 +)

PARENTS

17. FATHER'S NAME *(First, Middle, Last)*	18. MOTHER'S NAME *(First, Middle, Maiden Surname)*

INFORMANT

19a. INFORMANT'S NAME *(Type/Print)*	19b. MAILING ADDRESS *(Street and Number or Rural Route Number, City or Town, State, Zip Code)*

DISPOSITION

20a. METHOD OF DISPOSITION ☐ Burial ☐ Cremation ☐ Removal from State ☐ Donation ☐ Other *(Specify)* _____	20b. PLACE OF DISPOSITION *(Name of cemetery, crematory, or other place)*	20c. LOCATION—City or Town, State

21a. SIGNATURE OF FUNERAL SERVICE LICENSEE OR PERSON ACTING AS SUCH ▶	21b. LICENSE NUMBER *(of Licensee)*	22. NAME AND ADDRESS OF FACILITY

SEE DEFINITION ON OTHER SIDE

PRONOUNCING PHYSICIAN ONLY

Complete items 23a-c only when certifying physician is not available at time of death to certify cause of death.	23a. To the best of my knowledge, death occurred at the time, date, and place stated. Signature and Title ▶	23b. LICENSE NUMBER	23c. DATE SIGNED *(Month, Day, Year)*

ITEMS 24-26 MUST BE COMPLETED BY PERSON WHO PRONOUNCES DEATH

24. TIME OF DEATH M	25. DATE PRONOUNCED DEAD *(Month, Day, Year)*	26. WAS CASE REFERRED TO MEDICAL EXAMINER/CORONER? *(Yes or no)*

SEE INSTRUCTIONS ON OTHER SIDE

CAUSE OF DEATH

27. **PART I.** Enter the diseases, injuries, or complications that caused the death. Do not enter the mode of dying, such as cardiac or respiratory arrest, shock, or heart failure. List only one cause on each line.

Approximate Interval Between Onset and Death

IMMEDIATE CAUSE (Final disease or condition resulting in death) ➜ a. _____
DUE TO (OR AS A CONSEQUENCE OF):

Sequentially list conditions, if any, leading to immediate cause. Enter **UNDERLYING CAUSE** (Disease or injury that initiated events resulting in death) **LAST**

b. _____
DUE TO (OR AS A CONSEQUENCE OF):

c. _____
DUE TO (OR AS A CONSEQUENCE OF):

d. _____

PART II. Other significant conditions contributing to death but not resulting in the underlying cause given in Part I.	28a. WAS AN AUTOPSY PERFORMED? *(Yes or no)*	28b. WERE AUTOPSY FINDINGS AVAILABLE PRIOR TO COMPLETION OF CAUSE OF DEATH? *(Yes or no)*

29. MANNER OF DEATH ☐ Natural ☐ Pending Investigation ☐ Accident ☐ Suicide ☐ Could not be Determined ☐ Homicide	30a. DATE OF INJURY *(Month, Day, Year)*	30b. TIME OF INJURY M	30c. INJURY AT WORK? *(Yes or no)*	30d. DESCRIBE HOW INJURY OCCURRED
	30e. PLACE OF INJURY—At home, farm, street, factory, office building, etc. *(Specify)*		30f. LOCATION *(Street and Number or Rural Route Number, City or Town, State)*	

SEE DEFINITION ON OTHER SIDE

CERTIFIER

31a. CERTIFIER *(Check only one)*

☐ CERTIFYING PHYSICIAN *(Physician certifying cause of death when another physician has pronounced death and completed Item 23)* To the best of my knowledge, death occurred due to the cause(s) and manner as stated.

☐ PRONOUNCING AND CERTIFYING PHYSICIAN *(Physician both pronouncing death and certifying to cause of death)* To the best of my knowledge, death occurred at the time, date, and place, and due to the cause(s) and manner as stated.

☐ MEDICAL EXAMINER/CORONER On the basis of examination and/or investigation, in my opinion, death occurred at the time, date, and place, and due to the cause(s) and manner as stated.

31b. SIGNATURE AND TITLE OF CERTIFIER ▶	31c. LICENSE NUMBER	31d. DATE SIGNED *(Month, Day, Year)*

32. NAME AND ADDRESS OF PERSON WHO COMPLETED CAUSE OF DEATH (ITEM 27) *(Type/Print)*

REGISTRAR

33. REGISTRAR'S SIGNATURE ▶	34. DATE FILED *(Month, Day, Year)*

PHS-T-003

Left margin: NAME OF DECEDENT: For use by physician or institution

Left margin (vertical): DEPARTMENT OF HEALTH AND HUMAN SERVICES – PUBLIC HEALTH SERVICE – NATIONAL CENTER FOR HEALTH STATISTICS – 1989 REVISION

FIGURE 7. U.S. STANDARD CERTIFICATE OF DEATH (REVERSE SIDE)

INSTRUCTIONS FOR SELECTED ITEMS

Item 9.— Place of Death

If the death was pronounced in a hospital, check the box indicating the decedent's status at the institution (inpatient, emergency room/outpatient, or dead on arrival (DOA)). If death was pronounced elsewhere, check the box indicating whether pronouncement occurred at a nursing home, residence, or other location. If other is checked, specify where death was legally pronounced, such as a physician's office, the place where the accident occurred, or at work.

Items 13-a-f. — Residence of Decedent

Residence of the decedent is the place where he or she actually resided. This is not necessarily the same as "home State," or "legal residence." Never enter a temporary residence such as one used during a visit, business trip, or a vacation. Place of residence during a tour of military duty or during attendance at college is not considered as temporary and should be considered as the place of residence.

If a decedent had been living in a facility where an individual usually resides for a long period of time, such as a group home, mental institution, nursing home, penitentiary, or hospital for the chronically ill, report the location of that facility in items 13a through 13f.

If the decedent was an infant who never resided at home, the place of residence is that of the parent(s) or legal guardian. Do not use an acute care hospital's location as the place of residence for any infant.

Items 23 and 31 — Medical Certification

The PRONOUNCING PHYSICIAN is the person who determines that the decedent is legally dead but who was not in charge of the patient's care for the illness or condition which resulted in death. Items 23a through 23c are to be completed only when the physician responsible for completing the medical certification of cause of death (Item 27) is not available at time of death to certify cause of death. The pronouncing physician is responsible for completing only items 23 through 26.

The CERTIFYING PHYSICIAN is the person who determines the cause of death (Item 27). This box should be checked only in those cases when the person who is completing the medical certification of cause of death is not the person who pronounced death (Item 23). The certifying physician is responsible for completing items 27 through 32.

The PRONOUNCING AND CERTIFYING PHYSICIAN box should be checked when the same person is responsible for completing Items 24 through 32, that is, when the same physician has both pronounced death and certified the cause of death. If this box is checked, items 23a through 23c should be left blank.

The MEDICAL EXAMINER/CORONER box should be checked when investigation is required by the Post Mortem Examination Act and the cause of death is completed by a medical examiner or coroner. The Medical Examiner/Coroner is responsible for completing items 24 through 32.

Item 27. — Cause of Death

The cause of death means the disease, abnormality, injury, or poisoning that caused the death, not the mode of dying, such as cardiac or respiratory arrest, shock, or heart failure.

In Part I, the immediate cause of death is reported on line (a). Antecedent conditions, if any, which gave rise to the cause are reported on lines (b), (c), and (d). The underlying cause, should be reported on the last line used in Part I. No entry is necessary on lines (b), (c), and (d) if the immediate cause of death on line (a) describes completely the train of events. ONLY ONE CAUSE SHOULD BE ENTERED ON A LINE. Additional lines may be added if necessary. Provide the best estimate of the interval between the onset of each condition and death. Do not leave the interval blank; if unknown, so specify.

In Part II, enter other important diseases or conditions that may have contributed to death but did not result in the underlying cause of death given in Part I.

See examples below.

Figure 8. Super-MICAR Certificate Listing

```
------------------------------------------------------------------------------
                            Certificate Information
------------------------------------------------------------------------------
Certificate:  000466          Sex:   M              Date of Death:  03/24/1993
Age:          9               Unit:  MONTHS         State of Death:

                     Conditions Causing Death       Duration:
Ia:  CRANIO-CEREBRAL INJURIES                        MINUTES
Ib:
Ic:
Id:


II:  ACUTE ALCOHOLIC INTOXICATION


Manner of Death:  1           Date of Injury:  03/24/1993    Injury at Work?:  N
Injury Description:
FELL DOWN STAIRS
Place of Injury:              Date of Surgery:

State of Occurrence:          State-Specific Data:  02

------------------------------------------------------------------------------
```


Figure 9. Super-MICAR Certificate Listing

```
------------------------------------------------------------------------------
                            Certificate Information
------------------------------------------------------------------------------
Certificate:  000398          Sex:   F              Date of Death:  02/14/1993
Age:          6               Unit:  MONTHS         State of Death:

                     Conditions Causing Death       Duration:
Ia:  PROBABLE ASPHYXIA
Ib:  WATERBED ACCIDENT
Ic:
Id:


II:


Manner of Death:  1           Date of Injury:  02/13/1993    Injury at Work?:  N
Injury Description:
WATERBED ACCIDENT
Place of Injury:              Date of Surgery:

State of Occurrence:          State-Specific Data:  02

------------------------------------------------------------------------------
```

Figure 10. Super-MICAR Certificate Listing

```
-----------------------------------------------------------------------------
                          Certificate Information
-----------------------------------------------------------------------------
Certificate:  000438        Sex:   M              Date of Death:  03/26/1993
Age:          9             Unit:  MONTHS          State of Death:

                  Conditions Causing Death         Duration:
Ia:  MULTIPLE ORGAN FAILURE                         48 HOURS
Ib:  SEPSIS                                         48 HOURS
Ic:  50% TOTAL BODY SURFACE AREA BURN               7 WEEKS
Id:

II:

Manner of Death:  1         Date of Injury:  02/07/1993    Injury at Work?:  N
Injury Description:
PRESUMABLY CARELESS COOKING
Place of Injury:            Date of Surgery:

State of Occurrence:        State-Specific Data:  02

-----------------------------------------------------------------------------
```

Figure 11. Super-MICAR Certificate Listing

```
-----------------------------------------------------------------------------
                          Certificate Information
-----------------------------------------------------------------------------
Certificate:  000005        Sex:   M              Date of Death:  01/15/1993
Age:          77            Unit:  YEARS          State of Death:

                  Conditions Causing Death         Duration:
Ia:  HYPOTHERMIA
Ib:  ENVIRONMENTAL COLD (OUTDOOR) EXPOSURE FOLLOWING
     APPARENT FALL WITH MINOR HEAD INJURY
Ic:
Id:

II:

Manner of Death:  1         Date of Injury:            Injury at Work?:
Injury Description:

Place of Injury:            Date of Surgery:

State of Occurrence:        State-Specific Data:

-----------------------------------------------------------------------------
```

Experiences Using New Zealand's Hospital Based Surveillance System for Injury Prevention Research

by John Langley Ph.D.

Abstract

The focus of this paper is the Injury Prevention Research Unit's (IPRU's) experience in analysing New Zealand's national public hospital injury data set. The existence of the national inpatient data management system has enabled the IPRU to develop an injury morbidity data set for period 1979-1992. The IPRU thus, has data on over three quarters of a million injury events that were serious enough to warrant admission to a hospital. This data set has been used extensively by the IPRU to address a wide range of injury issues.

Apart from the demographic variables those variables that have proved most useful in our work have been: length of stay, readmission indicator, a personal identifier code number named the National Master Patient Index Number (NMPI), WHO International Classification of Disease coding for: diagnoses and external cause of injury (E-code), and written descriptions of external cause of injuries and location of injury event. Practical examples of IPRU's use of each of these variables are given. These examples demonstrate how invaluable New Zealand's inpatient injury data set is for: documenting resource utilisation, accurately determining the incidence of events, undertaking analytical epidemiological studies, and addressing shortcomings in E-codes.

A key aspect of the system is the narrative information. Evidence is produced that demonstrates the electronic recording of narratives of the circumstances of injury is an invaluable tool for conducting epidemiological research which has direct implications for injury prevention policy and practice. Given the numerous objections that are raised about E-coding, injury prevention personnel would be well served to encourage health authorities to electronically record narratives as a first step towards uniform coding.

The Importance of Morbidity Data

Traditionally, injury mortality has been used in determining priorities for prevention. While deaths are clearly a significant outcome of injury it is important to realize that non fatal injuries place a substantial burden on a community. For example, in New Zealand for each injury death there are approximately 32 admissions to a public hospital for the treatment of injury (Langley and McLoughlin 1989). Of greater significance is the fact that the distribution of injury events can vary markedly depending on the outcome of interest. The leading cause of injury death in New Zealand is motor vehicle traffic crashes (MVTC) (37 percent), followed by suicide (21 percent), whereas the leading injury event resulting in an admission to hospital is a fall (25 percent), followed by a MVTCs (19 percent), with self inflicted injury playing a minor role (Langley and McLoughlin 1989). Such variations have been shown to exist in other countries (Baranick et.al. 1983) and clearly need to be considered in determining priorities for prevention.

New Zealand National Hospital Based Data System

There is only one national hospital based 'injury surveillance' system in New Zealand. It is part of the national hospital morbidity data collection system that is managed by the New Zealand Health Information Service of the Ministry of Health. The hospital data base records detail, at discharge, on all persons who have been inpatients or daypatients in public general hospitals, maternity hospitals and registered private hospitals. Data on patient separations from psychiatric hospitals is recorded in a separate Mental Health data set.

For public hospital discharges the data system records information on a range of demographic, injury, and circumstances of injury data elements (see below). A substantially reduced range of data elements is recorded for private hospitals. Significant among those absent from those records are the ICD External causes of Injury and

Poisoning coding, otherwise known as E-codes (WHO 1978). The latter omission, in particular, has precluded the inclusion of private hospital data in studies undertaken by the Injury Prevention Research Unit (IPRU). This exclusion, however, is of little significance from a primary prevention perspective, however, when it is considered that most acute injury, is treated in public hospitals in New Zealand. This is demonstrated by the statistics for 1992 which show there were 59,918 injury inpatients, and 9,951 injury day patients discharged from public hospitals in New Zealand. The comparable figures for private hospitals were: 1,717 and 676. Reference to the injury diagnosis codes for the latter show that treatment is primarily for non acute injury (e.g., late effects of injury) (New Zealand Health Information Service 1993).

In addition to the national hospital injury data set there are a large number of local emergency department based surveillance systems. These, however, vary widely in their coverage, comprehensiveness and methods of recording (Irving 1994) and at present, are of limited use from an injury prevention perspective. The focus of this paper is thus on the IPRU's experience in analysing the national public hospital injury data set (hereafter referred to as the data set).

Summary of Public Hospital Data Elements

The following data are currently collected from public hospitals:

- gender
- age
- marital status
- date of birth
- **length of stay**
- referral source
- discharge date
- source of admission (routine, or from another hospital)
- admission date
- ethnicity
- type of admission (e.g., acute, arranged)
- **readmission indicator**
- type of discharge
- hospital of treatment
- hospital transferred from
- domicile
- **National Master Patient Index Number (NMPI)**
- hospital department treating patient
- event type
- **WHO International Classification of Disease coding for:**
  - **diagnoses**
  - **external cause of injury (E-code)**
  - operation
- **written descriptions of**
  - diagnoses
  - **external cause of injuries**
  - **location of injury event**
  - operations performed

The maintenance of this patient management system has enabled the IPRU to develop an injury morbidity data set for period 1979-1992. IPRU has thus, data on over three quarters of a million injury events that were serious enough to warrant admission to a hospital. This data set has been used extensively by the IPRU to address a wide range of injury issues. Aside from the demographic variables those variables that have proved most useful in our work are printed in bold type above. Applications of these are discussed below.

Length of Stay

In determining priorities for prevention one important consideration is the personal and societal costs of specific categories of injury. Although a class of events may not have a high incidence relative to others, the costs associated with it may be disproportionate to its incidence. Unfortunately, at present we have no simple way of determining all the personal and societal costs for specific classes of injury. One key element in any determination of the cost of injury would be health service utilisation costs. Length of stay in hospital in the acute phase of injury provides a crude indicator of these costs. In 1992 persons whose primary diagnosis was a fractured neck of femur represented 6.3 percent of all discharges from public hospital but 24 percent of the total injury bed day utilisation (NZHIS 1993).

Readmission Indicator

Most IPRU studies have sought to estimate the incidence of specific events. Given that persons are admitted to hospital for the treatement of their injury in the acute and rehabilitative phases it is important to be able to differientate the two. Failure to do so could produce a substantial error in instances where an individual has a series of readmissions for the ongoing rehabilitation of an injury (e.g., skin grafting following thermal injury). In the past reference has been made to the readmission indicator for this purpose. In the 1992 hospital data set there were 69,996 separations which had an E-code assigned to them, 20 percent of these related to readmissions. There has, however been increasing awareness that this field was not well reported and in some of the more recent IPRU studies (e.g., Collins et al 1993) reference has been made to a variety of other variables (e.g., date of injury) to determine incidence. The readmission indicator is no longer a mandatory field.

National Master Patient Index Number (NMPI)

It is important to note that the data system relates to episodes of care, not individuals. From 1988 onwards, all individuals admitted to hospital were assigned a unique identifier which was to be used for all their future contacts with the public hospital system. That identifier has enabled the IPRU to initiate analytical epidemiological studies. One such study, presently in progress, seeks to test the hypothesis that prior injury, especially that due to assault, is a risk factor for subsequent assault. Given that we have national data on admissions, we have been able to use a cohort study design using the total population of New Zealand to test this hypothesis. Very briefly, the method used was as follows. The "exposed" group consisted of all those who had been admitted to a hospital for the treatment of injury in a reference year. Using their NMPI the relevant files were searched to determine if they had been admitted for assault within a twelve month period from the date of their reference discharge date and a serious injury rate for the exposed group is calculated. Since the total population of persons who were admitted to hospital for assault for any specified period is known one is able by deduction to estimate the assault rate for the non-exposed group, that is, those who had not been hospitalised for the treatment of injury in the reference year.

Diagnosis Coding

All injuries are coded according to the ICD injury and poisoning codes, (WHO 1978). These enable us to more accurately identify cases of interest in a number of different respects.

It is not widely appreciated that E-coding is applied to morbidity other than injury and poisoning. The ICD-9 states "Certain other causes which may be stated to be due to external causes are classified in Chapters I to XVI of ICD and for these, the 'E'-code classification should be used as an additional code for multiple condition analysis only." In 1992, there were 69,996 persons who had an E-code assigned to their discharge summary. Of these, 10 percent had a non injury code as their primary diagnosis. Typical of such cases would be a person who suffered epilepsy followed by an immersion incident. In this case the submersion would be assigned an injury code of 994.1 as a secondary diagnosis. Another example would be at patient who suffered injury while being treated in hospital for another non-injury condition.

There are a number of injury events for which it is difficult, if not impossible, to accurately determine incidence by reference to specific E-codes. Submersion incidents provide a good example. The submersion codes in ICD are: E830 "Accident to watercraft causing drowning", E832 "Other accidental submersion or drowning in water transport", E910 "Accidental drowning and submersion", E954 "Suicide and self inflicted injury by submersion [drowning]", E964 "Assault by submersion [drowning]", and E984 "Submersion [drowning], undetermined whether accidentally or purposely inflicted." Reference to these codes alone will result in an underestimate of the incidence of drowning. For example, all submersion incidents which result from motor vehicle traffic crashes (e.g., driver losing control, car running off road and into lake) are coded within the motor vehicle traffic crash grouping (E810-E819). The use of the diagnostic code for submersion provides a solution to this. The code is 994.1 "Drowning and non fatal submersion." A search of the public hospital database for the period 1988-92 inclusive revealed that there were 567 discharges which had this diagnosis. There were nine cases which were the result of motor vehicle traffic crashes (E810-E819).

Similarly, reference to diagnostic codes also allows one to identify coding errors. For example, in the submersion investigation referred to immediately above, we also identified 22 cases which had the code E883 "Fall into holes or other opening in surface" assigned to them. The ICD specifically excludes submersion incidents from this code. It appears that coders in New Zealand have not adhered to ICD guidelines in this regard.

External Cause of Injury (E-code) and Written Descriptions of External Cause of Injuries

One key aspect of any injury surveillance system is information on the circumstances of the injury event. There have repeated calls, particularly in the USA, for uniform E-coding; that is, coding according to the External Causes of Injury and Poisoning Codes of the International Classification of Diseases (WHO) (Runyan et.al. 1992, Graciter 1987). Overseas observers will no doubt be envious of the fact that New Zealand has a national inpatient injury data system which is E-coded.

Runyan et.al. (1992) asserted that "Without E-code information, it is almost impossible to define directions for prevention or to evaluate adequately the success of prevention interventions." While IPRU supports the principle of uniform E-coding it should be noted that E-codes have several shortcomings from a prevention perspective (Langley 1982, Baker 1982). Moreover, it has been IPRU's experience that E-coding is not critical to prevention efforts and much can be achieved by the use of electronic recording of narratives of the circumstances of injury. This point deserves emphasising since it may well be easier in some countries or cities to initially encourage hospitals to electronically record the circumstances of injury in the form of a free text narrative, rather than argue for E-coding. The ideal, of course, is to have both and that is the situation in New Zealand.

Despite limitations associated with free text, this can be a very useful supplement to E-codes. The principal benefits are that: it can provide estimates of the incidents of events which do not have specific E-codes, enable misclassification errors to be detected, and provide more accurate estimates of the incidence of specific events within E-code categories. Below are examples of each of these points taken from the IPRU's experience.

<u>Determining the Incidence of Events Which Do Not Have Specific E-codes</u>

The E-codes attempt to summarize what is frequently a complex injury event by means of a single code. Given the variety of circumstances leading to injury, even within a relatively confined category, this is bound to be less than satisfactory for those concerned with injury prevention, since they often cannot obtain the degree of specificity which would allow prevention action to be initiated or evaluated. Once solution to this limitation is to conduct special surveys, but this can be expensive, time consuming, and in many instances where one is concerned with historical trends, of limited value. Free text descriptions can often address this shortcoming. A good example of this is the McLoughlin et.al. (1986) evaluation of New Zealand's Safety of Children's Night Clothes Act 1977 and the follow up study by Laing et.al. (1991). Critical to those evaluations was a determination of whether the clothing ignition burns recorded involved nightwear and, if so, the type of nightwear (pyjamas vs night dresses). The ICD E-codes do not provide for such a degree of specificity to be achieved. It was, thus, only by reference to narratives that the authors were able to determine the impact of the legislation.

Another good example was the study by Buckley et.al. (1993) which sought to determine the incidence of falls from horses. These events are coded under E828 "Accident involving animal being ridden." There is no fourth digit sub classification. Thus, in the absence of free text descriptions, it would not have been possible to identify the type of the animal being ridden or, indeed, whether the incident involved a fall.

Improving Estimates

Even where E-codes allow a high level of specificity, it is possible that case under-ascertainment can still occur due to shortcomings in the E-codes. Two examples illustrate the point.

"Unspecified Motorcyclists"

Begg et.al. (1994), in a recent study of motorcycle crashes, identified eighteen fatalities and 133 hospitalisations by examining the free text narratives for crashes where the road user was coded as "unspecified." Although provision is made in the E-codes for coding of drivers or pillion passengers of motorcycles, no such specific provision is made for those situations in which the victim is simply described as a "motorcyclist." These cases and analogous ones (e.g., "occupant of a car") are all coded as unspecified road users. Investigators in other countries who rely solely on ICD codings to identify cases will tend to underestimate the incidence of events involving specific classes of road user. Based on her findings Begg et.al. (1994) concluded that the underestimate is not likely to be substantial for mortality but could be significant for morbidity.

"Hidden" Firework Injuries

The ICD manual instructs that injuries due to fireworks should be coded under E923 "Accident caused by explosive material." A fourth digit makes specific provision for the coding of these events (E923.0 "Fireworks"). A recent investigation by the IPRU identified 170 fireworks events over an eleven year period by examining free text descriptions associated with E923. All the words and phrases which were associated with these events (e.g., firecrackers, fireworks, sky rockets), including those which were misspelt, were used to search the entire hospital injury morbidity files for any further cases. In total, an additional 36 cases were found. Sixteen injury events were classified as E917 striking against or struck by objects or persons; and 14 cases were attributed to fire and flames (E890-E899 "Accidents caused by fire and flames").

Written Descriptions of the Location of Injury Event

The ICD makes provision for the coding of ten categories of place of occurrence. This is a very limited classification and hinders prevention initiatives (Langley and Chalmers 1989). The ICD codes do not, for example, permit the identification of injury events which occur at school. These are typically coded as a public place. To complicate the issue further, injuries which occur in school 'playgrounds' are coded under places of recreation and sport. In New Zealand, specific provision is made to record a 12-character description of the place of occurrence. This facility has been used by Langley et.al. 1990 to produce an estimate of the incidence of school injuries. Fanslow et.al. (1991) also used this to produce an estimate of the incidence of assault events in hotels, taverns, and other licensed premises.

Conclusion

As the foregoing demonstrates New Zealand has a hospital data system which is invaluable for injury prevention research in terms of describing the incidence of specific events, undertaking analytical studies, and evaluating interventions. A key aspect of the system is the free text narratives. Evidence has been produced here to demonstrate that the electronic recording of narratives of the circumstances of injury is an invaluable tool for prevention. This point is critical since most emergency departments currently maintain hard copy of such information. The increasing role of computers in hospital administration provides the opportunity to electronically record this information. Given the numerous objections which will be raised about E coding (e.g., staff training, costs: Rivara et.al. 1990), injury prevention would be well served by the encouragement of health authorities to electronically record narratives as a first step towards uniform coding. This allows for the future possibility of subsequent coding although it is appreciated that the information currently recorded may be insufficient to E-code. This problem needs to be addressed by educating medical personnel. The accurate assessment of the mechanism of injury is as important on the medical record as are vital signs (Rivara et.al. 1990).

It has been the IPRU's experience that it would be valuable to have free text data fields tagged for specific items (e.g., occupation, location, event). Clearly, there is considerable scope beyond that which is recorded in New Zealand (e.g., activity, products). As has been shown here, the ideal would be to have both uniform coding and free text data.

References

1.   Begg DJ, Langley JD, Reeder AI. Motorcycle crashes in New Zealand resulting in death and hospitalisation I: Introduction, methods, and overview. Accid. Anal. & Prev. 26: 2:157-164. 1994.

2.   Buckley SM, Chalmers DJ, Langley JD. Injuries due to falls from horses. Australian Journal of Public Health. 17: 3:269-271. 1993.

3.   Buckley SM, Langley JD, Chalmers DJ. Falls from moving motor vehicles in New Zealand. Accid. Anal. & Prev. 25: 6:773-776. 1993.

4.   Chalmers DJ. (1991) Falls from playground equipment: An overview. A background paper prepared for the Child Accident Prevention Foundation's National Childhood Injury Prevention Forum, Wellington. Injury Prevention Research Unit, Dunedin.

5.   Chalmers DJ, and Langley JD. Epidemiology of playground equipment injuries resulting in hospitalisation. J. Paediatr. Child Health. 26: 6:329-334. 1990.

6.   Collins BA, Langley JD, Marshall SW. Injuries to pedal cyclists resulting in death and hospitalisation. NZ Med J. 106:514-517. 1993.

7.   Dixon GS, Danesh JN, Caradoc-Davies TH. Epidemiology of spinal cord injury in New Zealand. Neuroepidemiology. 12:88-95. 1993.

8.   Fanslow JL, Chalmers DJ, Langley JD. Injury from assault: A public health problem. Prepared for the Alcoholic Liquor Advisory Council. IPRU, Dunedin. 1991.

9.   Hume PA, Marshall SW. Sports injuries in New Zealand: Exploratory Analyses. NZ J Sports Medicine (in press).

10.   Johnston SE, Langley JD, Chalmers DJ. Serious unintentional injuries associated with architectural glass. NZ Med J. 103:117-9. 1990.

11.   Koorey AJ, Marshall SW, Treasure ET, Langley JD. Incidence of facial fractures resulting in hospitalisation in New Zealand from 1979 to 1988. Int. J. Oral Maxillofac. Surg. 21:77-79. 1992.

12.   Kotch JB, Chalmers DJ, Langley JD. Child day care and home injuries involving playground equipment. J. Paediatri. Child Health. Vol 29:222-227. 1993.

13.   Laing RM and Bryant V. Prevention of burn injuries to children involving nightwear. NZ Med J. 104:363-5. 1991.

14.   Langley JD. Description and classifications of childhood burns. Burns. 10:231-235. 1984.

15.   Langley JD. Frequency of injury events in New Zealand compared with the distribution of E-codes. Methods of Information in Medicine. 26:89-92. 1987.

16.   Langley JD. The incidence of dog bites in New Zealand. NZ Med J. 105:33-35. 1992.

17.   Langley JD. The International Classification of Diseases Codes for Describing Injuries and Circumstances Surrounding Injuries: A critical comment and suggestions for improvement. Accid. Anal. & Prev. 14:195-197. 1982.

18.   Langley JD, Begg DJ, Reeder AI. Motorcycle crashes in New Zealand resulting in death and hospitalisation II: Traffic crashes. Accid. Anal. & Prev. 26: 2:165-171. 1994.

19.   Langley JD and Chalmers DJ. Place of occurrence of injury events in New Zealand compared with the available ICD codes. Methods of Information in Medicine. 28:109-113. 1989.

20.   Langley JD, Chalmers DJ, Collins B. Unintentional injuries to students at school. J. Paediatr. Child Health. 26:323-328. 1990.

21.   Langley JD and Johnston SE. Purposely self-inflicted injuries resulting in death and hospitalisation in New Zealand. Community Health Studies. 1990; 15:190-199. 1990.

22.   Langley JD and McLoughlin E. Injury mortality and morbidity in New Zealand. Accid. Anal. & Prev. 21:243-254. 1989.

23.   Langley JD, Marshall S. The severity of road traffic crashes resulting in hospitalisation in New Zealand. Accid. Anal. & Prev. (in press).

24.   Langley JD, Phillips D, Marshall S. Inpatient costs of injury due to motor vehicle traffic crashes in New Zealand. Accid. Anal. & Prev. Vol 25:5:585-592. 1993.

25.   McLoughlin E, Langley JD, Laing RM. Prevention of children's burns: Legislation and fabric flammability. NZ Med J. 99:804-807. 1986.

26.   Marshall S, Kawachi I, Cryer C, Wright D, Slappendel C, Laird I. The epidemiology of forestry work-related injuries in New Zealand 1975-1988 fatalities and hospitalisations. NZ Med J (in press).

27.   Norton R, Langley JD. Firearm deaths in New Zealand, 1978-1987. NZ Med J. 106:463-5. 1993.

28.   Phillips DE, Langley JD, Marshall SW. Injury - The medical and related costs in New Zealand 1990. NZ Med J. 106:215-8. 1993.

29.   Waller AE, Marshall SW. Childhood thermal injuries in New Zealand resulting in death and hospitalisation. Burns. 19: 5:371-376. 1993.

30.   Baker SP. Injury Classification and the International Classification of Diseases Codes. Accid. Anal. & Prev. 14:199-201. 1982.

31. Baranick JI, Chatterjee BF, Greene YC, Michenzi EM and Fife D. North Eastern Trauma Study: I. Magnitude of the Problem. Am J Public Health. 73:746-751. 1983.

32. Graitcer PL. The development of state and local injury surveillance systems. Journal of Safety Research. 18:191-198. 1987.

33. Irving LM, Norton RN, Langley JD. Injury surveillance in public hospital emergency departments. NZ Med J (in press).

34. Langley JD. The International Classification of Diseases Codes for Describing Injuries and Circumstances Surrounding Injuries: A critical comment and suggestions for improvement. Accid. Anal. & Prev. 14:195-197. 1982.

35. New Zealand Health Information Service. Hospital and Selected Morbidity Data 1992 . Ministry of Health. Wellington, 1993.

36. Rivara FP, Morgan P, Bergman AB, Maier RV. Cost estimates for statewide reporting of injuries by E-coding hospital discharge abstract data base systems. Public Health Reports. 105:635-637. 1990.

37. Runyan CW, Bowling JM, Bangdiwala SI. Emergency department record keeping and the potential for injury surveillance. The Journal of Trauma. 32:187-189. 1992.

38. World Health Organisation, International Classification of Diseases, Geneva WHO, 1978.

Acknowledgements and Disclaimer

The Injury Prevention Research Unit is jointedly funded by the Accident Compensation and Rehabilitation Corporation and the Health Research Council of New Zealand. The views expressed here are those of the author and do not necessarily reflect those of the funding organisations. The comments and advice of Stephen Marshall, David Chalmers, Gail de Boer in the preparation of this paper are appreciated. The assistance and advice of the New Health Information Service in the provision of the injury data is appreciated.

Federal Injury Surveillance in Canada: Filling the Gaps

by G.J. Sherman, Ph.D.

Abstract

Health Canada's experience in injury epidemiology was almost nonexistent when, in May, 1989, representations to the Deputy Minister resulted in the formation of a 10–hospital surveillance system for childhood injury on a three year pilot basis. The first of the three years was devoted to investigating injury surveillance systems around the world for philosophical and technical merit and negotiating a working arrangement with the 10 Canadian pediatric hospitals. Eleven months later, in April, 1990, the first data from the *Children's Hospitals Injury Reporting and Prevention Program* (CHIRPP) were generated.

CHIRPP was based on the Australian national injury surveillance program (NISPP) and although a number of modifications have been made in both programs over the last four years they continue to share almost identical data collection strategies and record content. Both are Emergency Room–based systems which emphasize pre–injury event circumstances, as small a response burden on data providers as possible, a rapid processing turnaround for timeliness and a powerful software interface which is given to all program participants.

CHIRPP is now the *Canadian Hospitals... Program* because it now includes five general hospitals and has become, by default, an all–ages surveillance program although the emphasis remains on children. The presentation will concentrate on the strengths of the ER–based approach, some of the major difficulties that have been encountered and the usefulness of the program in the spectrum of activities that comprise injury surveillance and control.

Data Sources Prior to CHIRPP

Canada is a federal nation consisting of ten provinces and three territorial areas, each having its own government and a federal government, based in Ottawa. Provincial governments are responsible for the collection and maintenance of Vital Records and for the provision of direct health care services. Therefore, certain population–based information on "health" in a broad sense and on injury in particular are collected and collated at the provincial/territorial level, e.g., death certificates, hospital admission/discharge records. Under fairly long–standing and stable arrangements, copies (or in some cases, summaries) of these records are sent to the national statistical agency, Statistics Canada, for pooling into national datasets. For example, the national Mortality Database exists in machine–readable form back to 1950 (1927 for some provinces) and the national Hospital Morbidity Database dates back to 1979.

Both of these files are based on individual records (although person–based in the case of mortality and event–based in the case of morbidity) and both have been used by researchers and policy makers attempting to either summarize secular trend in injury occurrence, identify emerging injury hazards, carry out risk analysis–type exercises and even to attempt to monitor the effect of injury intervention programs.

Although neither dataset has been used to its full potential, these morbidity and mortality files have formed the basis for almost all of the injury epidemiology and prevention work that has been done in Canada when such activities have been "data driven".

There are two problems with this approach; one bears directly on my presentation today and the other only tangentially. The former has to do with the fact that hospitalization and death from injury, as important as they are, represent a relatively small proportion of the number of injuries that occur, i.e., the most serious or severe part. But this is a "clinical" or "medical" use of the term "serious", not a public health use. Injuries that are catastrophic (and possibly costly) to individuals tend not to be those that place the largest burden on populations. Concentrating on hospital admission and death from injuries reinforces the notion that the individual, "big injury" is the proper societal focus and this continues, in general, to be the case. It is also the case that the information on these records concentrates on post–event, patient management data.

The other problem is a constellation of difficulties and shortcomings created by historical inertia, logistics and bureaucratic compromises. Both hospital in–patient and mortality records are completed well after the injury event and sometimes, particularly in the case of mortality records, so long after that the event is not related to the outcome. Both record systems are primarily administrative in nature and contain little covariate information. Both are coded to the ICD revision of the day, the deficiencies of which for injury prevention planning purposes have been widely documented.[1] Both record systems concentrate on post–event, patient management and outcome data and are virtually lacking in any circumstantial information that might prove useful in planning interventions. Neither dataset is available less than two years from the date of the event and access is controlled by the provisions of the national *Statistics Act* and the cost–recovery mechanisms of Statistics Canada. The hospital in–patient records are not as yet linked to form records on individuals. The fact that these are *events* and not persons is a handicap to their usefulness.

In brief, mortality and hospital in–patient records provide a fairly selective window on injury in the population in a not particularly timely, informative or accessible way. They have been used to some advantage in the past and will continue to play a role in the development of our knowledge about injury but present sufficient shortcomings to predict a need for supplementary data sources.

Filling the Gap

Such a need was expressed by a group of professionals interested in injury prevention who met in 1988. Dr. Barry Pless of McGill University and one of Canada's few *bona fide* injury epidemiologists represented this group in meetings with Dr. Maureen Law, then Deputy Minister of Health Canada (at that time known as Health and Welfare Canada). One of Dr. Pless' messages was that Health Canada had a responsibility to conduct injury surveillance. His detailed arguments must have been unusually compelling and it was decided that the department would attempt to conduct a three–year pilot surveillance program in the ten Pediatric Hospitals in Canada. That was about the extent of the instruction I received five years ago in May, 1989.

We were generally aware of the limitations of mortality and in–patient morbidity records as a source of surveillance data. After a rather hurried review of some existing injury surveillance programs around the world we were put in touch with officials of the Australian national program which is now known as NISPP. The Australian program, although fairly recently established at that time, was attractive philosophically, technically proven and available. After an exchange of letters at the Ministerial level the software arrived from Australia, *gratis*. This software formed the basis for what is presently called the *Canadian Hospitals Injury Reporting and Prevention Program* (CHIRPP). Although the software itself has undergone several fundamental modifications in the interim and the organization of the national programs in Australia and Canada have developed along different lines, the NISPP ancestry of CHIRPP is easily seen and gratefully acknowledged.

Goals and Philosophy of CHIRPP

The primary tenet underlying CHIRPP is that many, if not most, injuries are preventable or can be minimized by the use of appropriate strategies.

By placing within communities collections of data acquired from surveillance in that same community and encouraging the community to use those data to develop and test intervention exercises is potentially the most cost–effective way of developing strategies to make the Canadian environment safer.

By doing this in multiple, dispersed and disparate locations, studies can be undertaken to identify the influence of factors unique to individual communities and the differing degrees of influence of common factors in different environments.

By maintaining a centralized national collection studies can be undertaken to identify population–wide influences and influences specific to age, gender, neighborhood, cultural background, emerging hazards from newly–introduced consumer products of all kinds and other factors.

CHIRPP is unique in that it is the only injury surveillance system in the world which contains cause and effect information on each of the accident and the injury components, precoded and available to the user by direct inquiry.

CHIRPP is designed to provide timely data. It is designed to operate effectively in the "real world" where data collection and completion rates fall below theoretically optimal targets and where significant but varying proportions of the data collected can be largely anecdotal. It is designed to allow non–specialist users separate important signals from noise in an environment where coding mistakes and diagnostic errors actually happen. In short, CHIRPP is designed, because the Australian concept allowed it, to be simple, cost–effective and useful.

Operational Details

Background

In somewhat more technical terms, CHIRPP is a hospital–based sentinel surveillance system. It is an "active" surveillance system in the sense that individuals are sought out (in the Emergency Room) and data are collected on a purpose–designed form, not abstracted from a form designed for a different purpose.

Participating hospitals are supplied with an IBM–compatible PC, the CHIRPP software and all relevant licences, data collection forms and funds, contracted on an annual basis to cover costs of long–distance telephone calls, hardware maintenance and the salary of a program coordinator based on a formula which incorporates a flat rate plus additional remuneration based on the number of records collected. The intention is to defray costs of the program to the hospital to the greatest extent possible. This is done at the price of accommodating more centers with a less generous compensation scheme or allowing more than one type of "membership" in the program.

Each hospital has a CHIRPP "Director" who is usually the Director of the Emergency Service. The Director, who is not personally compensated in any way, is the real "sponsor" of the program in each hospital and is expected to generate and foster enthusiasm for and acceptance of CHIRPP. Directors are also supposed to encourage the use of CHIRPP data locally both within and outside of the hospital.

Completed data forms are submitted to the national office at regular intervals for coding and keying. After keying, a copy of the electronic version of the records is returned to the hospital of origin to be merged into the local database. All records are also merged into the national dataset in Ottawa. All participating centers and the national office use exactly the same software.

Data Collection

The face of the data form is self–administered, i.e., it is completed either by the injured person or by a responsible person in attendance. In the case of children, this is usually a parent. The reverse of the form is supposed to be completed by the attending physician.

This data collection strategy has the great advantage of placing a minimum of responsibility on hospital staff but it requires a population literate in one of the two official languages. This requirement is a concern in the inner cores of some cities which have experienced heavy in–migration in recent years of peoples lacking language facility in either English or French. Moreover, about 10% of people receiving a form refuse to complete it. We have not as yet studied their characteristics but assume they are not "typical" of the general population of those who attend Emergency Rooms.

We have experienced considerably more difficulty with physician compliance. Although the reverse of the form should take no longer than 10–15 seconds to complete by someone who has seen it a few times, staff meetings, Grand Rounds, including the CHIRPP form in the Emergency Room chart and even the prospect of payment per form completed has proven to be insufficient incentive to achieve satisfactory physician compliance. In fact, most coordinators spend a good deal of their time completing the reverse of the CHIRPP form from details in the chart. This is not difficult but it is time consuming and it is not what we consider the best use of the coordinator's time.

Naturally, not all forms are completed equally. One wishes that everyone would fill all available space with clear, cogent, narrative done in 8–point Letter Gothic *sans serif*. That this is not the case can hardly be surprising. The fact that the amount of description varies from hospital to hospital might be. Nevertheless, the amount and richness of information that is passed on is impressive. An important part of the Coordinator's job is to ensure that the data capture rates and the quality of what is reported are as high as possible.

Data Coding, Keypunching

CHIRPP started with coding and keypunching done at the local level. This was abandoned after three years. One of the most difficult features of the Australian approach is in the attempt to summarize, in a few codes, the reasons why the injury occurred (i.e., the so–called "Breakdown" factors). This is a complex concept to impart, requiring, as we came to realize, intensive training and regular in–service refreshers. With (originally) 10 (now 15) hospitals scattered over a 4,800 km distance and 5 time zones we were simply not able to maintain the necessary contact with the coders.

Data forms are now coded and keyed in the national office by four full–time staff who work together, teaching and learning from each other. Coding consistency has increased considerably and the cost per record for data entry has decreased marginally. Approximately 2,400 records are processed and added to the national database each week.

Data Use

A surveillance system that is not used is useless. In the risk assessment/risk management model, surveillance data can and should be used at many points including hazard identification, risk estimation, option development and monitoring/evaluation.

CHIRPP data have not yet been used at either or local or national level to the extent originally anticipated. The program has been more or less preoccupied until the last year with collecting and coding data. However, analysis and dissemination activities have increased lately and are, of course, encouraged.

The federal–local nature of CHIRPP is somewhat unusual and it has taken two years of work to forge meaningful working relationships with the myriad of federal, provincial and non–governmental agencies with an interest in injury prevention which have appeared in the last five years. The direct application of CHIRPP data at the local level for program planning with subsequent program evaluation via CHIRPP has yet to happen but we are working toward it.

Program Management

Apart from four full–time data coders, CHIRPP is administered in the national office by a Section Head (Ph.D. in Epidemiology), an analyst (M.Sc. in Epidemiology), a Research Assistant and an Information Officer for communications functions. An additional analyst position is currently vacant. There is no in–house computer hardware or software support; it is contracted–in.

A consultative committee composed of professionals from a variety of disciplines and organizations was formed two years ago and meets twice a year to review the problems, progress and plans (including budget) of the program. In addition, the national office brings the CHIRPP Directors once a year for review and planning and brings the Coordinators together to compare notes on what works (and doesn't work) in each centre to improve data capture and quality. All of these meetings generate minutes with action items which are taken seriously and followed up.

The available staff complement seems about right to handle a program the size and design of CHIRPP as does the amount of contact we have with our consultative committee. The program would probably benefit from somewhat more frequent contact between and among CHIRPP Directors, Coordinators and national office staff but the distances and competing make this difficult.

Has the Gap Been Filled?

In the last five years CHIRPP has had its share of misplaced compliments and criticisms. It has been criticized for not being population–based when in fact it was never intended to be. It has been criticized for not "getting the message" out with some justification although that is now happening. It has been complimented as a technical marvel although we basically owe it to the Australians.

The important point is that the program seems to be working. Surveillance is more a psychological, sociological and diplomatic undertaking than a technical one and progress in the beginning is incremental. Nevertheless, a body of data is starting to emerge of a richness and detail that simply does not exist anywhere else in the country or the continent. The obverse is that this richness of self–reported human experience is "fuzzy" and a lot of data is necessary to extract the important information it contains.

CHIRPP is designed to make possible the extraction and interpretation of meaningful information by any reasonably educated person. Specialized subject–area knowledge is not a prerequisite. The potential exists to easily train large numbers of people to become CHIRPP data users at minimal cost. This potential encourages the formation of community–based, intersectoral injury prevention action groups which use CHIRPP data both to determine their goals and priorities and to evaluate their own intervention initiatives. CHIRPP is designed to encourage local experimentation. These will, individually, be data driven, tentative and inexpensive. Many will not succeed but knowing what doesn't work should be regarded as being of equivalent importance as knowing what did. Those programs that do succeed (as proven by the ongoing CHIRPP surveillance) can then be evaluated for national application. Little money will be spent in the experimentation overall and the potential for reducing costs of health care (including rehabilitation) and productivity due to potential years of life lost is considerable.

Reference

1. Langley, JD. (1982) The International Classification of Disease Codes for Describing Injuries and Circumstances Surrounding Injuries: A critical comment and suggestions for improvement. Accident Analysis and Prevention 14:195–197.

Trauma Registries and Public Health
Surveillance of Injuries

by Daniel A. Pollock, M.D.

Abstract

Trauma registries are a potential source of part of the data needed for comprehensive public health surveillance of injuries. Like other disease registries, those for trauma are used to collect, store and retrieve data describing the etiologic factors, demographic characteristics, diagnoses, treatments, and clinical outcomes of individuals who meet specified case criteria. In the U.S., the scope of trauma registry case criteria tends to be limited to the most seriously injured individuals who receive hospital care for blunt or penetrating traumatic injuries or burns. Trauma registries are used primarily to monitor and evaluate trauma care at the hospital, regional, and State levels. Multi-hospital trauma registries most often have emerged in geographic areas where emergency medical services (EMS) agencies are planning or administering regional trauma care systems. Several factors have impeded the use of regional trauma registries for calculation of population-based rates of traumatic injury. First, participation in multi-hospital registries often is limited to trauma center hospitals, and even at these specialized centers there are persistent concerns about the completeness of case ascertainment and data quality. Second, injuries that do not require hospitalization usually are excluded from these registries, as are prehospital deaths. Pressures on all acute care hospitals in the U.S. to collect and report standardized trauma care data are mounting, created in large part by hospital accrediting bodies and EMS agencies. These external pressures, coupled with a renewed interest in health care outcomes in general, have created opportunities to extend the coverage of trauma registries, thereby enhancing their potential value for public health surveillance and other purposes.

Introduction

A disease registry is a file of uniform data describing individuals who meet specified case criteria in which medical and demographic data are collected in an ongoing, systematic, and comprehensive way in order to serve predetermined purposes (Brooke, 1974). In the U.S., and in other nations with well-developed vital statistics systems, registration of causes of death provides the basis for the oldest and most successful diseases registries in existence. However, mortality data reveal only the proverbial tip of the iceberg of the public health impact of a disease, and they provide a limited measure of the availability, use, and effectiveness of health care services. Data from registries of nonlethal events, including those for traumatic injury, can provide much of the data needed for more comprehensive population-based surveillance of disease incidence and outcomes.

Emergency medical services (EMS) and trauma care professionals have been at the forefront of efforts to develop trauma registries in the U.S. and elsewhere (Burns, 1991). Much of the impetus for their efforts has come from a need for data with which to monitor and evaluate the quality of trauma care, particularly at trauma center hospitals that participate in trauma care systems. The increasing capacity of computers for storage and retrieval of large amounts of data has been an additional major stimulus to the development of trauma registries. However, these registries are expensive to maintain and they are beyond the means of most developing countries (Chiu, 1993). In this report, the development of computerized trauma registries in the U.S. is summarized, their major uses and limitations are described, and the opportunities further development are outlined.

The Development of Modern Trauma Registries (U.S.)

The first computerized trauma registry in the U.S. was introduced in 1969 at Cook County Hospital in Chicago, Illinois (Table 1) (Boyd, 1971). This registry served as the prototype for Illinois Trauma Registry (ITR), a multi-hospital registry that began operations in 1971. Each of 50 designated trauma center hospitals in the Illinois trauma care system contributed data to the registry, until the loss of federal funds led to the ITR's demise in 1976. A systematic analysis of the ITR experience provides still valuable insights into the operational requirements of trauma registries (Goldberg, 1980). A secure source of funding, a well-defined patient population, a minimum data set, adequate staffing and training, and a means to estimate the completeness and accuracy of case reporting remain critical operational imperatives.

State and local EMS agencies have had lead roles in developing multi-hospital registries, usually in conjunction with their responsibilities for initiating and maintaining trauma care systems. For example, the San Diego County, California EMS Division initiated a regional trauma care system in 1984, with participation by six designated trauma center hospitals. A multi-hospital trauma registry was established to facilitate a monthly quality of care audit and to measure each trauma center's performance against its contractual obligations with the county EMS agency (Shackford, 1987). Patients included in the registry are those who meet specified case criteria for "major trauma." Because few "major trauma" patients are thought to be transported to non-trauma center hospitals, EMS administrators maintain that the trauma registry database includes virtually all patients who meet the case criteria.

Findings from a recent survey of 50 state EMS directors showed that 24 states had established trauma registries as of 1993 (Shapiro, 1993). The typical state registry was 2 years old, most were established by legislation, and 67% required trauma center participation. Some EMS agencies have succeeded in extending trauma registry coverage to all hospitals in their state, regardless of their trauma center status. For example, Alaska's trauma registry, initiated as a pilot project at seven hospitals in 1988, was extended to all 25 acute care hospitals in Alaska by 1991 (Kilkenny, 1992). However, statewide coverage of all hospitals, and with it the capacity for population-based surveillance of traumatic injuries, remains an exceptional achievement.

Medical professional groups, often with the support of funds from federal agencies, have provided considerable impetus to trauma registry development (Table 1). The Major Trauma Outcome Study (MTOS) was a multi-center study conducted under the auspices of the American College of Surgeons (ACS) from 1982 through 1989 (Champion, 1990). Investigators at more than 140 hospitals used a standardized data collection form to submit data for analysis. Many of the data elements used in the MTOS and the outcome prediction methods developed during the study have been incorporated into trauma registries that remain in operation. At the conclusion of the MTOS, the ACS committed itself to the development of a national trauma registry. This registry began operations in 1993 (Strauch, 1992). The American Pediatric Surgical Association and the American Burn Association also have been active in trauma registry development (Tepas, 1989, Saffle, 1993).

Federal agencies, working with medical organizations and other groups, have helped catalyze and coordinate national-level standardization of trauma registries (Table 1). In 1989, the Centers for Disease Control and Prevention (CDC), the National Highway Traffic Safety Administration, the American College of Emergency Physicians, the ACS and the American Medical Association co-sponsored the first national trauma workshop (CDC, 1989). The deliberations at this workshop led to a set of CDC recommendations for trauma registry case criteria (Table 2) and a set of 95 data elements, including descriptors of the injury event (Table 3). The International Classification of Diseases codes in the case criteria are for injuries that are classifiable as blunt or penetrating trauma or burns. The recommended data elements, in addition to injury event descriptors, describe the patient's identity and demographic characteristics, prehospital care, emergency department care, surgical care, anatomic diagnoses, and outcome. The CDC trauma registry recommendations have been disseminated widely and have been incorporated into public-use and commercial software packages. The U.S. Health Resources and Services Administration (HRSA) is updating and revising CDC's recommendations for trauma registries as part of HRSA's implementation of the federal Trauma Care Systems Planning and Development Act.

Uses and Limitations of Trauma Registries

Trauma registries can serve multiple purposes, including public health surveillance of the causes and consequences of traumatic injury (Table 4). To fully understand the value of trauma registries for public health surveillance and other purposes, it is important to know how individuals and agencies responsible for trauma registry operations prioritize various registry functions. Trauma care professionals and EMS agencies generally place the highest priority on quality of care monitoring and evaluation, which is reflected in the decisions they make about trauma registry case criteria, data content, data collection procedures, data preparation and analysis, and report writing.

The selection of trauma registry case criteria reflects the primary use of registries as tools to help audit the care of patients who have sustained life- or limb-threatening injuries from exposure to excessive blunt or penetrating mechanical force. Patients with these injuries, after transport to the hospital and an initial period of evaluation and treatment in the emergency department, generally are admitted as inpatients. In some instances, these patients are transferred from one hospital to a second hospital for further evaluation or admission. In other instances, resuscitative efforts in the emergency department fail and these patients die prior to hospital admission or transfer to another facility. Regardless of treatment outcome, patients with life- or limb-threatening mechanical force injuries comprise what many clinicians refer to as "major trauma." This category does not include patients whose injuries resulted from other mechanisms, such as poisoning, exposure to extreme cold or other environmental extremes, or submersion in water. Nor does this category include individuals with blunt or penetrating traumatic injuries who are treated and released from emergency departments or those with fatal injuries who die prior to hospital treatment.

The emphasis on "major trauma" patients in trauma registry case criteria has advantages and disadvantages in terms of the value of these registries for public health surveillance of injuries (Tables 5 and 6). On the one hand, the focus on patients with life- or limb-threatening injuries resulting from excessive mechanical force means that clinicians, EMS administrators, health care policymakers, and the public, despite potential differences in how they view the problem of injury, can each comprehend in general terms the causes and severity levels of the injuries that are included in trauma registry databases. This common understanding can facilitate use of trauma registry data for public health surveillance and application of the data to community-wide injury prevention initiatives (Cales, 1989).

On the other hand, the exclusion of prehospital deaths and patients who are treated and released from emergency departments from the category "major trauma" means that the injuries included in trauma registries are not representative of all injuries in the population. This problem is compounded in multi-hospital trauma registries in which participation is limited to trauma center hospitals (Payne, 1989). Further, the category "major trauma" continues to lack a standard definition among clinicians (Valenzuela, 1990). In the absence of such a standard, controversy about case criteria for trauma registries persists (Brotman, 1991), leaving open the possibility that trauma registry databases will differ in the scope of their case coverage over time and across geographic areas.

The emphasis on quality of care also both enhances and limits the value of trauma registries for public health surveillance (Tables 5 and 6). Benefits include the availability of detailed data on injury severity levels and anatomic locations, particularly compared to data available from administrative databases such as hospital discharge files. However, the extensive amount of data collected and stored on individual patients means that trauma registry operations are labor intensive and expensive. Incomplete case finding and incomplete data in some registries continues to limit their value. Expanding the scope of coverage of multi-hospital trauma registries from trauma center hospitals to all acute care hospitals in defined geographic areas can lead to population-based incidence and outcome data. However, shortcomings in case finding and data quality must be resolved for trauma registries to reach their full potential.

Opportunities to Further Develop Trauma Registries

Trauma registries have undergone rapid proliferation in the U.S. in recent years and they now serve a variety of uses and users (Table 7). Still, differences in case criteria and data contents, persistent concerns about completeness and quality, and incomplete geographic and population coverage limit their value for quality of care improvement, public health surveillance, and other purposes. Despite rapid progress, trauma registries are at an early stage of development relative to other disease registries (Pollock, 1989). Experience with these registries, such as those for cancer, may help identify ways to further develop trauma registries. For example, in the U.S., several population-based state cancer registries were created by consolidating local hospital registries.

Several factors favor further progress in developing trauma registries. Hospital accrediting bodies and government agencies responsible for EMS are seeking trauma care data with which to monitor and evaluate trauma care. Professional medical groups active in trauma care are designing or have implemented plans for national trauma registries. Proponents of trauma care systems are advocating more inclusive systems, with participation by all acute care hospitals. These activities, coupled with the interest in health care outcomes generated by the movement for health care reform, have created opportunities to further development of trauma registries. Capitalizing on these opportunities will require a concerted effort by trauma care professionals, medical groups, public health agencies at the local, state and federal levels, health care services researchers, epidemiologists, specialists in medical informatics and other individuals and groups.

References

1. Boyd DR, Rappaport DM, Marbarger JP, Baker RJ, Nyhus LM. Computerized trauma registry: A new method for categorizing physical injuries. Aerospace Medicine 1971;42:607-615.

2. Brooke EM. The current and future use of registers in health information systems. Publication No. 8, Geneva: World Health Organization, 1974.

3. Brotman S, McMinn DL, Copes WS, Rhodes M, Leonard D, Konvolinka CW. Should survivors with an Injury Severity Score less than 10 be entered in a statewide trauma registry? J Trauma 1991;21:1233-1239.

4. Burns CM. The 1990 Fraser Garde Lecture: A Canadian trauma registry system - Nine years experience. J Trauma 1991;31:856-866.

5. Cales RH, Kearns ST, Jordan LS, and Division of Injury Epidemiology and Control, CEHIC, CDC. National survey of trauma registries--United States, 1987. MMWR 1989;38:857-859.

6. Centers for Disease Control. Report from the 1988 Trauma Registry Workshop, including recommendations for hospital-based trauma registries. J Trauma 1989;29:827-834.

7. Champion HR, Copes WS, Sacco WJ, Lawnick MM, Keast SL, Bain LW, Flanagan ME, Frey CF. The Major Trauma Outcome Study: Establishing national norms for trauma care. J Trauma 1990;11:1356-1365.

8. Chiu W-T, Dearwater SR, McCarty DJ, Songer TJ, LaPorte RE. Establishment of accurate incidence rates for head and spinal cord injuries in developing and developed countries. J Trauma 1993;35:206-211.

9. Goldberg J, Gelfand HM, Levy PS, Mullner R. An evaluation of the Illinois trauma registry: The completeness of case reporting. Med Care 1980;18:520-531.

10. Kilkenny SJ, Moore MA, Simonsen BL, Johnson MS. The Alaska trauma registry. Alaska Med 1992;34:127-134.

11. Payne SR, Waller JA. Trauma registry and trauma center biases in injury research. J Trauma 1989;29:424-429.

12. Pollock DA, McClain PW. Trauma registries: Current status and future prospects. JAMA 1989;262:2280-2283.

13. Saffle JR, Davis B, Kagan R, et al. Development of a Computerized registry for the patient with burns. J Burn Care Rehab 1993;14:199-206(Part I),368-375(Part II).

14. Shackford SR, Hollingsworth-Fridlund P, McArdle M, Eastman AB. Assuring quality in a trauma system--The Medical Audit Committee: Composition, cost, and results. J Trauma 1987;27:866-875.

15. Shapiro MJ, Cole KE, Keegan M, Prassad C, Thompson RJ. National survey of state trauma registries - 1992. J Trauma 1993;35:170.

16. Strauch GO. Trauma registry debuts. Bull Am Coll Surg 1992;77:57-58.

17. Tepas JJ, Ramenofsky ML, Barlow B, et al. National pediatric trauma registry. J Pediatr Surg 1989;24:156-158.

18. Valenzuela TD. What is "major trauma?" Ann Emerg Med 1990; 19:1470-1471.

Table 1. Development of Modern Trauma Registries (U.S.)

Year	Development
1969	Cook County Hospital trauma registry (Illinois)
1971	Illinois State trauma registry
1982	ACS Major Trauma Outcome Study (multicenter)
1985	National Pediatric Trauma Registry
1988	National Trauma Registry Workshop
1990	Trauma Care Systems Planning and Development Act
1993	ACS National Trauma Data Bank

Table 2. CDC-Recommended Trauma Registry Case Criteria

ICD-9-CM condition code 800-959.9
AND one or more of the following:
       Hospital admission
       Interhospital transfer
       Death in hospital

Table 3. CDC-Recommended Trauma Registry Injury Event Descriptors

Date, time, place of injury
Work-relatedness of injury
Protective equipment used
External cause of injury
Narrative description of injury
Blood alcohol and drugs detected

Table 4. Trauma Registry Purposes

Trauma care quality monitoring and evaluation
Public health surveillance
Injury research
Measuring economic impact of trauma

Table 5. Advantages of Trauma Registries for Surveillance

Primary focus is life- and limb-threatening injury
Extensive amount of data on individual patients
Timeliness of data collection, analysis, dissemination
Costs are shared, with major contribution by hospitals
Potential for population-based incidence and outcome data

Table 6. Disadvantages of Trauma Registries for Surveillance

Lack of standardized definition of major trauma
Registries are labor intensive and expensive
Incomplete case finding and incomplete data
Trauma center registries are not population-based

Hospitalized trauma does not represent all injuries

Table 7. Current Status of Trauma Registries (U.S.)

Rapid proliferation
Differences in case criteria and data contents
Persistent concerns about completeness and quality
Incomplete geographic and population coverage

Population-Based Surveys as Sources of U.S. Injury Data and Special Methodological Problems

by Mary Overpeck, Dr.P.H., Ann C. Trumble, Ph.D., Ruth A. Brenner, M.D., M.P.H.

In the United States, as in most countries, records of fatalities, hospitalizations, and treatment in trauma centers or emergency rooms are the standard sources of injury data.[1,2] These sources are frequently used to indicate relative magnitude of the injury problem with some potential ranking according to severity (Figure 1).[3] For fatalities, population-based census data for age, sex, residence and race are used as the denominator to determine injury death rates for specific demographic risk factors.[1,4]

Denominator data are problematical for non-fatal injury rates due to incomplete ascertainment at the medical treatment source for the population at risk.[5] Special studies are required to determine the population characteristics of persons using the treatment source.[6] Population data are needed as denominators to estimate the magnitude of the injury problem relative to the population at risk. In addition, population-based data are necessary to perform risk factor assessment according to either population or exposure characteristics in order to target interventions appropriately. Evaluation of intervention outcomes and planning for service area programs require knowledge of population characteristics for both injuries and risk factor distributions.

In addition, the many different disconnected sources of medical treatment in the U.S. result in a major gap for complete enumeration of injury data. The National Center for Health Statistics (NCHS) recently completed the first reports of emergency room and hospital outpatient department national surveys to supplement visit rate data previously based on hospital discharge and physician office surveys.[7,8,9,10] Denominators are based on U.S. Census data with estimates available only for broad age, place of residence and other demographic groupings due to sample sizes. These national surveys are limited to information available in medical records. Risk factor and exposure information is not available from these sources. Gaps exit for those persons who go untreated or are treated at home. Injury outcomes of most treated injuries, including severity and activity restriction, are generally unknown. Ability to compare population characteristics of the injured to the uninjured is limited. All of these factors reinforce the need for population-based injury data using some form of survey instrument. The following discussion of data sources and special methodological problems describes features that are pertinent for surveys used to obtain either injury or population risk factor data. Studies using census data as denominators for records from treatment sources are not discussed below.[11,12]

Population-Based Sources

Data sources may be generated by: (a) linking treatment or fatality records to survey data; (b) surveying special populations of interest; or (c) performing special studies to obtain risk factors for specific injuries. Some examples of each approach include the following:

- *linking treatment, fatality, and administrative records to survey data*:

    (1)   injured patients are identified at treatment source (emergency rooms, trauma centers, poison control centers) with additional information obtained about the patient and/or injury circumstances through a questionnaire, phone call or visit.[13,14,15]

    (2)   injury deaths are identified through death certificates with followback questionnaires to next-of-kin, treatment facilities and medical examiners or coroner reports such as in the 1986 National Mortality Followback Survey.[16,17]

(3)   administrative crash occupant-specific records on medical and financial data collected at the scene are linked to emergency room, hospitalization, rehabilitation, and long term care records to create population-based information for evaluation of exposure and longitudinal effects.[18]

- *surveying of special interest populations*:

    (1)   populations limited by age groups, such as children or the aging.[19,20]

    (2)   populations surveyed for occurrence of special events, such as crime victimization.[21]

    (3)   populations with small numbers and/or non-representative residential locations requiring tailored sample designs, such as farm injury surveys.[22,23,24]

    (4)   Longitudinal followups of cohorts yielding data for selected types of injuries such as occupational injuries,[25] falls in the aging,[20] or injuries by family characteristics in multigenerational studies.[26]

- *performing special risk factor studies for specific injuries*:

includes case control and/or field studies with cases identified at a treatment source or through fatality records and controls selected through survey of case or injury characteristics;[27,28,29] and cross-sectional or prospective surveys designed to identify risk factors for specific injuries.[30]

The common element among all approaches to population-based surveys is the incorporation of direct queries to individuals for additional information beyond that which is available from existing vital, administrative, or treatment records.

For the U.S. the primary source of estimates of total magnitude and rates of non-fatal injuries is the National Health Interview Survey (NHIS). Census denominators used for age- and sex-specific injury rates are similar to those available for fatalities with modification to reflect the civilian non-institutionalized population sample design.[31] The NHIS is a continuous survey covering approximately 50,000 households per year. The sample frame is a complex multistage design based on the U.S. census. The strength of the survey is the comprehensive representative design which allows national estimates for the resident civilian non-institutionalized population. Injury questions are based on both medically attended and/or activity restricting injury events yielding less biased estimates than data based on treatment sources alone. Analytic potential goes beyond the age, sex, race, and place information available on death certificate records to yield injury information on socioeconomic factors such as income. For example, Figure 2 shows the elderly poor are more likely to be injured at home than any other age group, which is useful information for targeting risk factor analysis.

While the sample size is adequate to estimate injury rates for broad age groups by income and place, the NHIS demonstrates that even such a large continuous sample has inadequate size to make such estimates for even five year age groups or for the nature of injuries on an annual basis. Many injury researchers are facing this sample size dilemma when designing studies of risk factors targeted to specific locations, ages, or exposures. The NHIS provides useful examples of methodological problems for population-based injury data because the sample size and information are complete enough to demonstrate the problem issues. Therefore, the following discussion of common methodological problems of injury surveys are based on NHIS data but are not specific to this national survey. Many survey methodological problem issues which are not specific to injury research are discussed elsewhere and are not addressed in this paper.[32,33,34]

Methodological Problems

<u>Sample Size</u>

As mentioned above, very large continuous surveys such as the NHIS may be of insufficient size to provide national estimates for even five year age groups or for the nature of injuries on an annual basis. In the case of the NHIS, the reference period used to accumulate injury episode occurrences is the previous two weeks, selected to reduce the amount of bias associated with respondent memory loss.[35] One solution to obtain an adequate sample size at the national level has been to accumulate the data from the prior two week reference period over a three year period. Resulting estimates have reliable precision for broad categories of injury types (or nature), smaller age groupings or impairments.[36,37]

Another solution for sample size limitations is to extend the reference period. To address the problem of the limited sample size for small age groups for injuries to U.S. children, the 1988 Child Health Supplement (CHS-NHIS) was added to the NHIS. The length of the recall period was extended to the previous 12 months to increase the probability of the child being injured in the reference period. However, injuries were limited to only those receiving medical attention.

Studies of specific populations of interest frequently require extra details. By obtaining injury data by month and year of age on a larger sample in the CHS-NHIS the effects of developmental stages and changing exposures are more clearly demonstrated to show how risk factors interact (Figure 3). Using year of age, differences in age-specific rates focus attention on injuries occurring in the places where children have the most exposures by age as their activities move from home to school.

Effects of Recall

Lengthening the recall period for the CHS-NHIS had the effect of decreasing the overall estimate of injury rates.[38] By asking when the injury occurred, attrition in injury rates was measurable by length of time from the interview to the injury event. Figure 4 shows that recall is affected by severity. Overall, the best recall period was one month with a continuing decrease after three months, particularly for minor injuries. Using the estimates according to the length of time from the injury event, overall injury rates estimates may be adjusted to what they would have been using a one month recall period. This is an important issue for most surveys currently in the field due to the need to balance recall effects against sample size needs. Adding the injury date allows corrections.

Medically-Attended and Activity Restricting Injuries

Analysis of NHIS data by injury type demonstrates the methodological strength of probing for injury episodes by asking about both medical attention and activity restrictions. Some types of injuries with high rates of medical attention do not result in high rates of activity restriction (Figure 5). Conversely, injuries serious enough to cause activity restriction do not always receive medical attention. Figure 5 demonstrates that head injuries (skull fractures and intracranial injuries) and open wounds or lacerations usually receive medical attention. Yet, less than half of medically attended head injuries and 30 percent of open wounds or lacerations result in any restriction of activity. A far greater proportion of lower limb fractures or sprains and strains cause restrictions of activity. Yet, between 10 to 20 percent of these latter injury types do not receive medical attention. Analytic results of studies may be strongly affected by differences in rates of medical attention.[39] In one study of the effect of access to medical care on estimates of injury rates, we found that about 30 percent of injuries serious enough to have an impact on the child did not receive medical attention when there was no medical care coverage (health insurance or Medicaid).[40]

Severity Measures

Since receipt of medical attention is not always a reliable indicator of severity or the impact on the injured person, it is important to obtain estimates on how the injury affected the person leading, in turn, to assessment of relative severity.[38] Analysis of small age groupings with information on effects of the injury on the child demonstrated that medically attended injuries of young children were more than twice as likely to be minor than severe (Figure 4). The proportion of total medically attended injuries that were considered severe increased with the age of the child.

Lay Terminology

Figure 5 also demonstrates the importance of using lay terminology to identify injury diagnoses in population-based surveys. Since some injuries have not received a medical diagnosis, lay terminology is needed to obtain an adequate description of the nature of the injury to facilitate coding of diagnostic categories. Even persons who received medical attention do not always understand the clinical terminology for the diagnosis or parts of the body affected. Probes about the part of the body affected, pictures of body parts, and alternate phrasing suggestions will help to identify the injury site.

Circumstances

The minimum basic data elements to obtain International Classification of Disease external cause of injury codes (E-codes) have been strongly recommended in the U.S.[41] Consistency at this minimum level has allowed comparison with other data that uses E-codes. For example, by obtaining the minimum information needed for e-coding in the 1988 NHIS-CHS, a comparison of nonfatal injury causes to fatal causes was possible (Figure 6).[19] An important finding for non-fatal injuries is that the leading causes are far different from the leading causes for fatal injuries. Combined with data on severity, such comparisons provide information to redirect attention to relative injury burdens. E-codes frequently are not specific enough for individual product exposures or activities. Population-based studies can be tailored to provide the amount of detail and degree of specificity needed for both risk factor and intervention analyses. This important information is often not available in existing administrative or treatment data sources. Some specific study needs include details on place of injury, activities at the time of injury, involvement of others and intent.

Summary

Methodological problems of population-based injury surveys include inadequate sample sizes, incomplete recall of injury events, lack of measures of severity, uncertain diagnosis on nature of injuries, and differential effects from varying degrees of access to medical care. One solution to eliminate sample size problems is expansion of the recall period to include more injury events. Adjustment for loss of information due to extended recall may be made by obtaining the date of the injury event to create correction factors for injury rates by time between interview and event. Obtaining information on duration and type of restrictions of activity due to injury provide severity measures that do not rely solely on access to medical care. Use of lay terminology to describe the nature of the injury facilitates coding of comparable diagnostic categories. Finally, obtaining age data by birth date provides the flexibility to analyze risks associated with changing developmental stages and exposures.

Realistic community perception of risk is needed to build support for appropriately targeted program priorities.[2,42] Community education on risks requires unbiased population-based data for comparisons across injury causes, severity and costs. Without the use of all available data sources linked to population descriptors, efficient resource allocation becomes extremely difficult, if not impossible.

References

1. Baker SP, O'Neill B, Ginsburg MJ, Guohua L. The Injury Fact Book. New York: Oxford University Press; 1992. Chap. 2, 4 & 22.

2. Waller JA. Injury Control: A Guide to the Causes and Prevention of Trauma. Lexington, Mass; Lexington Books, 1985. Chap. 6 & 7, pages 65-88.

3. National Committee for Injury Prevention and Control. Injury Prevention: Meeting the Challenge. New York: Oxford University Press; 1989. Chap. 2, 3, & 4, pages 37-84.

4. Fingerhut LA, Kleinman JC, Malloy MH, Feldman JJ. Injury fatalities among young children. Public Health Rep 1988;103:399-405.

5. Cooper A, Barlow B, Davidson L, Relethford J, O'Meara J, Mottley L. Epidemiology of pediatric trauma: Importance of population-based statistics. J Pediatr Surg 1992;27:149-54.

6. Schwarz DF, Grisso JA, Miles CG, Holmes JH, Wishner AR, Sutton RL. A longitudinal study of injury morbidity in an African-American population. JAMA 1994;271:755-60.

7. McCaig LF. National Hospital Ambulatory Medical Care Survey: 1992 Emergency Department Summary. Advance Data from Vital and Health Statistics, No. 245. Hyattsville, Md: National Center for Health Statistics. 1994.

8. McCaig LF. National Hospital Ambulatory Medical Care Survey: 1992 Outpatient Department Summary. Advance Data from Vital and Health Statistics, No. 248. Hyattsville, Md: National Center for Health Statistics. 1994.

9. Graves EJ. 1992 Summary: National Hospital Discharge Survey. Advance Data from Vital and Health Statistics, No. 249. Hyattsville, Md: National Center for Health Statistics. 1994.

10. Bryant E, Shimizu I. Sample design, sampling variance, and estimation procedures for the National Ambulatory Medical Care Survey. National Center for Health Statistics. Vital Health Stat 2(108). 1988.

11. Gallagher SS, Finison K, Guyer B, Goodenough SH. The incidence of injuries among 87,000 Massachusetts children and adolescents: results of the 1980-81 statewide childhood injury prevention surveillance system. Am J Public Health 1984;74:1340-7.

12. Barancik JI, Cramer CF. Northeastern Ohio Trauma Study: overview and issues. Public Health Rep 1985;100:563-5.

13. Nolan T, Penny M. Epidemiology of non-intentional injuries in an Australian urban region: Results from injury surveillance. J Paediatr Child Health 1992;28:27-35.

14. Rivara FP, Calonge N, Thompson RS. Population-based study of unintentional injury incidence and impact during childhood. Am J Public Health 1989;79:990-4.

15. Maiman LA, Yu KF, Hildreth NG, Liptak GS, Lawrence RA. Psychosocial and behavioral determinants of childhood poison ingestions. Presented at the Second World Conference on Injury Control, Atlanta, Ga: May, 1993 (abstract).

16. Seeman I, Poe GS, Powell-Griner E. Development, methods and response characteristics of the 1988 National Mortality Followback Survey. National Center for Health Statistics, Vital Health Stat 1 (29), 1993.

17. National Center for Health Statistics. National Death Index User's Manual. DHHS Pub. No. (PHS) 90-1148. Hyattsville, MD; 1990.

18. Walsh WH, Johnson SW. Crash outcome data evaluation system--Data linkage of medical patient records with highway crash data. Workshop presentation at the International Colloborative Effort on Injury. May 18-20, 1994, Bethesda, MD.

19. Scheidt PC, Harel Y, Jones D, Overpeck M, Bijur P. The epidemiology of medically-attended non-fatal injuries in children and youth from a nationally representative sample. Am J Dis Child 1992;146 (abstract).

20. Kovar MG, Fitti JE, Chyba MM. The longitudinal study of aging: 1984-90. Vital Health Stat 1 (28), 1992.

21.   Bureau of Justice Statistics. Criminal Victimization in the United States, 1992. Washington, DC: BJS Report No. NCJ 145125, March 1994.

22.   Stallones L, Gunderson P. Epidemiological perspectives on childhood agricultural injuries within the U.S. J Agro Medicine (in press).

23.   Pratt DS, Marvel LH, Darrow D, Stallones L, et al. The dangers of dairy farming: the injury experience of 600 workers followed for two years. Am J Industrial Medicine 1992;21(5):637-50.

24.   McKnight RH, Spurlock CW, Myers JR. Agricultural-injury surveillance in Kentucky. Presented at the Second World Conference on Injury Control, Atlanta, GA: May, 1993 (abstract).

25.   Bureau of the Census. Survey of Income and Program Participation: Users' Guide. Washington, DC: U.S. Dept. of Commerce, 1991.

26.   Center for Human Resource Research. The National Longitudinal Surveys of Labor Market Experience: Handbook, 1993. Columbus, OH; Ohio State University, 1994.

27.   Kellerman AL, Rivara FP, Somes G, et al. Suicide in the home in relation to gun ownership. N Engl J Med 1992;327:467-72.

28.   Kellerman AL, Rivara FP, Rushforth NB, et al. Gun ownership as a risk factor for homicide in the home. N Engl J Med 1993;329:1084-91.

29.   Brent DA, Perper JA Moritz G, et al. Firearms and adolescent suicide: A community case-control study. Am J Dis Child. 1993:147:1066-71.

30.   Anderson R, Dearwater SR, Olsen T, et al. The role of socioeconomic status and injury morbidity risk in adolescents. Arch Pediatr Adolesc Med. 1994;148:245-249.

31.   Massey JT. Design and estimation of the National Health Interview Survey, 1985-94. Vital Health Stat 2 (110), 1989.

32.   Kelsey JL, Thompson WD, Evans AS. Methods in Observational Epidemiology. New York: Oxford University Press, 1986.

33.   Rothman KJ. Modern Epidemiology. Boston, MA: Little, Brown and Co., 1986.

34.   Hulley SB, Cummins SR. Designing Clinical Research: An Epidemiological Approach. Baltimore, MD: Williams and Wilkins, 1988.

35.   Massey JT, Gonzalez JF, Jr. Optimum recall periods for estimating accidental injuries in the National Health Interview Survey. Proc Am Stat Assoc (Social Statistics Section) 1976:584-8.

36.   Collins JG. Types of Injuries by Selected Characteristics: United States, 1985-87. Vital and Health Stat 10 (175), 1990.

37.   Collins JG. Impairments due to Injuries: United States, 1985-87. Vital and Health Stat 10 (177), 1991.

38.   Harel Y, Overpeck MD, Jones DH, Scheidt PC, et al. Effects of recall on estimating annual non-fatal injury rates for children and youth. Am J Public Health 1994;84:599-605.

39.   Overpeck MD, Kotch JB, Trumble AC. Effects of maternal education and access to care on analysis of injury risk according to patterns of child care. Proceedings of the 1993 Public Health Conference on Records and Statistics. Hyattsville, MD: DHHS Pub. No. (PHS) 94-1214; 1994, pp. 67-72.

40.   Overpeck MD, Kotch JB. Effect of access to care on medical attention for injuries. Am J Public Health, in press.

41.   Center for Disease Control. Injury control in the 1990's: A national plan for action. Atlanta, GA: US Dept. of Health and Human Services, CDC, National Center for Injury Prevention and Control, 1993.

42.   Graitcer PL. Injury surveillance. In: Halperin W, Baker EL, Monson RR (eds.). Public Health Surveillance. New York, NY: Von Nostrand Reinhold, 1992, pp. 142-56.

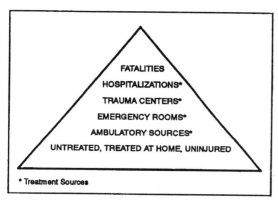

Figure 1. Data sources

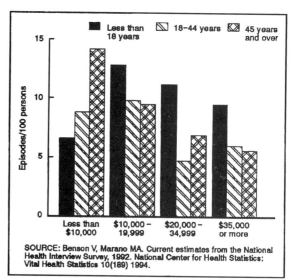

Figure 2. Injury episodes occurring at home by age and income

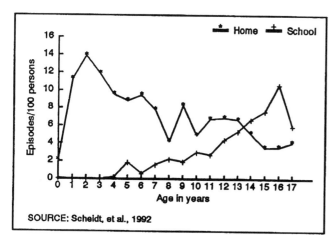

Figure 3. Place of injury by age of U.S. children

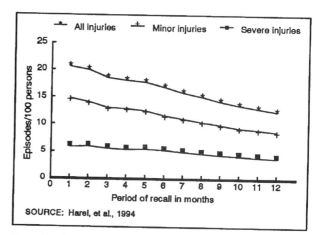

Figure 4. Estimated annual injury rates by severity and recall period

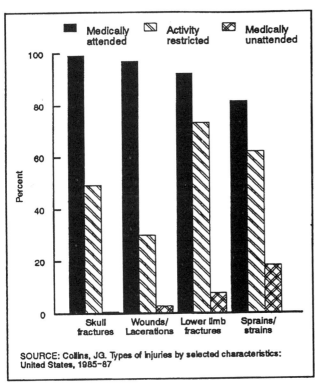

Figure 5. Medical attention and restricted activity for selected injuries

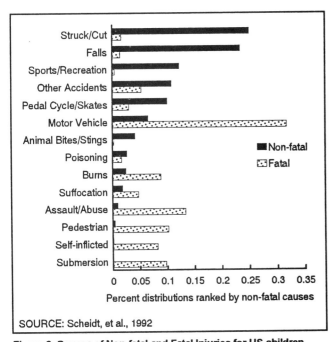

SOURCE: Scheidt, et al., 1992

Figure 6. Causes of Non-fatal and Fatal Injuries for US children

Current Problems in Producing Comparable International Mortality and Morbidity Statistics

International Comparisons of Injury Mortality:
Hypothesis Generation, Ecological Studies, and Some Data Problems

by Gordon S. Smith, M.B., Ch.B., M.P.H.,
Jean A. Langlois, Sc.D., M.P.H., and Ian R.H. Rockett, Ph.D., M.P.H.

Abstract

Injury rates vary widely from one country to another. Analysis of differences in rates may suggest important new areas of research. This paper brings together a series of studies looking at the use of injury mortality data both to illustrate the potential usefulness of such analyses and to point out some of the problems in interpreting comparative data, especially in the elderly.

In two separate studies, one comparing France, Japan, West Germany and the United Kingdom, and another comparing New Zealand, Australia and United Kingdom, low unintentional injury rates were reported for the United Kingdom. Female suicides were higher in Japan and homicide rates for both males and females were much higher in the U.S. One recent study examined the association of per capita alcohol consumption and population–based injury fatality rates in the U.S., Canada, France, Finland, the Netherlands, and Switzerland. While cirrhosis deaths were highly correlated with per capita alcohol consumption, injury rates were not, except for suicide in some countries. Another study however, adjusted for exposure and found a high correlation between alcohol consumption and motor vehicle fatalities when they were calculated on the basis of deaths per 100 million vehicle–kilometers traveled.

Although their findings are interesting, these studies do not account for the many other differences between countries in injury rates. In addition to obvious exposure differences, an important factor to consider in any cross–national comparison is the quality and comparability of the data, especially that on underlying cause. France, for example, classifies a much higher proportion of its injury deaths as due to unspecified causes when compared to other countries. In addition, injury death rates in the elderly may be difficult to compare, as illustrated by large differences in fall injury mortality between New Zealand and the U.S. More in–depth analyses found similar incidence of falls as measured by rates of fall and hip fracture hospitalizations. Other studies have shown considerable under–counting of injury deaths in the elderly in the U.S. Reporting of such deaths in New Zealand appears to be more complete. Detection of large international differences in other disease rates has suggested important new hypotheses and the resulting in–depth research has advanced our understanding of disease etiology and prevention. One example is the association of diet and some cancers. Similar studies of differences in injury rates may suggest important new areas of research. However, relationships may be very complex and differences in injury classification between countries must always be considered.

Introduction

Injuries remain an important cause of death in most countries and are usually the leading cause of premature mortality in most of the more developed countries. However, injury rates vary widely from one country to another (Rockett & Smith, 1989; Taket, 1986).

Detection of large international differences in rates for other diseases such as cancer have been important in both assessing the relative magnitude of disease burden between countries and in stimulating new research efforts (Reid, 1975). Such studies have suggested major new hypotheses which led to more in–depth studies to understand both disease etiology and prevention. In cancer research, for example, major differences in cancer rates between countries (Armstrong & Doll, 1975, Schrauzer et al., 1977) stimulated hypotheses on the relationship of diet and cancer and subsequently led to major insights into the importance of dietary factors in both causative and inhibitive roles (Wilett & MacMahon, 1984). Our earlier work has suggested that similar analyses of differences in injury rates between countries may also lead to important new insights for understanding the etiology and prevention of injuries (Rockett & Smith, 1989a, b).

What can we learn by conducting studies of differences in injury rates between countries? Are some countries more successful in injury prevention efforts than others? How can we learn from success stories in other countries? Are the observed differences real or simply due to differences in the way the data are collected and analyzed? Can cross–national studies suggest ways to improve our own data and make it more useful for prevention purposes? This study brings together a series of such studies in order to illustrate the potential usefulness of comparisons, to demonstrate the need to extend the research using more detailed models to explain differences, and also to point out some of the problems in comparing data from one country to another.

A number of the examples used to illustrate these points are based on our own earlier published research. This paper summarizes much of this work and relates it to work by other researchers. The reader should refer to the original articles for more detailed findings.

Cross National Injury Mortality Studies

All–Cause Mortality, Five Countries

The first in a series of three papers comparing injury mortality between countries compared cross–national all–cause injury mortality data in five countries: The United States, France, Japan, West Germany and the United Kingdom. Marked differences in both all–cause injury death and age–adjusted years of life lost (an indicator of premature mortality) were found among the five countries (Rockett & Smith, 1987). These five countries were chosen because they had large populations, were similar in terms of levels of development and had close social, political and economic links with the U.S.

Cause–Specific Mortality, Five Countries

The purpose of the second paper, which will be discussed here in more detail, was to describe the epidemiology of specific injuries in the five countries above as a basis for formulating hypotheses for potential differences between countries. Data for 1980 were abstracted from age–, sex– and cause–specific tabulations of injury published in the World Health Statistics Annual (WHO, 1982–84). Four separate causes of injuries were examined: motor vehicle fatalities, falls, homicide and suicide. Age and sex–specific rates were compared among countries.

Motor vehicle crashes were the leading cause of male injury death in all countries except for Japan (see Figure 1). For females, motor vehicle crashes were the leading cause only in the U.S. and were surpassed by suicide, falls or both in the other countries. Age–specific motor vehicle mortality rates were bimodal in all countries with peaks at ages 15–24 years and in the oldest ages.

Fall mortality rates were low in all countries except in the elderly, among whom rates are substantially higher (see Figure 2). They varied widely, with France exhibiting the highest rates and Japan the lowest. Rates in the U.S. were also low, as will be discussed later in this paper.

Suicide rates were highest among elderly French males and lowest in the U.K. (see Figure 3). Elderly females in Japan have much higher suicide rates than female counterparts in the other countries examined. Another study found elderly female suicide rates to be even higher in China (Lei & Baker, 1991). A striking finding is that the suicide rate in U.S. females declined after ages 45–54, while it increased in the other countries studied.

The most notable differences among countries were for homicide, with most countries except the U.S. having relatively low rates and little variation by age (see Figure 4). The marked excess in rates for young U.S. males has been well described in the literature, (Fingerhut & Kleinman, 1990; Kellerman et al., 1991). However, most studies concentrate on young males, yet homicide rates are markedly elevated in the U.S. at all ages, including for females.

Injury Mortality Australia, New Zealand, United Kingdom

Our third paper compared injury rates in Australia, New Zealand and the United Kingdom, three countries with similar origins (Rockett & Smith, 1989b). Mortality rates were relatively similar in Australia and New Zealand, however, their rates were almost double those in the United Kingdom. The biggest differences were for motor vehicle crashes and suicide, which explained about 75 percent of the variation in rates.

Overall Findings

Overall, the two studies comparing France, Japan, West Germany and the United Kingdom and the third comparing New Zealand, Australia and the United Kingdom found unintentional injury rates to be much lower in the United Kingdom and Japan. Female suicide rates for Japan were high and have subsequently been studied in more detail in a recent follow-up paper (Rockett & Smith, 1993). Very high rates were reported for homicide in the U.S., for both males and females. The role of firearms in U.S. homicides has been well described (Kellerman et al., 1991), including comparisons of homicide rates between Vancouver and Seattle, two similar cities but with very different handgun control policies (Sloan et al., 1988). To date, few studies have done similar comparisons to explain markedly divergent unintentional injury rates among countries.

Ecological Studies: Alcohol as a Case Study

While these comparisons of mortality data point out large differences in injury rates between countries, they can only suggest hypotheses for factors that may be important. The next step is to examine in more detail possible exploratory factors. One important risk factor for injuries is alcohol use (Smith & Kraus, 1988). Alcohol consumption is also known to vary widely across countries (Giesbrecht & Dick, 1993). Cirrhosis death rates, for example, have been shown to be highly correlated with alcohol consumption among countries (and within countries over time).

How do injury rates correlate with alcohol use between countries? One recent paper examined the association between per-capita alcohol consumption and injury fatality rates (or casualty statistics, as they called them) from 6 countries in Europe and North America (Finland, France, the Netherlands, Switzerland, Canada and the U.S.) (Giesbrecht & Dick, 1993). These countries were chosen because they represented a range of different patterns of alcohol consumption. Alcohol consumption patterns in the U.S. and Canada are very similar, with both countries being in the medium range compared to other countries, and both showed a steady, moderate increase in per capita consumption from 1961 – 1988 (the period being studied). Beer is the beverage of choice in both countries. Alcohol consumption increased markedly in Finland and the Netherlands over the same period, from low levels to moderate or high levels. Finland has higher levels of spirits consumption while people in the Netherlands drink more wine. In France, alcohol consumption levels have actually declined, although their current levels are still in the high range compared with other countries. In Switzerland, alcohol consumption patterns have remained high and stable. Switzerland has a similar drinking culture to France except, that beer is more popular than wine.

Mortality statistics from each of the six countries for the years 1962–88 were obtained from the same WHO Statistics Annuals described earlier (WHO – multiple years). The following categories were analyzed: "Chronic liver disease and cirrhosis, motor vehicle traffic accidents, other transport accidents, accidental poisoning, falls, fires and flames, drowning and submersion, machinery, and accidents caused by firearm missiles, all other accidents including late effects, suicide and self-inflicted injury, homicide and injury purposely inflicted by other persons, and other violence." Regression time series analyses, with "filtering" to account for auto-correlation, were used to compare trends of consumption and mortality rates (Skog, 1987).

The mean rates of cirrhosis deaths and "other accidental deaths" were highest in France. Finland had the highest mean rates of other transportation deaths, poisonings (including many alcohol poisonings) and drownings. As noted also in our earlier work, the U.S. had the highest level of homicide deaths. As found in other studies, liver cirrhosis rates were most highly correlated with alcohol consumption, but the strength of association varied widely by country, being highest in Canada with a correlation coefficient of 0.75 for males (see Table 1). The only other significant associations were for suicide in Finland (males and females) and in the Netherlands for females only (data not

13–3

shown), with weak associations with suicide in France for both sexes. There were no consistent associations found between per capita alcohol consumption and injury rates for the other injury causes examined.

While studies such as this can suggest potential correlations and areas for further research, they say nothing about the involvement of alcohol in particular injuries. There are also a wide variety of other factors that can influence injury mortality rates. More in depth studies are needed that examine the complex interactions among a wide variety of factors that determine injury risk. For example, the above study by Giesbrecht (1993) used only population–based mortality rates and made no attempt to adjust for important exposure differences between countries. This important methodological issue is illustrated well by another study that examined motor vehicle mortality rates using population–weighted, least–squares multiple regression rather than time series analysis (Lowenfels & Wynn, 1992). Using the same per capita alcohol consumption data as in the other study, Lowenfel and Wynn found a very strong correlation between per capita alcohol consumption and motor vehicle fatalities in 19 countries (Figure 5). An important difference however, was that the authors used the annual mortality rate per 100 million vehicle–kilometers travelled rather than just per 100,000 population. The relationship was moderately strong (r=0.62, p<.001) but was increased considerably when another potential confounder, percent of roads paved, was added to the regression equation (r=0.83, p<.001). These two factors alone were related to 70 percent of the variation in vehicular fatalities and the fit of the model was not improved measurably by the addition of other potential explanatory variables such as population density, blood alcohol level of the driver or percent of alcohol consumed as spirits.

The wide discrepancy of findings between the studies by Giesbrecht & Dick (1993) and that by Lowenfels & Wynn (1992) illustrate well the need to consider a variety of factors when attempting to explain differences between countries and illustrates some of the problems in doing ecological studies (Peek & Kraus, 1992). Are the differences in injury mortality rates due to differences in alcohol consumption or due to a variety of other factors that also vary in the same direction between countries – for example the use of seatbelts, airbags, improved highway design and better access to emergency care. The strength of the Lowenfels & Wynn article is that it attempts to address many of the potential confounding factors. However, like other ecological studies, it relies on available data and more in–depth studies collecting data on individual crashes are needed to examine other factors such as type of vehicle involved, emergency care provided and different types of driving exposure such as night versus daytime (Peek & Kraus, 1992). Never–the–less, as illustrated above, there are a wide variety of important factors that can be examined using currently available data, particularly when information from different sources are linked together.

Data Comparability Problems

Another potential problem in comparing injury deaths between countries may lie in coding differences such as variable conventions used in recording external causes on the death certificate. Are the differences between countries real or artifactual due to coding differences? We use two examples to illustrate how differences in coding can affect international comparisons. The first is the use of "unspecified accidents" in France, and the second involves international differences in the classification of delayed deaths subsequent to injury in the elderly. This paper does not claim to review all the problems in data collection, but rather to illustrate with these examples that the potential for artifactual differences in cross–national injury mortality rates must be considered.

Unspecified Accidents

In our analysis of French injury data, we found that the percentage of injury deaths coded as "other accidental deaths" was much higher in France. This was also noted by Giesbrecht (1993), who found that the injury mortality rate for the category "other accidental deaths" in France ranged during the years 1962–1988 from 16.7 – 29.2/100,000 for males, as compared with other selected countries where the rates ranged from 1.9 – 13.1/100,000 population (see Table 2). The average from 1962 – 1988 for French males was 23.1/100,000 population while the corresponding average figures for the U.S., Canada, Finland, the Netherlands, and Switzerland ranged only from 2.9 to 7.9. Upon further inquiry into possible reasons for this discrepancy, we learned that French physicians reportedly often write only "un accident" for motor vehicle crashes, and thus the unspecified accident group includes among them many undocumented motor vehicle fatalities (Dr. R.L. Salmi, Personal Communication Feb. 3, 1989). In addition, a number of injury deaths (especially in young people) are coded to this unspecified category because of strict confidentiality rules in France prohibiting use of more specific data from medico–legal investigations (which are done in a different government department from Vital Statistics) in revising the cause of death on the death certificate. In these cases, what in the U.S. would be initially coded as a pending cause will be classified as an unspecified accident and never updated even if the medicolegal investigation for example determines the death was a suicide. Similar problems are known to exist in a number of other countries such as Jamaica where many violent deaths investigated by the police are not even recorded by the vital statistics system. (Personal Communication, Dr. Cleone Rooney, Office of Population Census and Surveys, United Kingdom at I.C.E. meeting, May 18, 1994).

Injuries in the Elderly

Evaluation of disease–specific mortality data in the elderly, including injuries, may be even more problematic because deaths are commonly associated with a variety of co–morbid conditions, and a single underlying cause of death may not accurately reflect the true burden of a specific condition in the elderly. Because of these problems, analysis of multiple causes of death has been advocated to examine various factors related to the death (Israel et al., 1986). Previous studies have noted that injury death rates in the elderly are much higher in New Zealand than in Australia, the United Kingdom (see Figure 6) (Rockett & Smith, 1989b) and in the United States (Langley & McLoughlin, 1989).

The highest overall injury mortality rates are for elderly females and males in New Zealand, with rates much higher than corresponding rates in either Australia or the U.K. (see Figure 6). Paradoxically, injury rates were more similar in younger age groups where it is expected that differences in risk such as lifestyles and exposure to hazards are likely to be much greater than in the elderly.

We recently completed a study that sought to examine in more detail potential reasons for the apparent excess of injury mortality in the elderly in New Zealand (Langlois, Smith, Baker & Langley – submitted). Mortality data tapes were obtained from the New Zealand Health Information Service and the U.S. National Center for Health Statistics. Average annual rates were calculated for New Zealand from 1980–1987 and the U.S. from 1980–1986. Mid–range (1983) population estimates were used to calculate injury rates. Standard ICD E (External Cause) code groupings were used for specific injury groups. In order to compare injury incidence rather than just mortality rates we used hospital discharge data and data from other published studies to estimate differences in fall hospitalization rates between the two countries. Estimates of fall hospitalizations for the U.S. were available only from the "Cost of Injury" study (Rice, MacKenzie & Associates, 1989) due to incomplete E–coding of hospital data. Discharge rates for hip fractures (ICD 820) were also used as a proxy measure of fall injury incidence.

The most apparent difference between the two countries was the much higher proportion of injury deaths in New Zealand attributed to falls (52 percent) as compared to the U.S., where falls comprised only 28 percent of all injury deaths in the elderly (see Figure 7).

The age–adjusted (to U.S. 1983 population) fatal fall rate in New Zealand (92.0/100,000 population) was nearly three times higher than the U.S. rate (32.0/100,000) for both sexes combined. (see Table 3) For females, the discrepancy between the fall injury death rate in New Zealand, compared to the U.S., was much greater in the oldest age group. However, the age–adjusted fall and hip fracture hospitalization rates in New Zealand were relatively similar to the U.S. rates. There was however, an apparently higher in–hospital death rate from hip fractures in New Zealand, although the mean length of stay is more than double that of the U.S. reflecting in part very different patterns of hospitalization, rehabilitation and discharge patterns (such as to nursing homes). The data for males show a similar pattern, but with lower rates (data not shown).

The markedly different injury death rates for the elderly in New Zealand and the U.S. can be largely accounted for by the wide discrepancies in fall mortality rates, with falls comprising 52 percent of all injury deaths in those 65 years and over in New Zealand while comprising only 28 percent of injury deaths for the elderly in the U.S. The age–adjusted fall mortality rate was 92.0/100,000 population in New Zealand almost three times that of the U.S.

(32.0). Three potential factors could explain this excess – a higher risk of falls resulting in injury; a higher case fatality rate; or differences in classifying injury deaths.

Higher Risk of Injury Producing Falls in New Zealand?

Intrinsic factors appear to be an important determinant of the incidence of falls in the elderly. Community–based studies of the prevalence of risk factors report similar results in both New Zealand and the U.S. (Campbell et al., 1981, Tinetti et al., 1988). In addition, environmental factors such as housing and activities of the elderly, are likely to be relatively similar between countries. As measured by hip fracture discharge rates and estimates of fall injury hospitalizations, the incidence of fall injuries is very similar between two countries. Thus, differences in fall mortality do not appear to be due to a higher incidence of serious falls in New Zealand.

Higher Case–Fatality Rates?

Because of deficiencies in E–code data in the U.S., the figures for fall hospitalizations are only estimates, and it is not possible to analyze U.S. hospital discharge data tapes for in–hospital fall mortality (Rice, MacKenzie & Associates 1989, Sniezek et al., 1989). We analyzed hip fractures as a surrogate, since more than 90 percent of hip fractures are attributed to falls (Campbell et al., 1981, Tinetti et al., 1988, Nevitt et al., 1989, Sattin et al., 1990). However, only about 45 percent of fall hospitalizations among the elderly in New Zealand are due to hip fractures. The proportion of female hip fracture cases dying in–hospital was greater in New Zealand (8.8 percent) than in the U.S. (3.3 percent). (see Table 3) However, the mean length of stay was more than double in New Zealand (34.2 versus 14.2 days), which is likely to explain much of the difference in mortality. Compared with older Americans, older New Zealanders spend more time in a hospital rather than in other post–discharge settings because of greater pressure in the U.S. for early transfer to non–acute care hospitals for recuperation (Nevitt et al., 1989). Thus, New Zealanders are more likely to develop fatal complications in the hospital. It is also possible that reimbursement decisions, related to diagnostic–related groups (DRGs) (Cohen et al., 1987, Hsia et al., 1988), may also reduce the coding of hip fractures on discharges for in–hospital deaths. However, the magnitude of this association is unknown. It seems unlikely that differences in case–fatality rates could explain much of the cross–national difference in fall injury mortality rates.

Differences in Coding of Injury Deaths?

By comparing single cause–of–death information with multiple cause of death data, Fife (1987) determined that among those age 75 years and older, injury deaths may be underestimated by as much as 50 percent overall. The problem occurs when people die of multiple and often late complications of the injury, such as acute respiratory syndrome, cardiac failure or infection. Often these causes are listed in Part 1 of the death certificate, and the fall is only mentioned in Part II of the certificate. In many cases the fall may not even be mentioned on the death certificate (Waller, 1978). Injury causes listed in Part II can only be considered as the underlying cause under special circumstances (Fife 1987, NCHS 1984). Despite these limitations, international comparisons of injury mortality must rely on underlying cause data since few countries outside of the U.S. have data on multiple causes (Israel et al., 1986).

There are a number of factors that on further analysis suggest that variations in coding practices between the countries may explain at least in part the discrepancies in fall mortality rates between New Zealand and Australia. Fife (1987) found that the under–coding of fall deaths was common in the elderly and increased with age: 53 percent for ages 65–74, 61 percent for ages 75–84 and 65 percent for those 85 years and over (see Table 4). The discrepancy between injury deaths in the elderly between New Zealand and the U.S. also widened dramatically with increasing age, as indicated by increasing rate ratios as age increases. These findings suggest that coding differences may be a factor in the higher fall mortality among the elderly in N.Z.

There are several important differences between New Zealand and the U.S. in the recording and processing of mortality data that may explain potential differences in coding fall deaths in the elderly. New Zealand physicians probably have better knowledge of the coding of causes of death since training materials on how to complete death certificates are included as part of their medical education (Personal Communication, Geraldine White, N.Z. Information Service, Nov. 24, 1992). U.S. physicians on the other hand, receive little or no training in certifying causes of death (Comstock, 1986). In addition, the N.Z. Health Information Service coders routinely use medical examiner records, hospital charts and other sources of data to code the cause of death, and also frequently query physicians directly to check information on the cause of death. Such procedures are rare in the U.S. but have been shown to greatly enhance the identification of injuries as a cause of death, including falls (Hopkins et al., 1989; Kircher et al., 1985; Moyer et al., 1989). The training of the persons investigating injury deaths also varies widely from one state or county to the other in the U.S. Some jurisdictions have highly trained forensic pathologists while others only have lay coroners with no medical training. In the U.S., coders rely on information on the certificate, including the section "how injury occurs." The New Zealand certificate has no such a section, but relies on coders going back to original source documents for more information. In addition, autopsy rates in New Zealand are about double those of the U.S. High autopsy rates are known to improve the quality of cause of death certification for all causes of death including both the nature of the injury and the underlying cause. (Fife, 1987; Kircher et al., 1985).

In conclusion, we believe that improved coding practices for injury deaths in New Zealand are responsible for much of the apparent excess of fall deaths in elderly New Zealanders, especially since the rates for fall hospitalization appear to be similar. A number of other studies have shown that for other diseases differences in coding practices can be large, and result in wide variations in the certification of a single underlying cause (Jougla et al., 1992; Percy et al., 1981; Percy & Muir, 1989; Kelson & Farebrother, 1987). The potential for differences in coding practices between countries must always be considered when analyzing injury data.

Implications for Future Cross–national Studies

International comparisons of injury data between countries can be very useful for suggesting hypotheses for future studies. The apparently low injury rates in the United Kingdom, for example, needs further explanation. This in turn may suggest successful interventions, as yet unrecognized (Smith & Rockett, 1989b). There are wide variations in injury rates not only between developed countries, but also in the less developed countries (Smith & Barss; 1991 Taket, 1986; Li & Baker, 1991). Many of the less developed countries also have high injury rates and relatively good injury data which could be used in cross–national comparisons. This is especially true for Latin America countries. Variations in hospitalization rates are also an important but largely ignored area of research. Hip fracture hospitalization rates have been shown to vary widely from one region of the U.S. to another, for example (Bacon, Smith & Baker, 1989).

More in–depth cross–national studies are needed that examine differences in the factors that influence injury risk. Among these factors are societal norms, behavioral and socio–cultural factors activities, risk taking behaviors, and amount of exposure to hazardous situations. In addition, emergency medical care and prevention activities vary widely from one country to the next. The earlier mentioned study (Giesbrecht & Dick, 1993) comparing only one factor—alcohol consumption—is just one example of the potential problems of only examining a single factor. Very different results were obtained in the other study of motor vehicle fatalities and alcohol consumption that attempted to control for important differences in exposure (Lowenfels & Wynn, 1992). In order to provide more meaningful comparisons more complex models which incorporate multiple factors are needed. One example is that proposed by Holder (1989). His model includes factors for communities to consider in preventing alcohol–related injuries, which could also be used in comparing and interpreting differences in international mortality data. Among these factors are vehicle and driving conditions, environmental conditions, equipment characteristics, and a variety of other risk factors. He also includes more extensive alcohol variables such as cultural norms and control factors such as price and availability. Such factors should be included in future studies to more completely account for the obviously wide discrepancies in injury rates seen from one country to the other.

In any study comparing data between countries, care must be taken to ensure that similar coding practices are used in each country. A number of studies have shown wide variations in the practice of coding a single underlying cause for other diseases. The use of multiple cause of death data (Israel et al., 1986) can overcome some of these difficulties, and may improve the comparability of data between countries. However, few countries routinely use multiple cause coding. Comparative studies can also reveal problems in current data collection methods, and suggest areas for improvement. The use of multiple sources of information for cause of death certification, and better training and regular querying of physicians by nosologists in vital statistics offices, for example, may account for the much higher fall mortality rate in New Zealand compared to the U.S. The need for more general application of these methods to improve the quality of U.S. mortality data has also been recognized by others (Comstock & Markush, 1986; Rosenberg, 1989; Moriyama, 1989). Comparison of injury data in the elderly are likely to be especially problematic because of the difficulty of assigning a single underlying cause. However, despite the many potential problems, we believe that careful comparisons of injury data between countries can lead to important new insights into both the etiology and prevention of injuries.

References

1. Bacon WE, Smith GS, Baker SP. Geographic variation in the occurrence of hip fractures among the elderly white US population. American Journal of Public Health 1989;79:1556–8.

2. Baker SP, O'Neill B, Ginsburg MJ, Li G. The Injury Fact Book (Second Edition). New York: Oxford University Press, 1992.

3. Campbell AJ, Reinken J, Allan B, Martinez GS. Falls in old age: a study of frequency and related clinical factors. Age Ageing 1981;10:264–270.

4. Cohen B, Pokras R, Meads MS, Krushat WM. How will diagnosis–related groups affect epidemiologic research. American Journal of Epidemiology 1987;126:1–9.

5. Comstock GW, Markush RE. Further comments on problems in death certification. American Journal of Epidemiology 1986;124:180–1.

6. Fife D. Injuries and deaths among elderly persons. American Journal of Epidemiology 1987;126:936–41.

7. Fingerhut LA, Kleinman JC. International and Interstate Comparisons of Homicides Among Young Males. Journal of the American Medical Association 1990;263:3292–3295.

8. Fitzgerald JF, Moore PS, Dittus RS. The care of elderly patients with hip fractures: changes since implementation of the prospective payment system. New England Journal of Medicine 1988;319:1392–7.

9. Giesbrecht N, Dick R. Societal norms and risk–taking behavior: inter–cultural comparisons of casualties and alcohol consumption. Addiction 1993;88:867–876.

10. Holder H. Drinking, alcohol availability and injuries: a systems model of complex relationships. In: Giesbrecht, N. et al., (Eds) Drinking and Casualties: Accidents, Poisonings and Violence in an International Perspective. New York, Tavistock and Routledge, 1989, pp. 133–148.

11. Hopkins DD, Grant–Worley JA, Bollinger TL. Survey of cause–of–death query criteria used by state vital statistics programs and the efficacy of criteria used by the Oregon vital statistics program. American Journal of Public Health 1989;79:570–4.

12. Hsia DC, Krushat WM, Fagan AB, Tebbutt JA, Kusserow RP. Accuracy of diagnostic coding for medicare patients under the prospective payment system. New England Journal of Medicine 1988;318:352–5.

13. Israel RA, Rosenberg HM, Curtin LR. Analytical potential for multiple cause–of–death data. American Journal of Epidemiology 1986;124:161–181.

14. Jencks SF, Williams DK, Kay TL. Assessing hospital–associated deaths from discharge data: the role of length of stay and comorbidities. Journal of the American Medical Association 1988;260:2240–6.

15. Jougla E, Papoz L, Balkau B, Maguin P, Hatton F. EURODIAB Subarea C Study Group: Death certificate coding practices related to diabetes in European countries: the 'Eurodiab Subarea C' Study. International Journal of Epidemiology 1992;21:343–51.

16. Kellerman AL, Lee RK, Mercy JA, Banton J. The epidemiologic basis for the prevention of firearm injuries. Annual Review of Public Health 1991;12:17–40.

17. Kelson M, Farebrother M. The effect of inaccuracies in death certification and coding practices in the European Economic Community on international cancer mortality statistics. International Journal of Epidemiology 1987;16:411–14.

18. Kircher T, Nelson J, Burdo H. The autopsy as a measure of accuracy of the death certificate. New England Journal of Medicine 1985;313:1263–9.

19. Kleinman JC: Age–adjusted mortality indexes of small areas: applications to health planning. American Journal of Public Health 1977;67:834–840.

20. Langley JD, McLoughlin E: Injury mortality and morbidity in New Zealand. Accident Analysis and Prevention 1989;21:243–54.

21. Langlois JA, Smith GS, Baker SP, Langley J. International comparisons of injury mortality in the elderly: issues and differences between New Zealand and the United States. Submitted for publication, March 1994.

22. Li G, Baker SP. A comparison of injury death rates in China and the United States, 1986. American Journal of Public Health 1991;81:605–609.

23. Lowenfels AB, Wynn PS. One less for the road: international trends in alcohol consumption and vehicular fatalities. Annals of Epidemiology 1992;2:249–256.

24. Meade MS: Potential years of life lost in countries of Southeast Asia. Social Science and Medicine 1980;14D:277–281.

25. Moriyama IM. Problems in measurement of accuracy of cause–of–death statistics. American Journal of Public Health 1989;79–1349–50.

26. Moyer IA, Boyle CA, Pollock DA. Validity of death certificates for injury–related causes of death. American Journal of Epidemiology 1989;130:1024–

27. Nevitt MC, Cummings SR, Kidd S, Black D. Risk factors for recurrent nonsyncopal falls: a prospective study. Journal of the American Medical Association 1989;261:2663–2668.

28. National Center for Health Statistics. Instructions for classifying the underlying cause of death 1978 (part 2A). U.S. Department of Health Education and Welfare. Hyattsville, MD: National Center for Health Statistics, 1984.

29. Peek C, Kraus JF. International findings on alcohol consumption and vehicle crash fatalities: the role of the ecologic study. Annals Epidemiology 1992;2:339–341 (editorial).

30. Percy C, Muir C. The international comparability of cancer mortality data. American Journal of Epidemiology 1989;129:934–46.

31. Percy C, Stanek E, Gloeckler L. Accuracy of cancer death certificates and its effect on cancer mortality statistics. American Journal of Public Health 1981;71:242–50.

32. Reid DD: International studies in epidemiology. American Journal of Epidemiology 1975;102:469–76.

33. Rice DP, MacKenzie EJ, and Associates: Cost of Injury in the United States: Report to Congress. San Francisco, CA: Institute for Health and Aging, University of California and Injury Prevention Center, The Johns Hopkins University, 1989.

34. Rockett IRH, Smith GS. Covert suicide among elderly Japanese females: Questioning unintentional drownings. Social Science and Medicine 1993;36:1467–72.

35. Rockett IRH, Smith GS. Injuries in relation to chronic disease: An international view of premature mortality. American Journal of Public Health 1987;77:1345–1346.

36. Rockett IRH, Smith GS. Homicide, suicide, motor vehicle crash, and fall mortality: United States' experience in comparative perspective. American Journal of Public Health 1989(a);79:1396–1400.

37. Rockett IRH, Smith GS. Injuries and the Australian mortality mosaic: a comparison with the United Kingdom and New Zealand. Public Health 1989(b);103:353–61.

38. Romeder JM, McWhinnie JR. Potential years of life lost between ages 1 and 70: An indicator of premature mortality for health planning. International Journal of Epidemiology 1977;6:143–151.

39. Rosenberg HM. Improving cause of death statistics. American Journal of Public Health 1989;79:563–4.

40. Sattin RW, Lambert–Huber DA, DeVito CA, et al. The incidence of fall injury events among the elderly in a defined population. American Journal of Epidemiology 1990;131:1028–1037.

41. Skog OJ. Trends in alcohol consumption and death from diseases. British Journal of Addiction 1987;82:1033–41.

41. Sloan JH, Kellermann AL, Reay DT, et al. Handgun regulations, crime, assaults and homicide: a tale of two cities. New England Journal of Medicine 1988;319:1256–1262.

42. Smith GS, Kraus JF. Alcohol and residential, recreational, and occupational injuries: A review of the epidemiologic evidence. Annual Review of Public Health 1988; 9:99–121.

43. Smith GS, Barss PG. Unintentional injuries in developing countries: the epidemiology of a neglected problem. Epidemiologic Reviews 1991;13:228–266.

44. Sniezek JE, Finklea JF, Graitcer PL. Injury coding and hospital discharge data. Journal of the American Medical Association 1989;262:2270–2.

45. Taket A. Accident mortality in children, adolescents, and young adults. World Health Statistics Quarterly 1986;39:232–256.

46. Tinetti ME, Speechley M, Ginter SF. Risk factors for falls among elderly persons living in the community. New England Journal of Medicine 1988;319:1701–1707.

47. Waller JA. Falls among the elderly: human and environmental factors. Accident Analysis and Prevention 1978;10:21–33.

Table 1. Correlation of per capita alcohol consumption
with male cirrhosis and injury rates by country 1962–1988 (correlation coefficients)

Country	Cirrhosis	MVA	Drowning	Suicide	Homicide
Canada	0.75****	0.34*	0.16	0.04	0.27
Finland	0.09	0.21	0.05	0.48***	0.07
France	0.35*	0.06	0.35*	0.30*	0.23
Netherlands	0.28*	0.20	0.11	0.18	0.36
Switzerland	0.19	0.01	0.10	0.25**	0.23
U.S.	0.42***	0.26	0.11	0.07	0.26

****=p<.005, ***=p<.025, **=p<0.05, *=p<.10

Source: Giesbrecht, 1993. Addition

Table 2. Potential for misclassification among injury causes.
"Other accidents" mortality rates/100,000 for males from
1962–1988, WHO Statistics Annuals

Country	Average	(Range)
France	23.1	(16.7 – 29.2)
U.S.	7.9	(6.6 – 9.8)
Switzerland	7.1	(4.3 – 13.1)
Canada	6.9	(2.8 – 9.9)
Finland	6.5	(2.8 – 9.9)

Table 3. Comparison of elderly female fall death and hospitalization rates/100,000 population for falls and hip fractures, U.S. 1980–1986 and New Zealand

Injury rates/100,000	N.Z.	U.S.
Fall Deaths:		
Total (M & F)*	92*	32
Age: 65–74	14	8
75–84	100	34
85+	600	141
Hospitalizations:		
Falls	2,005*	1,678
Hip fracture	1,000	1,040
In hospital deaths	8.8%	3.3%
Mean length stay	34.2 days	14.2 days

*Age adjusted to U.S. Population, males included with females for this line only

Table 4. Under–counting of fall deaths in the U.S. compared to the rate ratio of fall deaths in New Zealand vs. U.S., by age

	Age (years)		
Fall Mortality	65–74	75–84	85+
Under–counting U.S. (Fife, 1987)	53%	61%	65%
Rate ratio N.Z. vs U.S.	1.8	3.0	4.2

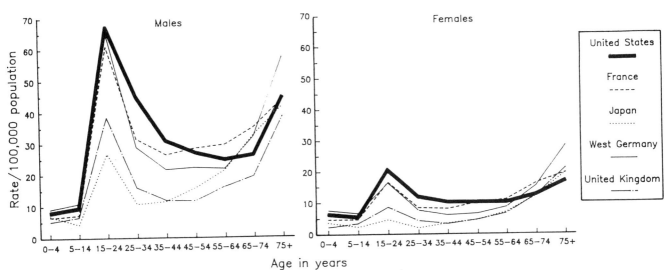

FIGURE 1—Age-Specific Motor Vehicle Crash Death Rates by Sex and Country, 1980

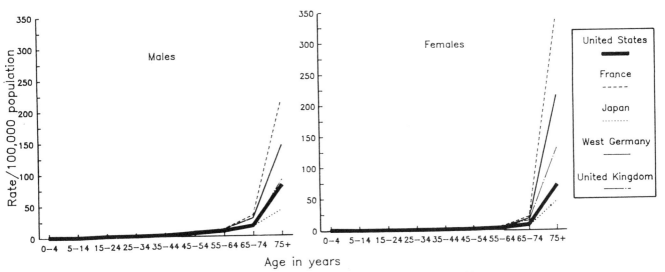

FIGURE 2—Age-Specific Fall Death Rates by Sex and Country, 1980

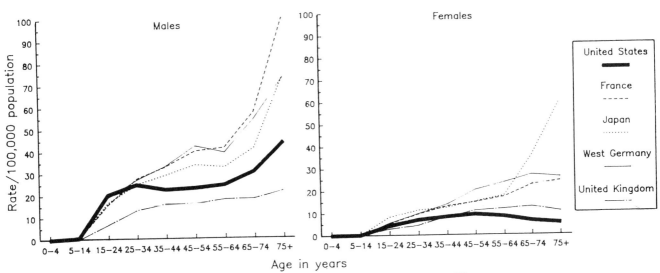

FIGURE 3—Age-Specific Suicide Rates by Sex and Country, 1980

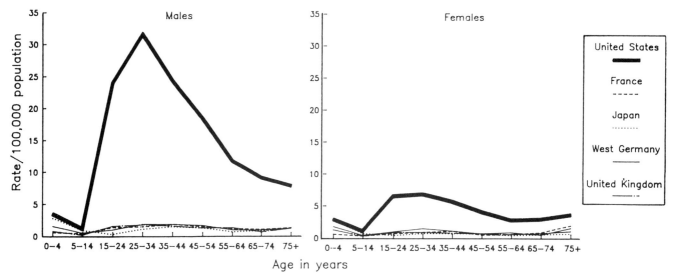

FIGURE 4—Age-Specific Homicide Rates by Sex and Country, 1980

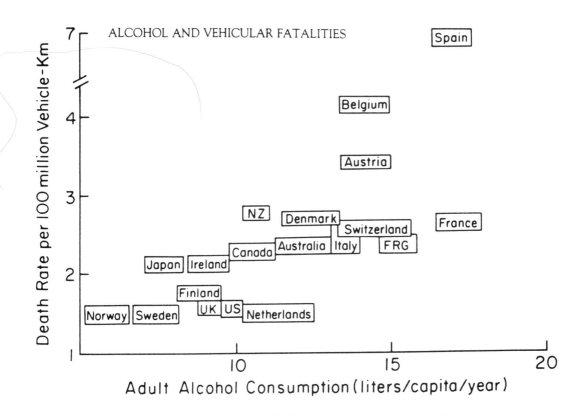

Figure 5. Scattergram showing relationship between death rate from vehicular accidents per 100 million vehicle-kilometers (Y) and adult alcohol consumption in liters per capita per year (1987 data or most recent available year).Source: Lowenfels & Wynn, Annals of Epidemiology 1992;2:249-256.

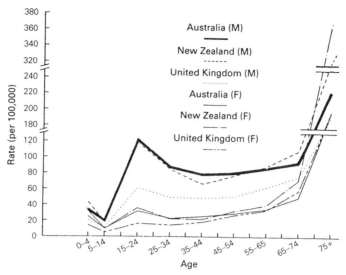

Figure 6 Sex/age-specific injury death rates for Australia, New Zealand, United Kingdom, c.1980.

Figure 7
Percent of Injury Deaths by Cause Among People Aged 65+ in New Zealand (1980-87) and the United States (1980-86)

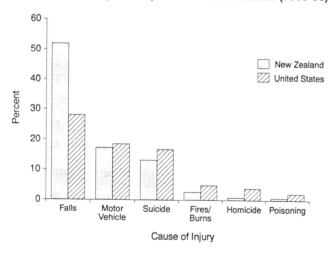

Methodologic Issues in Farm Injury Research

by Lorann Stallones, M.P.H., Ph.D.

Abstract

The hazards associated with farming have been well described for over 50 years in terms of the number of injuries. Despite this, there continue to be problems with interpretation of the patterns of injury and risk due to methodologic problems with the reported work. Specifically, use of denominators to clarify risk patterns are rare and sometimes not appropriate, definitions of farm work are usually absent, and coding on death certificate data is not adequate to identify farm work related injuries. Therefore, results of research cannot necessarily be compared. A number of researchers have worked to develop standard techniques for identification of farm or agricultural production work related injuries and to ensure use of appropriate denominators in the calculation of rates. The purpose of this paper is to discuss the methodologic issues, consequences of the choices researchers have made, and present information which will be useful in identifying methods which will allow comparisons of study results.

Introduction

The hazards associated with farming have been well described for over 50 years in terms of the number of injuries (Cogbill et al., 1985; Gordon et al., 1988; Simpson, 1984: Jones, 1990; McDermott et al., 1990; Demers et al., 1991; Saariet al., 1984; Hopkins, 1989; Cogbill et al., 1991; Calandruccio et al., 1949; Carlson et al., 1978; Cooper, 1969; Delzell et al., 1985; Gadalla, 1984; Goodman et al., 1985; Hatch et al., 1956; Hoskin et al., 1979; Huston et al., 1969; Jackson, 1983; Karlson et al., 1979; Kay, 1971; Knapp, 1966; Powers, 1939; Stallones et al., 1986). Farm injury research has been hampered by the lack of uniform definitions and classification schemes. Farms are places of business and residence (Murphy et al., 1990). Agriculture as an industry includes farm production work, agricultural services, and forestry. As an occupation, agriculture includes workers, owner/operators, managers and a host of other codes. Therefore, farm–related injuries and agricultural injuries are two overlapping, but not completely similar categories as occupational injuries. In addition, farms are places of residence and recreation. The farm–related home injuries and recreational injuries must be separated from the farm–work related injuries in order to present an accurate picture of the risks associated with working and living on a farm (Murphy et al., 1993). There is the additional complication of visitors and part time employees (Stallones,1990). All of these issues give rise to a wide array of estimates of farm related injuries. Murphy et al. (1993) have published a detailed classification system to address these issues. The researchers must begin to clarify what is being presented when farm injuries are studied, in fact if work related injuries are the study interest, a different approach is needed from the assessment of all injuries which occur in a farm setting (Murphy, 1992). The classification of an "at work" injury death is done by coroners or medical examiners (Runyan et al., 1994). There are not consistent, standard definition which apply to worker, a job or being on the job (Runyan, et al., 1994). In fact, Runyan et al. (1994) found that among medical examiners, only 52 percent would classify the death of a 16 year old who suffocated in a grain bin while loading grain on a family farm as a work–related death. In addition, a man who worked part time as a house painter killed by a tractor roll–over on his farm while harvesting hay was only classified as a work–related death by 36 percent of the North Carolina medical examiners surveyed (Runyan et al., 1994).

Denominators

Estimates of the number of agricultural workers there are in the United States vary drastically. In 1980, Bureau of Labor Statistics estimate was 943,000 agricultural workers while the National Safety Council estimate was 3,300,000 (Kraus, 1985). In 1984, the census estimate of the farm population was 3,435,000 persons aged 14 years or older employed in agriculture (US Department of Commerce, 1984). The differences in estimates of the number of agricultural workers has a direct effect on the estimated rates of injuries occurring on farms. Care in the selection of numerators and denominators which have been collected by different agencies is required to avoid artificially high or artificially low estimates of farm related injury rates.

Large discrepancies with regard to denominators is in part the result of different definitions used for farmers and farmworkers. National Safety Council does not apply an age category to the definition of workers, nor is it clear what is the source of the denominator (NSC, 1993). US Census data are based on Census Occupational codes and include farming, forestry and fishery workers 16 years of age and older (US Census, 1990). Whitener (1984) identified the additional problem of the large proportion of seasonal and migrant workers involved. A significant proportion of farm workers were not involved in farm work during the month of March. Farm work was defined as on–farm wage or salary work associated with producing, harvesting, and delivering agricultural commodities or managing a farm but excluding work by farm operators, unpaid family members, machine custom work, nonfarm work done on a farm or work performed for pay–in–kind (Whitener, 1984). The 1980 Decennial Census data indicated 792,000 wage and salary workers from five agricultural occupations (managers of farms and horticultural specialty farms, supervisors of farm workers, farm workers, and nursery workers) (Whitener, 1984). The 1981 Hired Farm Working Survey indicated 818,000 hired farm workers employed in March, but a total of 2,210,000 total farm workers (Whitener, 1984). The seasonal nature of farm work influences the accuracy of the count of farm workers, with only one third of all workers employed between January and March when the census is taken (Whitener, 1984). In addition, those workers who are on the farm in March work significantly more days than the workers who are not employed that month (average 105 days for all workers, 218 days for March workers) (Whitener, 1984). These differences have implications for the estimates of risk of farm work related injuries as well, particularly when using number of people as a denominator. The inclusion of only those who worked exceptional hours in the estimate of risk will give a different pattern of injury risk when compared with using the person hours worked as a denominator.

Finally, the United States Census of the Population does count the number of farm residents. In 1980, detailed tables of the age–race–gender information were not made available for states by county and had to be purchased as a special tabulation (Stallones, 1990). Availability of data from the 1990 Census on CD–ROM alleviates this problem, but the information is difficult to extract and requires a special program because the detail is not available on the summary files. This is the only source of data for the farm population who are under 16 years of age. A great deal of interest is evident in the literature, given the number of published articles on farm injuries among children (Pollack, 1992; Tormoehlen, 1986; No author, 1988; Field et al., 1982; Doyle et al., 1989; Weiser, 1968; Grand; 1985; Rivara, 1985; Salmi et al., 1989; Stallones, 1989; Waller et al., 1989; Cogbill et al., 1985; Lucas, et al. 1963; Swanson et al., 1987; Stueland et al., 1991; Davies et al., 1988; Edmonson, 1987; Anderson et al., 1980; Brennan et al., 1990; Purschwitz, 1990; Stallones et al., 1993). Use of an inappropriate denominator will influence the estimate of rates per 100,000 for farm related boys injuries as well, as indicated by the results reported by Salmi et al. (1989) (2.3 among 0–4 years; 2.2 among 5–9 years) compared to others (Rivara, 1985)(14.9 for 0–4 years; 13.9 for 5–9 years) (Stallones, 1989) (14.8 for 0–4 years; 27.4 for 5–9 years). Salmi et al. (1989) used the rural resident population as the denominator for the injury rates. The rural resident population is much larger than the rural farm population and will consistently give an underestimate of injuries (Table 1).

Table 1 contains estimates of the number of farm workers from differing sources. Clearly the selection of a denominator will influence the rate of injury estimated for the population. In addition, the inclusion or exclusion of operators and family members has an influence on the actual counts of the agricultural working population. Also included in the table are the counts for the rural farm population and the rural nonfarm population. The use of rural farm and nonfarm combined as a denominator will lead to a gross underestimate of the risk of injuries among farm residents.

Numerators

Another issue in the evaluation of farm related injuries is the definitions which are used to identify the farm relatedness of an event. Based on death certificates only, there are several useful fields which may or may not be coded within a state. A place of occurrence code can be used with the ICDA external cause of death codes (E–codes) using a fifth digit sub–classification. There is also a field on the death certificate which may be coded separately. The choices are shown in Table 2. When the information is not detailed, coding can be ambiguous and the ability to determine the farm–relatedness of an injury is affected. For example, if a drowning occurs in a farm pond, but the information obtained is not specific for farm, than the death would be coded to the other specified places rather than a farm. Another example would be a death occurring while mowing the hedge row near the farm house. This might be coded as occurring on the home premises rather than on the farm. This may or may not be viewed as a farm work related injury. Depending on the direction of the decisions, the rate of farm injuries can be increased or decreased.

Occupation and industry codes are also potentially useful in identifying farm related injuries, however are not uniformly available from state computer files. Since the occupation and industry which are coded are the usual occupation and industry, in areas where there is a large percentage of part–time farmers who have another primary occupation, this field will not give an accurate assessment of the magnitude of the problem.

The National Traumatic Occupational Fatality (NTOF) system was developed by the National Institute for Occupational Safety and Health (NIOSH) to monitor occupational fatalities (Murphy et al., 1990). The method for classification which is used to identify injuries is based on being coded as an at work injury, then the usual occupation and industry of the decedent (Murphy et al., 1990). Murphy et al. (1990) compared this classification scheme with one based on death certificates, a newspaper clipping service database and supplemental information obtained from next of kin in Pennsylvania. The investigators provided evidence of a 30 percent error in the NTOF method which resulted in a 20 percent undercount of agricultural work injury deaths and an overcount by the National Safety Council's system of approximately 35 percent (Murphy et al. 1990).

Results of such comparisons may differ from one state to another, being dependent on the proportion of part time farm operators within a state. For example, in Kentucky, a high percentage of farmers work at other occupations. In a detailed search of death certificates, a large percentage were not classified as at work (43 percent of farmers, 47 percent of farm workers, 61 percent of those with other occupations on the death certificate and 70 percent of students and family members) despite the fact that the description of the injury on the death certificate indicated a farm work related injury had occurred (Stallones, 1990). The error then will lead to an underestimate of the number of farm work related injuries which will be more significant in states where farm operators have multiple occupations. The most useful source of information in this study was the field which described how the injury occurred, but this information is not usually available from computer files and is only accessible through the hard copy of death certificates in most states.

Issues related to the definition of farm–relatedness are as similar when using medical records data as when using death certificates. The detailed information needed for assessing the injury episode rather than the type and significance of the injury may not be well documented. For this reason, the use of newspaper clippings, a traditional approach used by agricultural safety specialists, has been adopted by some investigators (Gunderson et al., 1990). Farm related trauma was defined as any injury occurring to individuals on any farm in Minnesota or any injury on a public road where farm equipment was involved (Gunderson et al., 1990). Limitations noted included the fact that only severe or catastrophic events were reported and data needed for research were not always included in the newspaper report (Gunderson et al., 1990). Not included in the discussion, but also a potential problem is the fact that two newspaper clipping services may actually obtain information on different groups of injuries, that is not all injuries found by one service will also be found by a different service.

Gunderson et al. (1990) reported that in Olmsted County, fewer than 5 percent of all farming–related injuries involved hospitalization, however 87 percent involved contact with a health care provider. These data indicate the need for surveillance mechanisms beyond hospital records to accurately count the number of nonfatal injuries which occur. Gunderson et al. (1990) reviewed reports based on data from the Occupational Safety and Health Administration (OSHA) and Workers' Compensation records and concluded that due to the fact that farmers are self–employed and frequently hire fewer than 11 employees, the majority of US farms would be excluded from a count of these records.

The Ninth Revision of the International Classification of Diseases–Adapted (ICDA) codes offer little assistance in the classification of farm related injuries. Codes are available for injuries where agricultural machines are involved, but these are only identifiable when the E–codes are used. In fact, many E–codes are involved when an injury occurs on a farm including the codes for falls, slips and trips, burn, drowning, fractures, carbon monoxide or other utility gas, excessive heat or cold, being struck by objects, injuries from electrical current, and injuries from firearms. In order for the injury to be identified as farm–related other information must be available (e.g., where the injury occurred, details about circumstances of the injury). In Kentucky, all death certificates which contained an E–code were hand searched to identify farm–related and farm–work related deaths (Stallones, 1990). A total of 17,821 records were searched for the period 1979–1985 (Stallones, 1990). In that survey, the distribution of ICDA Ninth

Revision codes was as shown in Table 3. Table 4 contains the same distribution for children under age 15 years of age who died from unintentional injuries on farms in Kentucky from 1979–1985 (Stallones, 1989). Table 5 contains the same ICDA code distribution for nonfatal work related injuries which occurred on farms in Colorado in 1993 based on a telephone survey being conducted among farm families in that state. While differences in the overall distributions are evident comparing fatal and nonfatal injuries and injuries occurring to children and adults, overall a wide variation in the ICDA codes is represented and the selection of the most important codes to identify farm injuries is complex.

Conclusions

Perhaps the most important issues to resolve in farm related injury research are those of definitions. The most critical are the separation of injuries to family members and operators who are injured in the course of daily activities unrelated to agricultural production. This will help in the selection of an appropriate denominator for a given study. The separation of farm residents from workers is critical for the evaluation of occupational related farm injuries as compared to injuries which occur on a farm related to home or leisure activities. Children at young ages (5–6 years) do work on farms and therefore should be included in evaluating work related injuries when appropriate. They can also be injured bystanders in the work setting and this also needs to be evaluated, but separated from those injuries which occur while a child is actually doing the work. These same circumstances apply to visitors to farms who may have an injury but will never be counted in the available denominators. The inclusion of this group will tend to inflate the estimates of injury risk to workers.

Finally, a uniform definition of a farm needs to be developed and applied by researchers. Census farm resident populations are self defined. The Census of Agriculture defines a farm as a place where in a normal year, $1,000 in agricultural produce is sold. If there are major discrepancies in the self defined farm population and the specific definition used by the Census of Agriculture enumerators, there is no valid way to compare the results of studies using the two data sources. This has not been examined in detail and has implications for expanding to international comparisons of farm injuries. This issue has particular significance for countries where subsistence agriculture is the norm and $1,000 in sales is not a normal year, but rather an abnormally high sales year for a small farmer.

The separation of farm workers from other workers who have been included in the classification (forest and fishery workers) will help in the clarification of the population at risk. The identification of individuals who live on farm separately from those who are employed on farms will also improve the estimate of the risk of farm work as distinct from farm living injury risk. This applies to the classification of both numerators and denominators. The use of person hours worked as a denominator may assist researchers in better understanding the magnitude of risk on farms, since the work hours vary widely from one season to another. In addition, a pressing question is whether there are different risks with different types of farming, as has been shown in a few studies (Gadalla, 1962; Stallones, 1990). The collection and presentation of injuries by type of agricultural production is important for evaluating injury risk.

References

1.   Anderson JM, Schutt AH. Spinal injury in children: a review of 156 cases seen from 1950 through 1978. Mayo Clinic Proceedings, 55:499–504, 1980.

2.   Brennan SR, Rhodes KH, Peterson HA. Infection after farm machine–related injuries in children and adolescents. American Journal Diseases of Childhood, 144:710–713, 1990.

3.   Calandruccio RA, Powers JH. Farm accidents: A clinical and statistical study covering 20 years. American Journal of Surgery:652–660, 1949.

4.   Carlson ML., Peterson GR. Mortality of California agricultural workers. Journal of Occupational Medicine 29(1):30–32, 1978.

5.   Cogbill TH, Busch HM. The spectrum of agricultural trauma. Journal of Emergency Medicine, 3:205–210, 1985.

6.   Cogbill TH, Steenlage ES, Landercasper J, Strutt P. Death and disability from agricultural injuries in Wisconsin: A 12–year experience with 739 patients. The Journal of Trauma, 31(12):1632–1639, 1991.

7.   Cogbill TH, Busch HM, Stiers GR. Farm accidents in children. Pediatrics, 76(4):562–566, 1985.

8.   Cooper DKC. Agricultural accidents: A study of 132 patients seen at Addenbrooke's hospital, Cambridge, in 12 months. British Medical Journal 4:193–198, 1969.

10.   Davis JB, Howell CG, Parrish RA. Childhood farm injury: The role of the physician in prevention. American Surgeon, 54:192–194, 1988.

11.   Delzell E, Grufferman S. Mortality among white and nonwhite farmers in North Carolina, 1976–1978. American Journal of Epidemiology 121 (3):391–402, 1985.

12.   Demers P, Rosenstock L. Occupational injuries and illnesses among Washington state agricultural workers. American Journal of Public Health, 81(12):1656–1658, 1991.

13.   Doyle Y, Conroy R. Childhood farm accidents: A continuing cause for concern. Journal of the Society of Occupational Medicine. 39(1):35–37, 1989.

14.   Edmonson MB. Caustic alkali ingestion by farm children, Pediatrics, 79(3):413–416, 1987.

15.   Field WE, Tormoehlen RL. Analysis of fatal and non–fatal farm accident involving children. ASAE Paper No. 82–5501, Winter, 1982 Meeting, Chicago, IL.

16.   Gadalla SM. Selected environmental factors associated with farm and farm home accidents in Missouri. Research Bulletin 790 University of Missouri College of Agriculture. Columbia, Missouri, Rural Health Series Publication 16, 1962.

17.   Gallagher RP, Threlfall WJ, Spinelli JJ, Band PR. Occupational mortality patterns among British Columbia farm workers. Journal of Occupational Medicine 26(12):906–908, 1984.

18.   Gerberich SG, Gibson RW, Gunderson PD, French LR, Melton J, Erdman A, Smith P, True J, Carr WP, Elkington J, Renier C, Andrenssen L. The Olmsted agricultural trauma study (OATS): A population–based effort. A report to the Centers for Disease Control, March, 1991. The estimate was developed using data from pages 38–40 by staff at the National Farm Medicine Center, and uses denominators constructed from baseline data compiled from U.S. Department of Commerce and U.S. Department of Agriculture, Rural and Rural Farm Population: 1988. August, 1989. Page 14.

19.   Gerberich SG. Overview of agricultural injury surveillance. Presentation at the Agricultural Injury Intervention Strategy Workshop, Minneapolis, MN, July 15–17, 1992.

20.   Goodman RA, Smith JD, Sikes RK, Rogers DL, Mickey JL. Fatalities associated with farm tractor injuries: An epidemiologic study. Public Health Reports 100(3):329–340, 1985.

21.   Goodman RA, Smith JD, Sikes RK, Rogers DL, Mickey JL. Fatalities associated with farm tractor injuries: An epidemiologic study. Public Health Reports. 100(3):329–333, 1985.

22.   Gordon G, Indeck M, Bross J, Kappor DA, Brotman S. Injury from silage wagon accident complicated by mucormycosis. Journal of Trauma. 28(6):866–867, 1988.

23.   Grand FJ. Children killed in tractor accidents in Denmark 1973–1977. Journal of Traffic Medicine/IAATM Newsletter. 8:2–6, 1985.

24.   Gunderson P, Gerberich S, Gibson R, Adlis S, Carr P, Erdman A, Elkington J, French R, Melton J, True J. Injury surveillance in agriculture. American Journal of Industrial Medicine, 18:169–178.

25. Haddon W. A logical framework for categorizing highway safety phenomena and activity. Journal of Trauma. 12:193–207, 1972.

26. Hatch CS, Jones RM. Unusual farm machinery injuries. American Journal of Surgery 91:501–505, 1956.

27. Hopkins RS. Farm equipment injuries in a rural county, 1980–1985: the emergency department as a source of data for prevention. Annals of Emergency Medicine, 18(7):758–761, 1989.

28. Hoskin AF, Miller TA. Farm accident surveys: A 21–state summary with emphasis on animal related injuries. Journal of Safety Research 11(1):2–13, 1979.

29. Huston AF, Smith C. Farm accidents in Saskatchewan, Canada. Medical Association Journal 100:764–769, 1969.

30. Jackson FC. Farm and ranch injuries in West Texas. Texas Medicine 79:51–54, 1983.

31. Jones MW. A study of trauma in an Amish community. Journal of Trauma, 30(7):899–902, 1990.

32. Karlson T, Noren J. Fatal tractor fatalities: The failure of voluntary safety standards. American Journal of Public Health 69(2):146–149, 1979.

33. Kay K. Agricultural health and hygiene–with special reference to the Canadian population. Environmental Research 4:440–468, 1971.

34. Knapp LW. Occupational and rural accidents. Archives of Environmental Health 13:501–506, 1966.

35. Kraus JF. Fatal and non–fatal injuries in occupational settings: A review. Annual Reviews of Public Health 6:403–418, 1985.

36. Letts RM. Degloving injuries in children. Journal of Pediatric Orthopedics, 6(2):193–197, 1986.

37. Lucas GL, Wirka HW. Farm accidents occurring in children. Wisconsin Medical Journal, October:405–409, 1963.

38. McDermott S, Lee CV. Injury among male migrant farm workers in South Carolina. Journal of Community Health 15(5):297–305, 1990.

39. Murphy, DJ. Safety and health for production agriculture. ASAE Textbook 5, St Joseph, MI. 1992.

40. Murphy DJ, Seltzer BL, Yesalis CE. Comparison of two methodologies to measure agricultural occupational fatalities. American Journal of Public Health 80(2):198–199, 1990.

41. Murphy DJ, Purschwitz M, Mahoney BS, Hoskin AF. A proposed classification code for farm and agricultural injuries. American Journal of Public Health 83(5):736–738, 1993.

42. Murphy D. Working unsafely on the farm. Applied Agricultural Research 1(1):2–5, 1986.

43. No author. The killing and maiming of American farm kids (and adults) Part II. Health Letter, June, 1988.

44. Powers JH. The hazards of farming. Journal of the American Medical Association 113(15):1375–1379, 1939.

45. Powers JH. Farm injuries. New England Journal of Medicine 243(25):979–983, 1950.

46. Purschwitz MA. Fatal farm injuries to children. Wisconsin Rural Health Research Center, May 1990.

47. Rivara FP. Fatal and non–fatal farm injuries to children and adolescents in the United States. Pediatrics 76(6):567–573, 1985.

48. Robinson TCM. Gathering and evaluating accident data with respect to farm people and farm workers. American Journal of Public Health 39:999–1003, 1949.

49. Runyan CW, Loomis D, Butts J. Practices of county medical examiners in classifying deaths as on the job. Journal of Occupational Medicine 36(1):36–41, 1994.

50. Saari KM, Aines E. Eye injuries in agriculture. Acta Ophtalmologica Supplementum. 161:42–51, 1984.

51. Salmi LR, Weiss HB, Peterson PL, Spengler RF, Sattin RW, Anderson HA. Fatal farm injuries among young children. Pediatrics, 83(2):267–271, 1989.

52. Simpson SG. Farm machinery injuries. Journal of Trauma, 24(2):150–152, 1984.

53. Stallones L, Gunderson PD. Epidemiological perspectives on childhood agricultural injuries within the United States. Journal of Agromedicine. (accepted), 1993.

54. Stallones L, Pratt DS, May JJ. Reported frequency of dairy farm–associated health hazards, Otsego County, New York, 1982–1983. American Journal of Preventive Medicine 2(4):189–192, 1986.

55. Stallones L. Fatal unintentional injuries among Kentucky farm children: 1979–1985. Journal of Rural Health. 5(3):246–256, 1989.

56. Stallones L. Surveillance of fatal and non–fatal farm injuries in Kentucky. American Journal of Industrial Medicine 18:223–234, 1990.

57. Stueland D, Layde P, Lee BC. Agricultural injuries in children in central Wisconsin. Journal of Trauma, 31(11):1503–1509, 1991.

58. Swanson JA, Sach MI, Dahlgren KA, Tinguely SJ. Accidental farm injuries in children. American Journal Diseases of Childhood, 141:1276–1279, 1987.

59. Tormoehlen R. Fatal farm accidents occurring to Wisconsin children, 1970–1984. ASAE Paper No. 86–5514, 1986 Winter Meeting, Chicago, IL.

60. US Department of Commerce. Farm population of the United States 1984. Current Population Reports Series. Page 27, no 58. Bureau of the Census. US Department of Agriculture. Economic Research Service. 1984.

61. Waller AE, Baker SP, Szocka A. Childhood injury deaths: National analysis and geographic variations. American Journal of Public Health, 79(3):310–315, 1989.

62. Weiser J. Tractors and children. Acta Medica Belgica, 26(3):216–221, 1968.

63. Whitener LA. Counting hired farm workers: Some points to consider. US Department of Agriculture Economic Research Service Agricultural Economic Report Number 524, 1984.

Table 1: Number of Agricultural Workers by Source of Data

Source of Data	Year	Number
National Safety Council[1]	1992	3,200,000
Census of Agriculture[2]	1982*	4,855,857
Bureau of Labor Statistics[3]	1992	3,207,000
US Census Summary[4]	1990	2,839,010
Hired Farm Worker Survey[5]	1981	2,210,000
Rural farm residents[6]	1990	3,871,583
Rural nonfarm residents[6]	1990	57,786,747

[1]Includes all persons gainfully employed, including owners, managers, other paid employees, the self–employed, and unpaid family workers, but excludes private household workers (NSC, 1993).

[2]Most recent estimate available because 1987 Census of Agriculture eliminated the number of hired farm and ranch workers (Census of Agriculture, 1987, A–2 Appendix A).

[3]Employed civilians 16 years of age and older (BLS, 1993).

[4]Available on CD–ROM 1990 Census Summary, includes farming, forestry and fishing occupations, employed persons 16 years and over.

[5]Interim Census of workers age not specified, not operators of farms (Whitener, 1984).

[6]Available on CD–ROM 1990 Census Summary Tape File 3C

Table 2: Place of Occurrence of Injury Codes

Home	Apartment, Boarding house, Farm house Home premises, House, Noninstitutional place of residence, Private (driveway to home, garage, garden to home, walk to home), swimming pool in private house or yard, yard to home Excludes: home under construction but not yet occupied; institutional place of residence
Farm	Buildings, land under cultivation Excludes: farm house and home premises of farm
Mine and quarry	Gravel pit, sand pit, tunnel under construction
Industrial place and premises	Building under construction, dockyard, factory, garage etc.
Place of recreation/sport etc.	Amusement park, Baseball field, Basketball court, Beach resort
Street/highway	
Public building	Airport, bank, cafe, post office etc. Excludes: home garage, industrial building or workplace
Residential Institution	Children's home, dormitory, hospital, prison, old people's home, orphanage, prison, reform school
Other specified places	Beach, canal, caravan site, derelict house, desert, dock, forest, pond or pool (natural), prairie, river, stream, sea, lake, mountain, parking lot, parking place etc.

Table 3: On–farm unintentional injury deaths in Kentucky by ICDA code, 1979–1985*

ICDA Ninth Revision	Number	Percent
E810–E819: Motor Vehicle Traffic	35	6.5
E820–E825: Motor Vehicle Nontraffic	15	2.8
E826–E829: Other Road Vehicle	5	0.9
E830–E838: Water Transport	3	0.5
E860–E869: Accidental poisoning by other solid and liquid substances, gases and vapors	9	1.7
E880–E888: Accidental falls	25	4.7
E890–E899: Accidents caused by fire and flames	65	12.1
E900–E909: Accidents due to natural and environmental factors	20	3.7
E910–E915: Accidents caused by submersion, suffocation and foreign bodies	51	9.5
E919.0: Agricultural equipment	198	37.0
E916–E928: Other accidents, excluding E919.0	109	20.4
TOTAL	535	99.8

*Note: this includes all deaths on Kentucky farms without regard to work–relatedness. This also represents unintentional deaths and those for which intent had not been determined.

Table 4: On–farm unintentional injury deaths among children under 15 years of age in Kentucky by ICDA code, 1979–1985*

ICDA Ninth Revision	Number	Percent
E810–E819: Motor Vehicle Traffic	1	2.1
E820–E825: Motor Vehicle Nontraffic	5	10.4
E826–E829: Other Road Vehicle	2	4.2
E830–E838: Water Transport	1	2.1
E860–E869: Accidental poisoning by other solid and liquid substances, gases and vapors	0	0.0
E880–E888: Accidental falls	0	0.0
E890–E899: Accidents caused by fire and flames	1	2.1
E900–E909: Accidents due to natural and environmental factors	0	0.0
E910–E915: Accidents caused by submersion, suffocation and foreign bodies	14	29.2
E916–E928: Other accidents	24	50.0
TOTAL	48	100.1

*Note: this includes all deaths on Kentucky farms without regard to work–relatedness. This also represents unintentional deaths and those for which intent had not been determined.

Table 5: On–farm unintentional work related injuries in Colorado by ICDA code, 1993

ICDA Ninth Revision	Number	Percent
E810–E819: Motor Vehicle Traffic	0	0.0
E820–E825: Motor Vehicle Nontraffic	1	1.3
E826–E829: Other Road Vehicle	5	6.3
E830–E838: Water Transport	0	0.0
E860–E869: Accidental poisoning by other solid and liquid substances, gases and vapors	2	2.6
E880–E888: Accidental falls	14	17.5
E890–E899: Accidents caused by fire and flames	0	0.0
E900–E909: Accidents due to natural and environmental factors	11	13.7
E910–E915: Accidents caused by submersion, suffocation and foreign bodies	0	0.0
E919.0: Agricultural equipment	5	6.2
E916–E928: Other accidents, excluding E919.0	42	52.5
TOTAL	80	100.1

Injury Mortality and Morbidity Reporting Systems in France
(Unintentional Injuries of Children and Adolescents)

by Anne Tursz, M.D.

In spite of increased attention given to traffic injuries, and, because of their high frequency and lethality, the passing of road safety legislation in the 1970's, a global interest in accidents as an important public health problem is of recent date, as is an epidemiological understanding of non–traffic related injuries. Before 1980 the only usable data for purposes of prevention were mortality statistics and some limited studies, the latter carried out almost exclusively on in–patients, primarily in surgery departments and intensive care units.

Between 1970 and 1980, injury mortality rates decreased dramatically in neighboring countries, whereas this decrease was very slow in France, especially in the case of deaths related to home and leisure injuries. For the past ten years, injuries have been the first cause of hospital admission of children, ranking ahead of respiratory infections.

Therefore, in the early 1980's, the Ministry of Health sponsored morbidity surveys in the field of childhood injuries, children being considered as the highest risk group [1, 2, 3]. These surveys concentrated on measuring the magnitude of the problem, identifying the most frequent injury circumstances, and assessing the feasibility of a permanent surveillance system. Since that period, several different systems for gathering morbidity data have been put in place, but none of them can pretend to being truly representative at a national, or even a regional level. For this reason, the analysis over time of changes in injury pathology in relationship to prevention programs has relied primarily on mortality data. However, these data, in spite of their being exhaustive, valid nationally and relatively reliable, raise a number of methodological problems, which make certain international comparisons risky.

This paper deals only with unintentional injuries, and the data presented concern almost exclusively children and adolescents. Both the terms "accident" and "injury" are used. In France, as is the case in other European countries, the word "accident" is still used in a scientific and epidemiological context, and in French does not have the pejorative connotation it has acquired in English (fatalistic, unavoidable, therefore not preventable).

Finally, this paper emphasizes methodological issues in the collection and analysis of mortality and morbidity data. It is for this reason that reference is made to fairly early morbidity data [1, 4, 5], because they are the only data analyzed from the dual perspectives of their statistical and epidemiological quality and of the difficulties in data collection.

Mortality

The data presented here come from two sources: national statistics published by INSERM* [6], and, in the case of international comparisons, the WHO World Health Statistics Annual [7]. The figures are for 1990 whenever possible. E–codes from the WHO International Classification of Diseases (ICD), used for the tables of figures, are listed in the annex.

Level of Accidental Mortality among Children and Youths

Injuries (and most particularly unintended injuries) in France, as in the rest of the developed world, are the primary cause of death from the age of one year and for all of childhood and adolescence. In 1990, 840 children aged 1 to 14 years died accidentally (representing 33.4 percent of all deaths for that age), and 3,527 youths aged 15 to 24 died accidentally (53.0 percent of deaths). This interest in unintentional injuries only is justified by the fact that

---

*National Institute for Health and Medical Research

intentional injuries in France are a problem of much less magnitude; for example, among 15 to 24 year olds in 1990, 791 suicides were recorded (12.1 percent of the causes of death) and 70 homicides.

The analysis of rates by age and sex (Table I) shows characteristics found in most of the countries:

–   higher rates among the youngest children, adolescents and young adults than among children aged 5 to 14 years;

–   a higher mortality among males at all ages;

–   the increasing of this higher male mortality with age (sex ratio = 1.6 at ages 1 to 4 years, and 3.1 at ages 15 to 19 years).

It is difficult to interpret the very high rates observed among children under one year of age because of obvious methodological problems (with the certification of cause of death) which will be discussed below.

Rates of accidental mortality in France are among the highest observed in European countries (Table II). Among children 1 to 14 years old, higher rates than those in France are noted in two North European countries—Germany and Belgium—and in three southern countries: Greece, Spain and Portugal. (It should be noted in the case of Luxembourg that rates calculated for a single year are not usable because of the very small size of the population).

Causes of Accidental Death

Beginning at age one year, traffic accidents predominate (Table III) and represent 78 percent of fatal accidents among adolescents aged 15 to 19 years. The second most important cause of accidental death is by drowning. The very high number of fatal suffocations before the age of one year poses methodological problems which will be discussed below.

Main Methodological Issues

The analysis of accidental death before the age of one year is difficult.

This problem is due especially to possible confusion between "sudden infant death" and "suffocation". As previously noted, the accidental death rate in children less than one year old is very high, higher than in all other European countries, except Greece and Portugal (Table II), and the rate of suffocations is also abnormally high. The possibility of confusing suffocation with sudden infant death stands out clearly in the comparative analysis of the change over time of these two conditions between 1970 and 1980 (Table IV). (Sudden infant death as an entity was recently identified and diffusion of the diagnosis has only been occurring since the 1980's). Most probably, rather than a change in the distribution and rate of these conditions, there has been a change in the diagnostic and coding habits. When certifying the cause of death of a child found dead in his bed, the physicians who used to code "suffocation" are now coding "SID" (with only about 30 percent of SID diagnoses being established after an autopsy). It is also likely that an unknown proportion of "suffocations" and "sudden deaths" are in fact infant homicides.

There is a higher percentage of "injuries undetermined whether accidentally or purposely inflicted" than in other Northern European countries.

This is particularly the case for children under one year of age. It is likely that physicians, when coding the death certificate, are quite reluctant to record a diagnosis of intentional traumatic death. Furthermore, there are a number of deaths (certified as "accidents", "suicides" and "homicides") where the intention to cause death is not clear and misclassifications are made either by mistake or deliberately, because the diagnosis of intentional death seems socially and culturally unacceptable (primarily in the case of adolescent suicide or infant homicide). Some cases of adolescent suicide are probably coded as accidents, as shown by the trends over time of these two categories of death, the current decrease in accident rates corresponding to a similar increase in suicide rates [8]. This is most probably related to changes in coding habits rather than to real changes in rates.

There are a certain number of accidental deaths (whose importance varies with age) classified among deaths of undetermined cause and considered as belonging to the category of "symptoms, signs and ill–defined conditions."

This is especially true in the case of violent and suspicious deaths which are the object of a medico–legal investigation, the results of which cannot be communicated at the time of the compiling of mortality statistics. In 1983–1985, the percentage of these cases among all deaths was 2 percent for all ages, but reached 6 percent in the 15–24 year old group at the national level, and 35 percent in the city of Paris [9].

The cause of the accident is often not specified.

In the French language, and in the minds of most people, including the physicians in charge of coding death certificates, the word "accident" is more or less synonymous with "traffic accident". Therefore, most of these accidental deaths of unknown cause are probably deaths from traffic injuries. This proportion of "undetermined cause of accidental death" is more or less constant for age (from 7 to 10 percent between the ages of 1 to 24 years; Table III).

This "linguistic issue" most probably leads to an underestimation of traffic injuries, and also to an overestimation of home and leisure injuries when the latter percentage is calculated by subtracting traffic and occupational accidents from all accidental deaths.

In cases of accidental death delayed beyond the date of the accident, the death may be certified as being from other causes (complication of infection, for example).

In the case of traffic accidents, there is a standardized European definition which considers as having died accidentally "any person killed outright or dying from the sequelae of the accident within 30 days". In France, the accepted period is 6 days [10]. Such large differences make international comparisons hazardous.

There are discrepancies between information sources.

The results may show different figures for the same type of accidental death. This is the case for traffic accidents for which deaths are identified from death certificates and recorded by INSERM in the annual statistics on medical causes of deaths [6], but are also registered by the police from accident reports, then recorded in the statistics of the National Interministerial Observatory for Road Safety [10].

Morbidity

Any analysis of morbidity data should be carried out within the context of the French health system, a complex system associating a large public sector, composed primarily of hospitals, and an important private sector with hospitals and physicians' offices. Both sectors are reimbursed for care by the national public health insurance system, and both sectors care for injury victims.

The 1981 Studies

These studies originated with and were financed by the Ministry of Health within the framework of discussion in Europe on the development of a European accident surveillance system. They were carried out in three geographically–defined areas: in a health care district of the Paris region (Yvelines, [1]); in the north of France (Lens and Montmédy [2]); and in a city in the east of France (Bar le Duc, [3]). They dealt with medically treated injuries of out–patients, and data collection involving the entire health care system, including private medical facilities. Based on well–defined populations, they enabled the calculation of frequencies (Table V). There has not been a more recent survey of this type, as the calculation of frequency is a difficult objective to attain in a complex health system.

The largest study, the Yvelines survey, was used as the feasibility study for the French Accident Surveillance System. It raised various methodological issues which are described below.

Multiplicity of information sources needed for the calculation of frequency.

The private health care sector is an important source of cases in the Yvelines study (principally private hospitals; Table VI), as in the one at Bar le Duc where 22 percent of cases were found in the offices of private physicians [3].

In the Yvelines study, limiting the registration to the public hospitals would have led to calculating an annual rate of incidence of 5.1 percent, instead of the final observed rate of 8.33 for 100 subjects under 15 years of age.

Under the assumption that all severe cases are registered in public hospitals, most epidemiological surveys disregard private facilities. In the Yvelines study, the fracture rate was the same in private and public hospital cases, and some cases registered in the private sector were quite serious.

On the other hand, inclusion in the registration of school infirmaries and day care centers (which explains the higher rates noted in the study at Bar le Duc, Table V), led to gathering data on what were essentially benign cases.

Finally, it should be noted that the comparison of the cases recorded in public facilities with those from private facilities showed significant differences as concerns the characteristics of injuries, with a higher percentage of sports related injuries in the private hospitals.

Underreporting

The comparison of reported and missing cases showed significant differences and selection bias. Cases were not missed at random, and for example, the rate of poisoning was higher among missing cases. Because cases of child poisoning were rapidly admitted to the hospital, in a high percentage of cases the form was not filled out in the emergency room. Therefore, there is a need for regular verification of registration (emergency room and out-patient department log books).

The reporting level was lower in private hospitals (50 percent) than in public ones (75 percent). This is but one of the problems found in collaborating with the private sector (poor quality of the log books; poor quality, or even the absence of medical records). The response rate of private practitioners (investigated through a postal survey) was 47 percent (34 percent for GPs and 52 percent for pediatricians).

Missing Data

The percentage of missing data is especially high for those related to the accident circumstances and causative agents (site of accident, activity of the victim, products involved), and especially when the information has to be retrospectively searched for in the medical files (the location of accident was missing in 12 percent of the reporting forms filled out in hospital emergency rooms, and in 44 percent of the cases retrospectively recorded in medical files). These data are essential to prevention programs.

Coding Problems

Ad hoc codes had to be designed for describing the circumstances of accidents and identifying the causative agent of injuries, since the E-code of ICD (9th revision) was not designed for describing home and leisure injuries of children.

Severity Scoring

In the Yvelines study, the AIS and ISS were used, but these scales had poor discriminatory power and low predictive value for long-term functional prognoses in cases of domestic, school and sports injuries.

Current Sources of Information and Methodological Issues

Current knowledge of injury morbidity in France comes from four main sources of information: 1) routine statistics (hospital discharge diagnoses, road traffic accident statistics, anti-poison center data); 2) surveillance systems: the French survey of EHLASS (European Home and Leisure Accident Surveillance System, hospital based and product oriented) and the national household survey run by the French national public health insurance system, the CNAMTS("Caisse Nationale d'Assurance Maladie des Travailleurs Salariés"); 3) alert systems; 4) research (mainly epidemiological).

Routine Statistics

Hospital statistics cover only hospitalizations in public facilities and in-patients. The three principal problems encountered in the utilization of morbidity statistics compiled from discharge diagnoses are: not taking into account out-patients, especially in emergency services; not using the E-code from the ICD manual; and counting hospitalizations and not subjects, which over-represents serious injuries which have resulted in several hospitalizations.

As concerns traffic accidents, data furnished by SETRA (Service d'Etudes Techniques des Routes et Autoroutes [10]) include, besides the number of deaths, the number of seriously injured persons, mildly injured and uninjured persons, by age, sex, urban/rural milieu, time of day, user category (driver or passenger of a four-wheeled vehicle, pedestrian, driver or passenger of a two–wheeled vehicle, other), type of vehicle, type of road, weather conditions. The main problem posed by these statistical data is that of under–reporting of cases, inversely proportional to the seriousness of the injuries. This is especially a problem in the case of mildly injured and uninjured persons.

Surveillance Systems

EHLASS (European Home and Leisure Accident Surveillance System)

The decision to finance a European system for recording accidents of daily living was made in 1985 by the Council of European Ministers. In France, the system is run by the ministers of health and of consumer affairs. It depends on participation by hospitals which record emergency room consultations and who send these data on a monthly basis to a national Center. It is managed by the Ministry of Health (Direction Générale de la Santé).

This system was put in place gradually starting in the Summer of 1986, with three hospitals starting in 1987 and eight hospitals beginning in 1988. In 1993, seven hospitals furnished 28,597 accident cases, of which 46 percent concerned children under the age of 15 years [11].

Monographs are regularly produced on a particular age group (children), a type of accident (burns, poisonings . . .), a particular causative agent (for example, slides, toys, baby and child equipment), a specific place (playground, farm . . .), an activity (sports . . .), or a type of lesion (hand, eye . . .).

The principal methodological problems are linked to the choice of public hospitals only, to the exclusion of any private facilities, leading to numerous missed cases, and the sampling method. Hospitals are recruited on a voluntary basis and the sample is not representative at a national level; the catchment area of each hospital is not well defined nor is the size of the background population. It is therefore not possible to calculate frequencies or to publish national estimates.

Results are presented in the form of tables showing distribution in percentages, not rates. The coding of causative agents allows exchange of information between European countries. Unfortunately, as is also the case in the other European countries, data concerning products involved in accidents are generally presented in the form of a simple listing, without the possibility of relating the frequency of accidents linked to a particular product to the actual risk exposure (number of users of a product and length of time of utilization, in particular at a national level).

Recently, a synthetic score of gravity was developed, describing the dangerousness of a product and combining the following variables: number of cases involving the product, rate of hospitalization, length of stay, number of deaths.

The quality of data, especially those related to accident circumstances, has improved considerably since the implementation of the system. In 1993 the percentage of information not supplied on the reporting forms was 3.9 percent for the location of accident, 4.6 percent for the activity of the victim, and 4.7 percent for the causative agent (Table VII). In 1987 these percentages were respectively 11.3, 16.0 and 26.7. Furthermore, present percentages are lower than those of the Dutch and British systems [12, 13] and comparable to those of EHLASS in Denmark which has the best quality data [14].

CNAMTS Survey of Home and Leisure Accidents ("Les accidents de la vie courante")

This is a retrospective postal survey of beneficiaries insured by departmental offices of the national public health insurance system, which has been carried out every year since 1987. The studies are done by the local offices recruited on a voluntary basis. Each office agrees to participate during several consecutive years in the study (3 to 4 years normally). Thus the data base of offices participating in the national study varies over time, in number and in geographic distribution. The rate of response to the questionnaires of around 75 to 80 percent also varies according to the offices and over time. Starting with the participation of 6 departmental offices, the system included 21 in 1991. But in 1994, only 3 offices are participating and the study will doubtless be suspended, but should be restarted in 5 years in order to evaluate changes in accident frequencies.

The representativeness at a national level was doubtless better than for EHLASS during maximum operation of the system, but nevertheless questionable because: 1) the recruitment of the offices is done on a voluntary basis; 2) the agricultural sector is not included because it has its own health insurance system (therefore farm accidents to children, for example, are not recorded, though known as a major problem); 3)though rather high, the response rate is 75 percent to 80 percent (probably inducing selection bias).

The questionnaire sent to families deals with all types of injuries, including those which were not medically treated. The recall period is one year, probably inducing recall bias, especially for the most benign injuries. The information on accident circumstances is of better quality than in EHLASS, but the reliability of medical information is questionable.

Rates are calculated and national estimates are given. Within the period 1987–1992, 148,000 persons were investigated and 42,000 accidents recorded, 14,000 concerning children and adolescents under the age of 17 years. The annual incidence rate for this age group was estimated to be 12 percent and it was estimated that, at a national level, 1,157,000 home and leisure accidents to children occur every year in France, leading to 144,000 hospital admissions [12].

Specific studies are published (children's accidents between 1987 and 1991; accidents in the elderly, 1987–1990; sequelae of accidents, 1989; accidents in immigrant children, 1987–1990; animal related injuries, 1987–1988; sports injuries, 1987–1988; injuries in the kitchen, 1987–1988).

Comparability of the Two Systems

EHLASS and the CNAMTS survey have the same scope (home and leisure injuries), and record the same information (age and sex of the victim, location of the accident, activity of the victim, mechanism of injury, type and site of lesions, outcome and treatment, causative agents). In both systems, circumstances and causative agents are described in a free text.

In spite of very different methodologies and levels of representativeness, there is an obvious consistency in the findings regarding the problem of childhood injuries. Both surveys show higher male morbidity (around 65 percent of the cases), the predominance of home injuries in young children, of sports injuries in adolescents after the age of twelve, a fracture rate around 25 percent, a hospitalization rate between 12 and 15 percent.

Alert Systems

Most of these systems are primarily designed to detect and notify the proper authorities of hazards and dangerous products, but may occasionally describe related accidents and their associated injuries as well. These systems are regional, national or access information at the level of Europe.

– Local alert systems are managed by Departmental Directorates for Consumer Products, Competition and the Repression of Fraud (DDCCRF). They facilitate the diffusion of bulletins on hazards.

– the system "3614–Sécuritam" uses the Minitel service (telephone/home computer combination and data base). It registers complaints on hazardous products and reports of injuries, and gives out information to any consumer on injuries and products, including morbidity data, using for this purpose EHLASS data and data from ad hoc studies. This system is run by the Consumer Safety Commission and the CNAMTS.

– The "European system of rapid exchange of information" is set in motion in the presence of serious and immediate danger. It may request that studies be done among manufacturers and potential victims, the results being transmitted to the appropriate authorities in Brussels.

Research

Epidemiological research on injury morbidity has been and is still being conducted by hospital departments, schools of medicine, "Regional Health Observatories", departmental committees for health education, and INSERM.

Recently, studies have been designed to identify long term consequences of accidental injury [16, 17, 18], with special emphasis on sports related injuries in children and adolescents which appear to have possible consequences in terms of functional prognosis [17, 18, 19].

It should be noted that all studies on children of migrants, a high risk group, are rendered difficult by strict laws on confidentiality.

Psychological and sociological research on risk factors and consequences of accidents is poorly developed, as are studies on economic aspects, although there is a recent interest in the cost of injuries, not only financial cost, but also social cost, including "invisible" components of this cost (changes in professional activities of parents, moving, schooling . . .).

Examples of the analysis of financial costs, as well as of certain social costs, may be found by studying reimbursement schemes used by insurance companies. Indeed, in addition to costs directly related to medical care involved in an accident, insurance companies, in their reimbursement process, take into account aspects of social costs such as those caused by suffering, inconvenience, anguish (*pretium doloris*, aesthetic damages, damages caused by inconvenience).

In France, a study was done using a reference population of 1411 subjects under 19 years of age injured in traffic accidents and reimbursed in 1986. It was estimated that traffic injuries to children in the sample cost insurance companies 152 million Francs ($28,700,000), or a cost of 107,526 Francs ($20,290) per child [20]. It was noted in the study that reimbursement varied by sex and that, for equivalent disability, it was always higher for boys. This phenomenon is very probably related to estimating techniques based on an evaluation of the probable future level of income of the accident victim.

Recommendations and Conclusions

Better epidemiological knowledge of accidents in France may be gained by improving routine statistics and by developing new studies and tools.

Improvement of Routine Statistics Through

- Better certification of the causes of death through physician training. These health professionals usually consider certifying and coding the cause of death as a boring administrative task and probably do not realize its importance, nor the use made of their work. Medical students should receive education on the importance of mortality statistics as a public health tool.

- Better identification of death from domestic and leisure injuries. In France, it is very difficult to introduce changes in the death certificate form, which is a legal document, and to add items for determining the place of occurrence of fatal accidents in cases other than traffic accidents. It would therefore be advisable to develop complementary documents allowing the description of deaths due to domestic accidents, as is the case in England with HAAD (Home Accident Deaths Database) [13].

- Systematic use of E-codes for hospital discharge diagnoses.

Use or Development of New Tools

–   Use of the tenth revision of the ICD which includes optional codes for the place of accident and the activity of the victim.

–   Development of severity scales adapted to sports, leisure and home injuries and of scoring systems for accident–related disabilities and handicap.

Development of Research

–   In the field of long term consequences of all types;

–   In economic aspects;

–   Aimed at identifying the best preventive strategies targeted to specific groups, which presupposes studies of social, cultural and psychological risk factors.

In conclusion, before the 1980's, there was nearly complete ignorance of the problem of home injuries in France and much effort has been made to increase knowledge and improve prevention. Though the present level of the epidemiological research and the quality of morbidity statistics are not yet satisfactory, the evolution of mortality shows very positive trends.

In children aged 1–4 years, age group with the highest rate of home injuries, the non–traffic related accident mortality rate has been reduced by half between 1980 and 1990 (Table VIII). This has been accomplished without preventive measures or laws as numerous and visible as those enacted in the field of traffic safety in the 1970's. Obviously an awareness has been created among both communities and professionals. Of course, these figures raise the question of the linkage between epidemiological data and preventive efforts when the action has been broad, not targeted, and when no evaluation indicators more refined than mortality data have been developed.

Finally, we should note that, as is the case with all the European countries, France should now adapt its statistical information gathering systems to a European scale.

References

1.   Tursz A, Crost M, Guyot MM, Pivault M. Childhood accidents: a registration in public and private medical facilities of a French health care area. *Public Health 1985*; *99*: 154–164.

2.   Davidson F, Maguin P. Les accidents chez les enfants. Etude épidémiologique d'une zone rurale et d'une zone urbaine. *Arch. Fr. Pédiatr. (English abstract). 1984*; *41*: 67–72.

3.   Spyckerelle Y, Des Fontaines–Merckx VH, Gervaise F, Royerp, Legras G, Deschamps JP. Etude de l'incidence et des caractéristiques des accidents de l'enfant dans une ville de 20,000 habitants. *Rev. de Péd. (English abstract). 1984*; *20*: 159–166.

4.   Tursz A, Crost M, Pivault M, Guyot MM, Rumeau–Rouquettec. Enregistrement des accidents de l'enfant dans les structures de soins et de prévention d'un secteur sanitaire. *Rev. Epidém. et Santé Publ (English abstract). 1984*; *32*: 286–294.

5.   Tursz A. Epidemiological studies of accident morbidity in children and young people: problems of method. *World Health Statistics Quarterly. 1986*; *39*: 257–267.

6.   INSERM. Statistiques des causes médicales de décès. Paris: INSERM. Publication annuelle.

7. World Health Organization. World Health statistics annual. Geneva : WHO. Yearly publication.

8. Tursz A, Souteyrand Y, Salmi R. Adolescence et risque. Paris: Syros, 1993; 266 p.

9. Carre JR, Zucker E. Mortalité et morbidité violentes dans la population des jeunes de 15 à 24 ans. Paris, Haut conseil de la population et de la famille. Paris : La documentation française, 1989.

10. Observatoire National Interministeriel de Securite Routiere. Accidents corporels de la circulation routière. Bagneux: Service d'Etudes Techniques des Routes et Autoroutes (SETRA). Publication annuelle.

11. Duval C, Nectoux M, Darlot JP EHLASS. Rapport France 1993. Direction Générale de la Santé. Paris, 1994.

12. Stichting Consument en Veiligheid. PORS 1988–89 Review. Home and Leisure Accident Surveillance System. Amsterdam. 1990; 79 p.

13. HASS. Home Accident Surveillance System. Home and Leisure Accident Research. 16th Annual Report. 1992 data. London : Department of Trade and Industry. Consumer Safety Unit. 1993; 75 p.

14. EHLASS. European Home and Leisure Accident Surveillance System. Annual Report. Denmark: National Consumer Agency, National Board of Health, 1993.

15. Caisse Nationale d'Assurance Maladie des Travailleurs Salaries. Les accidents de la vie courante des enfants de 0 à 16 ans. Résultats 1987 à 1991. Dossier "Etudes et Statistiques" n°24. Paris: CNAMTS. 1994; 71 p.

16. Tiret L, Garros B, Maurette P, Nicaud V, Thicoipe M, Hattonf, Erny P. Incidence, causes and severity of injuries in Aquitaine, France: a community based study of hospital admissions and deaths. Am J Publ Health. 1989; 79: 316–321.

17. Tursz A, Crost M. Séquelles des accidents d'enfants. In: Tursz A. Epidémiologie et prévention des accidents dans l'enfance et l'adolescence. Symposium franco–israëlien (English abstract). Paris. INSERM. 1989; pp 55–71.

18. Yacoubovitch J, Lelong N, Cosquer M, Tursz A. Etude épidémiologique des séquelles d'accidents à l'adolescence. Arch Péd (English abstract). In press.

19. Tursz A, Crost M. Sports related injuries in children. A study of their characteristics, frequency and severity with comparison to other types of accidental injuries. Am J Sports Med 1986;14 : 294–299.

20. Lamy H. Les conséquences financières des accidents de la voie publique chez les enfants: la prise en charge par les compagnies d'assurance. Mémoire de DESS "Economie et gestion du système de santé". 1988; 99 p.

Table I: Accident Mortality Rate per 100,000 Children and Young People Aged 0-24 Years, According to Sex and Age, in France, in 1990

	Age (Years)					
	< 1	1-4	5-9	10-14	15-19	20-24
Male	45.3	14.6	7.8	8.7	46.6	86.2
Female	30.3	9.1	4.7	4.9	15.2	16.3
Total	38.0	11.9	6.3	6.9	31.3	51.6

Source: INSERM

Table II: Accident Mortality Rate per 100,000 Children and Young People Aged 0-24 Years, According to Age and Sex, in the 12 Countries of the European Union in 1990

	Age (Years)							
	< 1		1-4		5-14		15-24	
	M	F	M	F	M	F	M	F
Belgium*	26.5	26.3	14.7	9.3	11.5	6.3	63.8	17.5
Denmark	9.2	0	9.4	6.3	11.4	7.0	34.4	11.1
France	45.3	30.3	14.6	9.1	8.3	4.8	66.5	15.7
Germany	24.5	18.2	17.7	9.6	9.2	5.6	51.2	13.8
Greece	42.0	40.2	12.5	6.2	12.5	6.2	70.3	17.3
Ireland	10.9	3.9	13.8	8.1	9.5	5.4	44.0	15.4
Italy**	20.6	9.4	7.9	5.2	8.0	3.1	52.6	10.6
Luxembourg	77.5	42.5	21.3	11.0	9.1	9.5	73.3	20.2
Netherlands	15.8	9.3	11.8	8.8	8.5	5.5	26.0	8.1
Portugal	70.1	47.8	19.7	14.0	16.5	9.6	84.8	12.9
Spain**	35.5	22.3	14.7	10.5	11.4	5.6	73.0	18.5
United Kingdom	12.5	7.4	9.7	6.1	8.0	4.4	39.7	8.8

Source: WHO
*Belgium: 1987
**Italy, Spain: 1989

Table III: Cause of Accidental Death According to Age in Children and Young People Aged 0-24 Years in France, in 1990

Causes	< 1		1-4		5-9		10-14		15-19		20-24	
	N	%	N	%	N	%	N	%	N	%	N	%
Traffic	36	13	127	35	134	61	177	68	1,029	78	1,759	80
Poisonings	1	0	8	2	2	1	4	1	12	1	19	0.5
Falls	2	1	29	8	13	6	10	4	15	1	66	3
Fire and Flames	5	2	36	10	11	5	12	5	14	1	13	0.5
Drowning	7	2	63	18	17	8	19	7	46	3	43	2
Suffocations and Foreign Bodies	223	78	46	13	11	5	6	2	11	1	20	1
Other Including Late Effects	1	0	26	7	11	5	12	5	62	5	83	4
Undetermined	10	4	26	7	20	9	20	8	129	10	206	9
Total	285	100	361	100	219	100	260	100	1,318	100	2,209	100

Source: INSERM

Table IV: Evolution of the Number and Rate (per 100,000 Live Births) of Suffocations and Sudden Infant Death in Children under 1 Year of Age in France Between 1970 and 1990

	Total Number Of Deaths	Suffocations		Sudden Infant Death	
		N	Rate per 100,000	N	Rate per 100,000
1970	15,437	521	61.3	217	25.5
1975	10,277	632	84.8	211	28.3
1980	8,010	596	74.5	823	102.8
1985	6,389	237	31.9	1,231	165.8
1990	5,599	223	29.7	1,369	182.4

Source: INSERM

Table V: Annual Incidence Rate of Injuries in Children According to Sex and Age in France

Incidence Rate (%)

Survey	Males			Females		
	0-4	5-9	10-14	0-4	5-9	10-14
Yvelines, France 1981-1982	11.7	9.4	10.1	8.0	5.3	6.0
Lens, Montmédy, France. 1981	12.6*	8.9	11.0	9.1*	6.6	7.0
Bar-le-duc, France.	16.2	14.1	21.7**	12.9	8.8	17.7**

*Children Aged 1-4 Years
**Children Aged 10-15 Years

Table VI: Yvelines Survey (1981-1982):
Number of Cases Registered According to the Source of Information and the Survey Length

Sources of Information	Number of Cases	Survey Length
Public Hospitals and SMUR* of the Survey Area	5,483	1 Year
Private Hospitals of the Survey Area**	2,550	1 Year
Dispensaries	15	1 Year
Private Practitioners	32	7 or 14 Days
Public Hospitals of Areas next to the Survey Area	197	1 Year (Retrospective Study)
Anti-poison Center	323	1 Year (Retrospective Study)
Death Certificates***	5	1 Year (Retrospective Study)

*SMUR: Service Mobile d'Urgence et de Réanimation (Mobile Emergency and Resuscitation Unit)
**Excluding Cases Also Registered in Public Hospitals (N = 29)
***Excluding Fatal Cases Registered in the Medical Facilities of the Survey (N = 8)

Table VII: Percentage of Information Not Supplied on the Reporting Forms Filled Out in the French "EHLASS" and in the Accident Surveillance Systems of Other European Countries

	EHLASS France 1993 (28,597) %	PORS Netherlands 1988-1989 (146 363) %	HASS United-Kingdom 1992 (115 257) %	EHLASS Denmark 1993 (67 531) %
Sex of the Victim	0	0.1	0.1	0
Age of the Victim	1.2	0	0.2	0
Location of the Accident	3.9	13.5	47.6	5.9
Type of Accident	0.7	0.8	9.3	1.9
Activity of the Victim	4.6	32.5	45.2	3.2
Causative Agent	4.7	--	19.0*	1.4
Type of Lesion	1.5	0.1	1.6	0
Outcome and Treatment	0.3	0.1	0.6	0

*1991

Table VIII: Evolution of the Rates of Overall and Accidental Mortality per 100,000 Children Aged 1-4 Years In France Between 1960 and 1990

	Overall Mortality	Accidental Mortality	Traffic Accident Mortality	Non-traffic Related Accident Mortality
1960	119.2	25.6	---	---
1965	91.8	25.7	8.0	17.7
1970	79.6	27.2	7.7	19.5
1975	67.4	24.7	6.5	18.2
1980	58.3	21.2	5.8	15.4
1985	45.4	13.0	4.2	8.8
1990	38.2	11.9	4.2	7.7

Source: INSERM

Annex
Catégories from Who's International Classification
of Diseases (ICD) Included in Analysis of Accident Data

E 810-819 +	E 820-829	=	Transport Accidents
E 830-832 +	E 910	=	Water Transport Accidents + Accidental Drowning and Submersion
E 850-858 + (Including E 868)	E 860-869	= =	Accidental Poisoning (Carbon Monoxide-accidental Poisoning)
E 880-888		=	Accidental Falls
E 890-899		=	Accidents Caused by Fire or Flames
E 911-915		=	Accidents Caused by Suffocation and Foreign Bodies
E 916-929 + E 800-807 + E 830-838 (minus 830-832) + E 840-848 + E 900-909		=	All Other Accidents and Late Accidental Injury

Excluded are:

E 870-879	=	Misadventures to Patients During Surgical and Medical Care
E 930-949	=	Drugs, Medicaments and Biological Substances Causing Adverse Effects in Therapeutic Use

Comparability of Injury Related Questions From National Population–Based Surveys

by Jacqueline P. Davis

Introduction

In 1983, the Office of International Statistics, National Center for Health Statistics developed and published the first International Health Data Reference Guide which, on a biennial basis, has been updated six times. This guide provides information from 40 nations on the availability of selected national vital, hospital, health personnel resources and population–based survey statistics. The information is obtained from the government and the official agencies of the represented countries.

The latest edition of the Guide was published in March of this year, and expanded upon the information previously provided on national population–based health surveys. From a profile of each survey, information was obtained on the objective, scope, collection method, data content, frequency of the survey, and availability of the data. Copies of the questionnaires were also obtained from which we were able to extract the data variables from the surveys and present them in matrix format. For the countries that did not have questionnaires to provide to us, we asked that they complete the matrix indicating the data variables in their surveys.

Of the 40 nations that provided information about their population–based surveys, 23 indicated that they collected some injury related data on one or more surveys of their country.

It is from these 23 countries that some comparability issues will be described in this paper..

Objectives of the Surveys

Most of the surveys that contain injury related data have similar objectives. Basically they provide national baseline and trend data on:

- the population's status of health,
- the prevalence of acute illnesses and chronic diseases, and;
- the use and need of health services and facilities.

These data are used to:

- provide measures of the prevalence and incidences of illness,
- measure level of activity restriction due to short–term illness or injury (missed work or school days, days of reduced activity),
- measure consequences of injuries, and;
- develop health and use indicators.

Methodology

Typically, the implementing agency for the surveys is a national statistics office or a government ministry. The surveys are national in scope, mostly probability samples, with the sampling activities carried out by highly experienced and trained staff.

The target population is usually the civilian noninstitutionalized population residing in the country, although the countries of Italy and Switzerland sample the total resident population. All of the surveys are administered face–to–face by a well trained personal interviewer in the home with the exception of the Czech Republic. The Czech survey is of treated morbidity and therefore, the data are gathered by the general practitioner who has treated the patient. In most cases, all family members of the household 15 years of age, or in some countries 16, 17 or 18 years of age and older are interviewed. A few countries have upper age limits such as Iceland, age 75, Sweden, age

16–1

84, and the National Nutrition and Health Examination Survey of the United States, age 74. An adult family member usually provides data for persons not at home and for children. A few countries such as Canada, the Netherlands and New Zealand interview only one member of the household who is randomly selected.

Frequency of Data Collection

Surveys differ in timing and frequency. There are two distinct patterns: those surveys that are continuous or annual, and those surveys carried out at 4 to 5 yearly or longer intervals. Overall, about 1/4 of the surveys are conducted on an annual or continuous basis. These are from the countries of Korea, the Netherlands, Sweden, Ukraine, United Kingdom, and the United States.

The countries of Australia, Canada, Czech Republic, Denmark, Germany, Israel, Japan, and Switzerland collect injury related data on surveys conducted every 2 to 5 years; and Hungary collects injury related data on a survey conducted every 7 years. France and Norway collect injury related data on a survey conducted every 10 years, while Austria conducts a special accident survey every 10 years. The countries of Iceland, New Zealand, Poland, Spain and Switzerland have conducted only one survey each that contains injury related data.

Lack of Standardized Terms and Definitions of Terms

A review of the questionnaires clearly showed that there is no consensus on the wording and phrasing of questions about injuries and accidents. The term "illness and injury" is used interchangeably on many surveys while "injury and accident" is used interchangeably on others.

In the National Health Interview Survey of the U.S., an _injury_ is defined as a condition as classified in the International Classification of Diseases (ICD) code numbers (800–999). In addition to fractures, lacerations, contusions, burns, and so forth, which are commonly thought of as injuries, this group of codes includes effects of exposure, such as sunburn, adverse reactions to immunization and other medical procedures; and poisonings. Unless otherwise specified, the term "injury" is used to cover all of these. Statistics of acute injury conditions include only those injuries that involved at least one–half day restricted activity or medical attendance.

In the U.S., accidents show up as injuries, injured persons, and resulting days of disability which are grouped according to the class of accident. Most of these events are accidents in the usual sense of the word, but some are other kinds of mishaps, such as overexposure to the sun or adverse reactions to medical procedures, and others are nonaccidental violence, such as attempted suicide. The classes of accident are:

1. moving motor–vehicle accidents;
2. accidents occurring while at work;
3. accidents occurring at home; and,
4. other accidents.

In the Australian surveys, data are collected using an "actions" based approach. Respondents are asked: During the two weeks prior to the interview, did they take certain actions in relation to their health?
These actions include consultations with doctors and other health professionals, use of medications, days away from work or school, and hospital episodes terminating in that two week period. For each action taken, additional questions are asked to determine the medical condition termed as an illness/injury.

In one Canadian Survey, injury data is captured when it has been caused by an accident during the year prior to the interview. In the Czech Republic survey, injury data is only captured when medical care is required.

Reference Period

In the majority of surveys, the reference period for an injury condition is the two weeks prior to the interview, whereas, the accident reference period is usually within the past year of the interview. However there are a few countries that use different time references or do not specify any timeframe for when the injury or accident occurred.

Injury Related Questions from Different Surveys

There is a great variation in the number of questions and the wording of the questions that are asked about injuries and related topics in the surveys. Some countries (U.S.,Australia, Canada, Denmark, Japan, New Zealand, and Norway) asks a battery of questions regarding injuries:

1. During the past two weeks, did the respondent miss any time from work or school due to any illness or injury?

2. During the past two weeks, how many days did the respondent miss more than half of the day from his job or school because of illness or injury?

3. During the past two weeks, did the respondent stay in bed more than half of the day because of illness or injury?

4. During the past two weeks, how many days did the respondent stay in bed more than half of the day because of illness or injury?

5. What was the illness or injury?

6. What caused the illness or injury?

7. Was medical treatment sought due to the illness or injury?

Other countries, Israel, the Netherlands, and the United Kingdom ask a minimum set of questions

1. Did respondent have any restricted activities due to injury/illness?

2. What was the injury/illness?

3. Were there any bed days due to the injury?

Canada's newest health survey which is being conducted this year, prefaces the injury questions with this statement: The following questions refer to injuries, such as a broken bone, bad cut or burn, sore back or a sprained ankle, which occurred in the past 3 months and were serious enough to limit normal activities ... The questions that follow ask what type of injury, part of the body injured, how it happened, etc.

Accidents

Some countries (Australia, Austria, Canada, Hungary, Spain, U.S.) asks a battery of questions regarding accidents.

1. Did the respondent incur an injury from an accident in the past year?

2. What type of accident?

3. Where did the accident occur?

4. When did the accident occur?

5. How did it happened?

6.   What part of body was injured?

7.   Was medical care required including hospitalization?

Other countries such as Denmark only ask

1.   If any accidents occurred in the past year?

2.   What type of accident?

Violence

Sweden was the only country that asked a battery of questions specifically geared towards violence.

1.   During the past 12 months was the respondent subjected to any violence that lead to some type of injury that required medical attention?

2.   Did the respondent receive any visible scars or marks or bodily injury due to the violence that did not require medical attention?

3.   Did the respondent receive any threat of violence that caused concern?

4.   What type of threat e.g., knife, firearm, etc.?

5.   Did this threat affect the daily living of the respondent?

6   Where did the violence occur?

7.   Were the police notified?

8.   Was the assailant know to the respondent?

Summary

In conclusion, it can be said that while there are injury related data being collected in many countries, there are sufficient differences in the national systems that may somewhat hamper international comparisons. These differences are the age old ones and are not unique to injury–related data.

Therefore, before comparability is considered, there are several methodological differences that must be addressed. Namely,

•   there are base population differences, the non–institutionalized population versus the total resident population.

•   there is a need for more standardization of questions and definition of terms.

•   there is a need for a minimum core set of injury–related questions worded similarly.

•   and there is a need for comparable periodicity of the surveys.

Levels and Trends in Infant and Child Injury Mortality in Selected Countries

by Bob Hartford, Ph.D.

The purpose of this presentation is to describe levels of child injury mortality in selected countries, and changes in those levels between 1980 and 1990, or the latest available year.

We will be looking at not only overall mortality but five major causes, paying particular attention to possible problems of compatibility of the data.

These data are derived from vital statistics and census data. The World Health Statistics Annual is the source of the international data. Because conditions are so different between blacks and whites in the United States, I have used NCHS data, in order to present the United States data by race.

Because of the small numbers involved in these cause categories in most countries, data have been aggregated in three year periods around the target years. As you see, the latest data available at best were 1988 to 1990 (See Table 1). Ideally, we should separate the presentation or the examination by age and by sex; by age because of the relative importance of various causes is so different in the infant year—that is, under one year of age—and in the one to four year period.

Analysis by sex, even at these young ages, is important. A substantial male excess is already noticeable, even in the infant period. This was also noted by Anne Tursz.

Unfortunately, the small numbers preclude this level of detail. In future analyses, however, we should aggregate data for longer periods, such as 10 years, and look more closely at age and sex differentiation.

Mortality rates presented are deaths per 100,000 population. The ICD–9 version was used in all instances to code cause of death, except for Sweden in the 1979 to 1981 period, at which time, ICD–8 was still in effect.

Child mortality as it is used in this presentation, refers to the population under five years of age.

As seen in Table 2, there are wide differences among countries in the levels, and as well in the rates of change in those levels. For example, the overall mortality among blacks in the United States is about three times the rate in Sweden for 1990. The differences are even greater—more than six fold—for injury mortality.

Mortality due to injury has declined. It is about 4 to 5 percent annually in most countries, except among blacks in the United States, where the decline was only about two–and–a–half percent, and in Israel, where the rate rose slightly.

Injury mortality constitutes five to ten percent of mortality under five, although the relative importance in the one to four year period is much greater, on the order of 25 to 35 percent, showing the importance of differentiating these two age groups in future analyses.

Figure 1 shows the major causes of child mortality in 1990. Motor vehicle traffic accident, falls, fires, drownings, homicide, and the "other," or residual category. (Rates of less than 1 per 100,000 are not shown.) Of particular note is the high homicide rate in the two U.S. populations. Also notable are the high rates due to drownings in Canada, among U.S. whites, and in New Zealand. Also of particular note is the extremely high rate of the other category, the category of a problematic nature mentioned by Gordon Smith, particularly in Israel.

Pnina Zadka, one of our colleagues here from Israel, tells me that this is probably the result of a change in coding practices.

Figure 2 presents the same data, but on a percentage basis, to illustrate the relative importance of the various causes.

As seen, the "other" category comprises one fourth to two fifths of injury mortality in the other countries.

It is my impression that the various causes comprising the "other" category vary substantially from one country to another, as well as within a single country over time.

The next series of graphs focus on levels and changes in the various major cause categories. Figure 3 shows that motor vehicle traffic accidents are very high, among blacks in the United States and in New Zealand. The range in mortality levels is approximately three–fold between lowest and highest. As seen, the declines achieved by Canada, England and Israel are substantial. The rates in New Zealand and among blacks in the United States are quite high and showed much less of a decline than in the other countries. In fact, motor vehicle accident traffic mortality in these two populations are more than all accident and injury mortality rate of 7.2 in Sweden in the 1990s.

While mortality due to falls (See Figure 4.) is generally the least important contributor to overall injury mortality, the declines reported are rather impressive.

We wonder what led to the declines. Are they are real? Are there any lessons to be learned from these experiences.

Figure 5, showing mortality due to fires and flames, shows substantial reductions. However, the extremely high rate among blacks in the United States is disturbing—it is more than three–and–a–half times the rate of whites in the United States, and 13 times the rate in Sweden. It would be interesting to learn how Sweden has achieved such a low rate.

While the rates have declined for drownings in four countries to under one per 100,000, the situation in New Zealand, while improving, is puzzling. (See Figure 6.) Why is it so much higher there? Is the difference real, or are there problems of comparability of the data?

Figure 7 illustrates an ongoing tragedy in the United States, the homicide mortality of blacks, even to children under five. The rate in 1990 was 10.6, slightly higher than in 1980. There are also increases reported in Israel, and Scotland, and among whites in the United States. The rest of the countries registered some sort of decline, but generally not as strong a decline as in other injury categories. One never likes to see an increase in any kind of mortality, but an increase in homicide mortality is particularly disturbing.

Figure 8 summarizes the changes in injury mortality. Except for Israel, all the countries reported substantial declines in the overall injury mortality. While declines were reported in most of the cause categories, there were, as previously mentioned, increases in the homicide rates in Israel and Scotland and the United States.

Canada reported an increase in the "other" category. As similar increase reported in Israel, is thought to be a data coding artifact.

Hopefully, the answer to these questions, and others that are being raised will come to light in the evolution of the ICE project. Thank you.

Table 1. Data years

Country	Data years around 1980	Data years around 1990
Canada	1979–81	1988–90
England and Wales	1979–81	1989–91
Israel	1979–81	1987–89
New Zealand	1979–81	1987–89
Scotland	1970–81	1989–91
Sweden	1979–81	1989–91
United States—blacks	1980	1990

Note: Deaths are classified according to ICD–9 except for Sweden, which classified deaths according to ICD–8 in 1979–81.

Table 2
Child and child injury mortality in selected countries: 1980–90
deaths per 100,000 population

	1980		1990	
	All causes	Injury	All causes	Injury
Sweden	167.4	11.7	152.1	7.2
United States—whites	283.4	27.7	198.9	19.2
England and Wales	298.9	16.1	193.3	10.2
Scotland	302.8	23.8	190.2	14.0
New Zealand	309.8	36.0	260.0	26.6
Canada	346.8	27.5	180.1	15.9
Israel	432.5	20.6	250.9	20.9
United States—blacks	590.7	53.7	478.3	42.0

Source: WHSA and NCHS

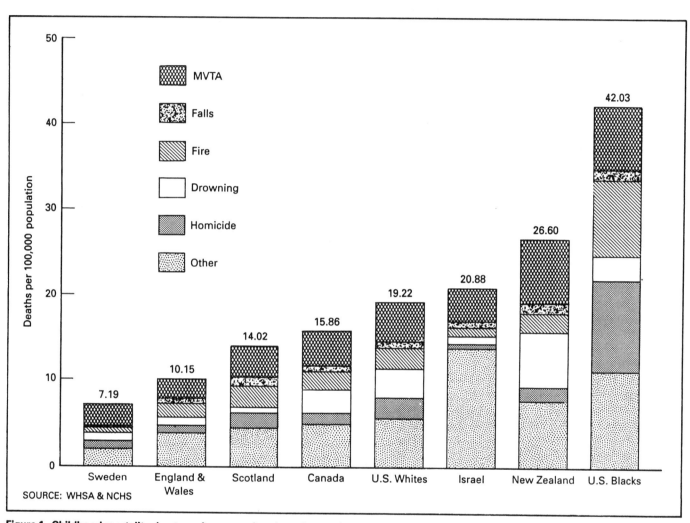

Figure 1. Childhood mortality due to major causes in selected countries: 1990

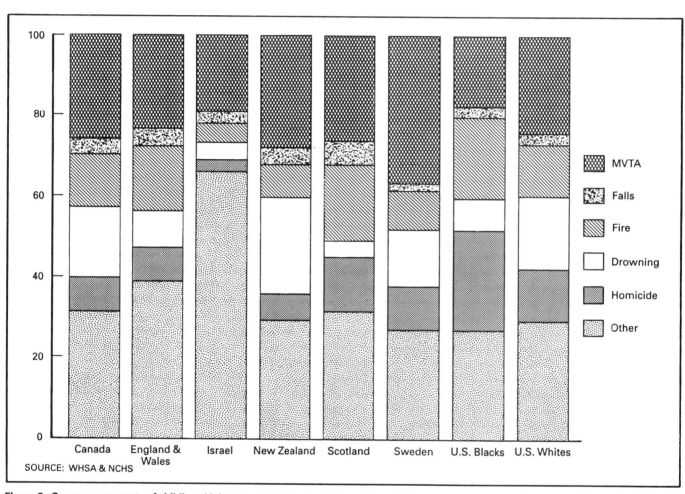

Figure 2. Cause components of childhood injury mortality in selected countries: 1990

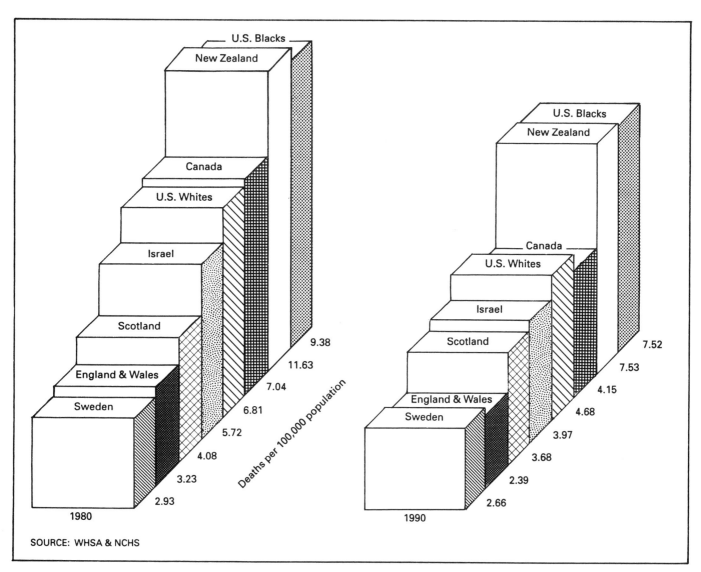

Figure 3. Child mortality due to motor vehicle traffic accidents in selected countries: 1980 and 1990

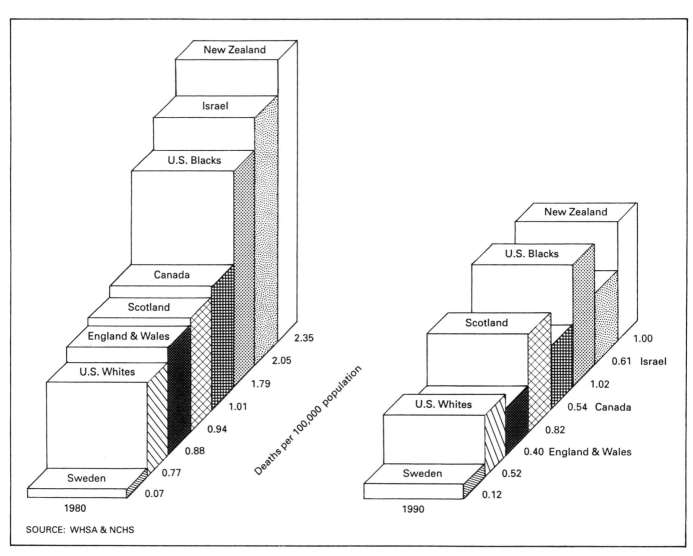

Figure 4. Childhood mortality due to falls in selected countries: 1980 and 1990

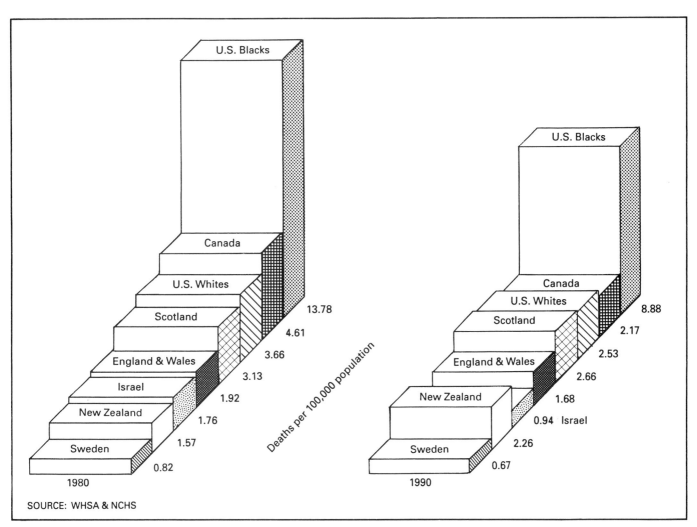

Figure 5. Child mortality due to fire and flames in selected countries: 1980 and 1990

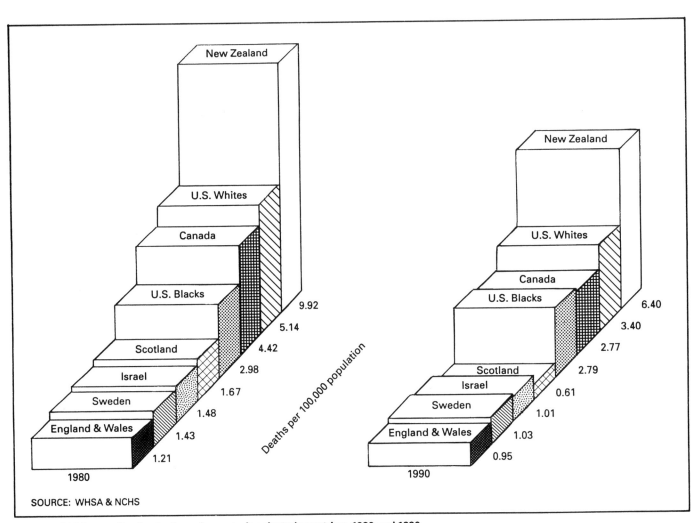

Figure 6. Child mortality due to drownings, etc. in selected countries: 1980 and 1990

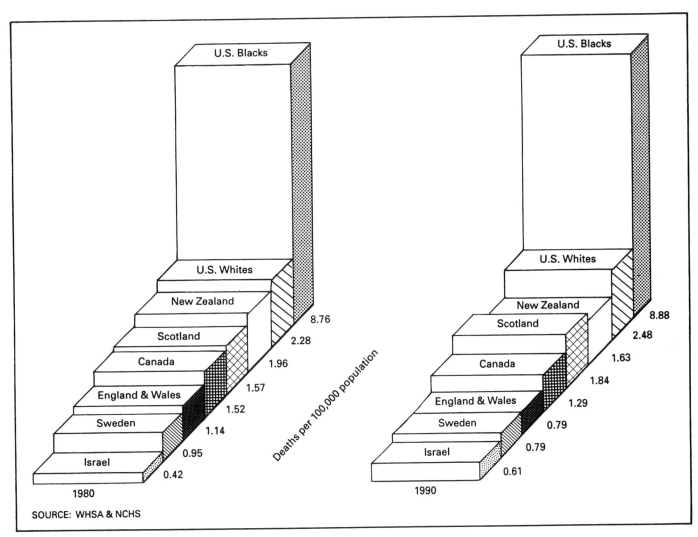

Figure 7. Child mortality due to homicide in selected countries: 1980 and 1990

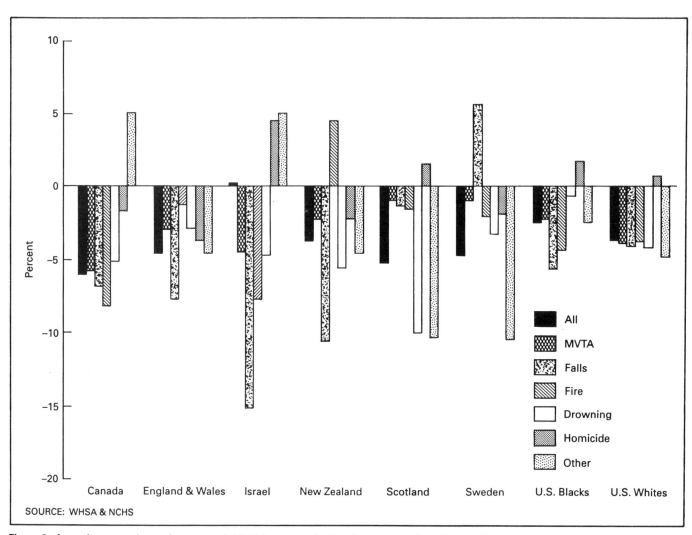

Figure 8. Annual percent change in causes of child injury mortality in selected countries: 1980–1990

Data Needs and
Linkage Issues

Data Needs for Injury Prevention and Control Programmes

by Wim Rogmans, Ph.D.

Introduction

In most Industrialized economies, the fundamental rights of citizens with respect to safety are well recognized. These include:

1.   The rights of workers to being protected from injury and health risks at the workplace and to continuous improvement of working conditions;

2.   The constant improvement of road and traffic infrastructure, of the basic safety features of vehicles and of road users' behavior;

3.   Consumers' rights to expect that consumer goods and home environment are safe under conditions of normal use and of foreseeable misuse.

In particular the latter aspect of consumers' rights has gained substantial interest in past decade and has led to new initiatives in accident prevention policy and related research efforts, which will be briefly described in this paper.

Consumer Safety Policy

Consumer safety policy covers the entire body of statutory and voluntary measures aimed at protecting the consumers' health and safety in physical contact with consumer products or built environment. These measures include:

–   preparatory actions by surveying consumer products on the market, monitoring incidents that lead to injuries and/or damages;

–   regulatory actions such as the development of safety regulations and safety standards;

–   corrective actions by intervening in case of detection of significant hazard;

–   education and information strengthening consumer awareness of risks at home and in leisure–time and encouraging adaptive behavior.

Consumer safety is not absolute but relative: the degree of safety that can be reached in a given society depends on a number of varying social, economic and cultural factors. This leads to the conclusion that with ever changing life–patterns and socio–economic development, the levels to be set for consumer safety will never be fixed and set forever. Reliable data on the risks involved will certainly facilitate the process of decision making regarding which hazards to address and the priorities to be allocated for further enhancement of current standards.

However safety policies and priorities are only to a limited extent influenced by statistical data. In most countries the influence of mass media, interest groups and incidental events frequently take precedence over rational statistics. Nevertheless, on the long run these statistics prove to be indispensable for adequately defining key areas of interest and strategies to be followed. These statistics can be obtained from specialized data collection systems or from broader surveillance programmes.

Current Information Needs

It is evident that information management should be geared by the basic information needs expressed by those in charge of prevention policy. In practice this has been addressed from two different angles of perspective:

- One inspired by a systematic approach towards accident research and in particular the Haddon– approach in accident analysis;

- another inspired by day to day practice, taking into account the availability of data and data utilization.

In the first approach it is found useful to think of a 'causal chain of events' leading to injuries. Each link in the chain is a potential starting point for injury prevention and control. By studying the circumstances in which injuries occur, the dynamics and causes of accidents can be understood. The well–known model developed by Haddon analyses injuries according to three factors (host/agent/environment)and three phases (pre–event/ event/ post–event). From this perspective one can conclude that information systems for injury control should cover all these relevant factors and phases of the process. The WHO 'basic data set' (WHO.1988) is based on such an approach. A brief look at the available sources and systems, taking into consideration the Haddon–framework, reveals that they all lack details on the early phases of the process, which limits severely prevention potentially (Lund, 1990) [Figure 1]. Fortunately, new initiatives have been guided by this approach, as for instance in the development of the nordic classification (NOMESCO, 1990).

The second approach is followed by a number of operation researchers while in process of developing practical systems for consumer policy implementation. Most of their designs are based on an inventory of existing information needs among those in charge of consumer safety policy and its implementation and on their data utilization (Bourgolgnie e.a., 1992; Irving, 1994). It is evident that judgments on the availability and informative value of existing data are implicitly in these evaluations. In general one can conclude from these studies that most policy makers have limited demands as regards the availability of continuous data and are satisfied with basic information. However the utilization of information increases significantly as the availability improves and the facilities for in–depth studies growths. This has been for instance the case in the European countries that participated in the European Home and Leisure Accident Surveillance System (Rogmans & Mulder, 1990): a majority of Member States reported an increased and more efficient policy programming and implementation owing to their participation in the system.

Sources of Information

Information on injuries and injury–related events can be obtained from various sources, for example [Figure 2]:

- mortality statistics which are readily available in most countries;

- hospital discharge statistics, which are in only a few countries nationwide available;

- statistics collected in the course of medical examinations among a great part of the population (for instance in entering the military service);

- national and regional epidemiological research programmes (for instance cohort studies);

- sentinel systems in primary health care;

- records of absenteeism and sick leave, usually collected by insurance bodies;

- general surveys and inquiries based on retrospective questionnaires.

There is a strong interdependence between the sources where the information is tapped from and the nature of injury (in particular with respect to its severity) reported [Figure 3]. The method of ascertainment of cases is intimately associated with the severity of the injury and to a certain extent to the nature of the injury. The minor ones being reported in the office of general practitioners and the most severe injuries being reported in trauma centers for instance.

Assessment of Available Information

In a number of countries mortality statistics have proved to be an invaluable source of information, in spite of its shortcomings in depth of information collected and timeliness of reporting. It should also be noticed that countries differ in their methods of recording which complicates comparative studies. In only a few countries data on hospital admittance, including a consistent coding of diagnosis) are being aggregated at national level. In many countries, however, the technology of patient administration is advancing and as information technology is rapidly expanding its impact also in hospital administration, one may expect improved availability of injury data, provided by the health care sector, in the near future. However, for the time being, one has to rely on information provided by specially designed surveillance systems, among which those collecting injury data in accident and emergency units at hospitals. So far, data collecting in these emergency rooms have proved to be the most cost–effective means of fulfilling the information needs of policy makers. The very high number cases that can be recorded at hospitals provide the volume of data needed for accurate assessment of specific areas of interest and of trends. Part of the data is already being collected through the regular administrative procedures within hospitals, without placing an extra burden upon hospital staff. The information can be provided timely and with reasonably precision. Such systems also provide for follow–up studies at a later stage, targeting at selected populations of cases.

References

1.   Bourgolgnie PT, e.a. Utilization of accident data, as summary report on the application of information collected on accidents in view of product safety policy, Consumer Safety Institute, Amsterdam, 1992.

2.   Irving LM. Injury Surveillance in public hospital emergency departments, Injury Prevention Research Centre, Auckland, 1993.

3.   Lund J. Integrated data collection systems at hospitals, In: W. Rogmans & M. Schuurman, Proceedings International Seminar on Accident Data, Universitätsverlag, Wien, 1990.

4.   Rogmans W and Mulder S. Evaluation of activities undertaken in the framework of the EC–demonstrations project EHLASS, Consumer Safety Institute, Amsterdam, 1990.

5.   World Health Organization, Prevention of accidents – a basic data set and guidelines for its use, Geneva, 1988.

Figure 1. Data sources and the amount of information provided
with respect to the accident scenario
Accident/injury Process

	Pre-Injury Phase	Injury Phase	Outcome Phase
Health surveys	-	+	+
Medical exam	-	+	+
G.P.	-	+	-
Absenteeism Rec.	+	-	+
			-
Hospital Rec.	-	+	+
			-
Death certificate	+	+	+
	-		
Surveillance systems	+	+	-

+	RATHER RICH INFORMATION
+,-	THIN
-	POOR INFORMATION

Figure 2. Sources of Information

* Mortality Statistics
* Hospital discharge Statistics
* General medical examinations
* Screening programmes
* Sentinel systems (G.P.)
* Absenteeism/sickleave records
* General health surveys

Figure 3. Data sources and their interdependence with severity of injury and representativeness of information provided

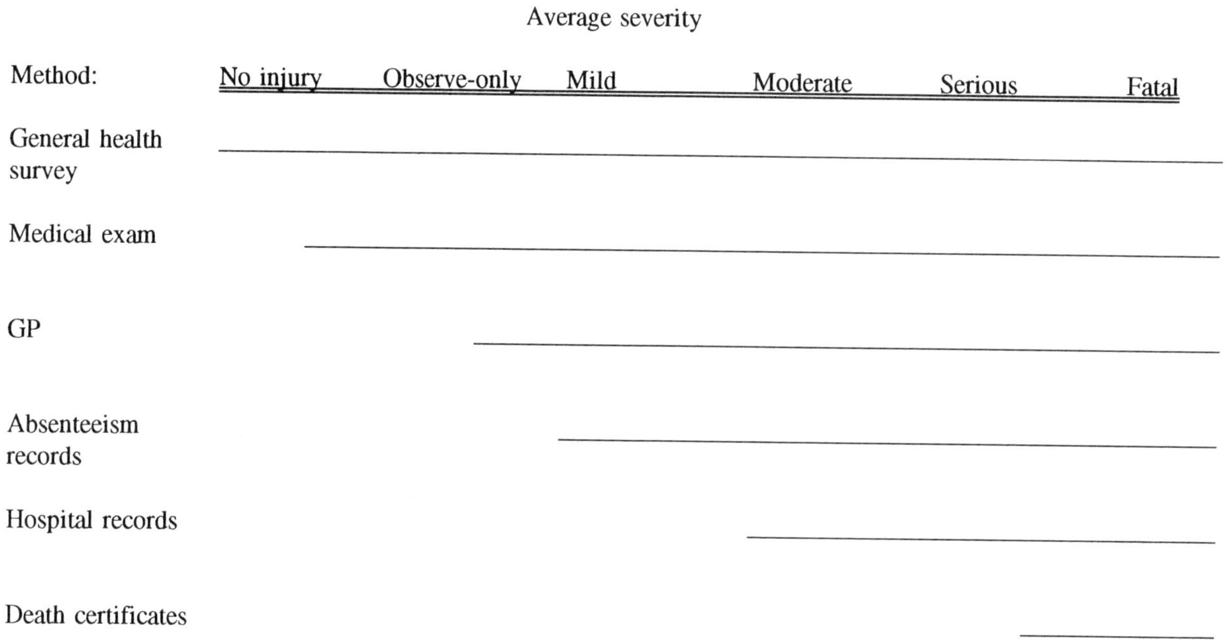

Average severity

Method:	No injury	Observe-only	Mild	Moderate	Serious	Fatal

General health
survey

Medical exam

GP

Absenteeism
records

Hospital records

Death certificates

Data Needs for Evaluation of Injury Prevention Programs – Experiences From Sweden

by Lars Berg, M.D., Anders Åberg, Lothar Schelp, Leif Svanström, Ph.D.

Abstract

Evaluation of injury prevention programs demands data from different sources. This includes data about input and exposure of preventive activities, and the influence on knowledge, attitudes and behavior of the population and to injuries as such. In this paper we will emphasize the measurement methods and validity problems of injury surveillance.

Sweden by tradition has good access to register data with good quality. Since 1951, Swedish cause–of–death statistics have been collected and classified according to ICD with few coding errors and missing data. A national hospital discharge register was established in 1964, including injury data with a low drop–out rate.

The National Injury Prevention Program starting 1986 promotes local injury out–patient registration activities. Almost every county council has been monitoring injuries, but mostly for parts of the counties covering one or more hospital areas. There is a great variation in the level of missing data and a lack of studies on reliability and validity.

Surveys including a few injury–related questions are performed both at local, regional and national level.

Information about injuries is collected at different levels in the health care systems. By tradition and technical reasons these different data are stored and analyzed apart from each other. By linking the injury cases of the causes of death, the hospital discharge and the local out–patient registers more comprehensive injury patterns can be described. The surveys cannot be linked to the registers due to lack of a civil registration number.

The about 5,000 fatal and 160,000 hospital–treated in–patients with injuries are coded according to the external causes of morbidity and mortality (E–number) of the ICD classification.

The current challenge is the possibility of getting national representative information of the about 800,000 injuries treated in out–patient care by physicians. The NOMESCO classification of injuries is used in almost all local out–patient registrations, and has shown to be the most applicable data collection instrument.

Data Needs for Evaluation of Injury Prevention Programs – Experiences from Sweden

The strategy of the Swedish Injury Prevention Program stress the responsibility for injury prevention in different sectors in the community and at the national level [1]. Prevention may focus on the individuals in order to change behavior and attitudes, but also on the environment by supervision and legislation.

Preventive activities are performed at different levels and with different messages aimed to influence the individual behavior or the environment. Models can be used to show the relationship between these structures.

Preventive work is mainly based on two dimensions – the primary target levels, and the nature of the message (Figure 1). At one extreme the message can be of the single–factor type and aimed at the individual, e.g., "use bicycle helmet". At the other extreme, the National Institute of Public Health may work on prevention on the national level. Such an intervention may consist of a lot of varying things – legislation, guidelines for advertising, information, etc. Between these extremes you may find a multi–factor accident and injury prevention program on the local community level—a "community intervention"—or perhaps accident prevention work within a business firm—an organizational intervention. The general nature of the message will differ substantially for each of these examples because of different focus.

The model in Figure 1 is used as a base for another model (Figure 2) [2, 3]. This second model is developed in connection with an evaluation of a cancer prevention project in Stockholm County. A third dimension is now added—individual/environmental conditions. The individuals risk are affected by knowledge, attitudes and practice/behavior (KAP), and related to norms in the society or in the groups/organizations to which the individual belongs. The environmental condition consists of the physical local environment, safety equipments, but also the laws, policies, supervision, etc. and the sociopolitical structure.

When influence of preventive activities is discussed a fourth dimension has to be considered—intervention components/links. The input of intervention creates or modifies activities that determine the level of exposure. This affects the individuals knowledge, attitudes and behavior, and hopefully decrease the risk for injury, and in turn reduce injury morbidity/mortality. This logical chain of events serves as a
point of departure for a discussion of problems with evaluating injury preventive work.

In Figure 3, the different components in this chain of events have all been assigned their own box—all with their specific, and in certain respects, general measurement problems to discuss [3].

In this paper we will emphasize the injury surveillance and the validity problems (the box to the right). A more complete discussion of all these boxes and the evaluation problems are presented in the proceedings from a conference about Child Safety in Sweden 1987 [4].

The presentation will be divided in three parts—the demographic data (as a denominator and for linkage), survey data on injury and mortality/morbidity data. Available data sources are described with comments on validity problems.

Demographic Data

Demographic data can be used as a denominator, for linkage to injury registers to add valuable information.

Population Statistics in Sweden

Population statistics for the counties and municipalities of Sweden are published in an annual report—Population Statistics [5]. The population reports are based on the Register of the Total Population (RTB) kept by the National Central Bureau of Statistics (SCB or Statistics Sweden). Every person living in Sweden has a unique civil registration number, which is used as an identifier. The vital statistics are based on the notifications of births, deaths, migrations etc., which the RTB obtains each week from the Tax Authorities. Between 1686 and July 1, 1991, the local work was a task for the Church of Sweden and was carried out by the parish offices.

The County Councils update their own population registers every second week. These registers are used for linkage to health care data registers to add information about address and check for correct civil registration numbers. The local registers for use in the health care systems are updated about every month with data from the County Councils.

The quality of the population register is considered to be good. Births and deaths cause very small under- and over-coverage problems. Undercounting is less than 0.1 percent for newborns and children under one year of age. Immigration causes some under-coverage because the time-lag between entry in Sweden and population registration is generally about four months. Emigration causes over-coverage because the population register is not always informed about departures. At the time of the 1985 Census the over-coverage was 0.1 percent of the population.

Population and Housing Census

Sweden has a long-standing tradition of population censuses, the first being performed as early as 1749. The importance of the censuses as population counts has now decreased, and the principal significance is instead as the only national source about household, occupation and housing conditions. Since 1960 the Swedish population and housing censuses (FoB) have been combined in one census carried out every fifth year [6].

The value of the census was questioned before the latest performance 1990. The census was strongly supported by the Swedish epidemiologists and new censuses are supposed to be performed in the future. The information was at the latest census collected to November 1, 1990 by using questionnaires and by adding information by linkage to administrative records (SCB RTB, Register of Employment, Central register of Enterprises and Establishments, register on income–tax).

The census 1990 has been validated by a random sample of 17,000 persons, included in a special working craft investigation where different variables have been checked against the census. The classification quality is good, e.g., the marriage/consensual union groups with 1.3 percent is not correctly classified in the census 1990.

Survey Data on Injury

National Survey of Living Conditions

The National Surveys of Living Conditions (ULF) studies started 1974 with a sample of 11 – 14,000 persons from the whole of Sweden in the ages 16–74 year [7]. The data are collected by interviews. From 1980 the sample also includes persons 75–84 and reduced to a sample of 7–9,000 each year. In the analysis two years is used as a basis. From 1988 also people above 85 are included.

ULF contains questions about health and social data especially from 1981–82 and 1988–89 and every year from 1975 a question about long term disease or a consequence of an injury within the latest 12 months. A follow–up question about type of problem and if an injury coding by ICD9 is done. According to this definition of an injury about 4 percent of the population had such injury in the ULF studies from 1988/89.

The drop–out rate is between 14 to 20 percent. The influence of the interviewer has to be considered.

Community (Regional/Local) Surveys

Regional or local population surveys have been conducted in many Counties during the last decade. Some of these surveys include questions about injuries.

In Stockholm County population surveys are performed every third year as a basis for a public health report and for preventive purposes. The latest surveys are conducted 1993, one survey for the adults and one performed in school classes in the ages 11,13 and 15 year.

Injury Mortality and Morbidity Data

Cause of Death Register

Swedish data on causes of death have been collected on a national basis since 1749. For the period 1831–1910, however, the collected data are incomplete and include only selected causes of death.

Since 1951, Swedish cause–of–death statistics have been collected, classified, and edited according to the International Classification of Diseases (ICD). The ninth revision of the ICD was implemented in 1987 [8].

Before July 1, 1991 a death certificate including information about the cause of death, had to be issued by a qualified physician within a week. The certificate was sent to the local parish offices and forwarded to the Statistics Sweden (SCB). From July 1, 1991 the death certificate is divided in two parts: a certificate and a cause–of–death statement. The death certificate must be issued and sent to the local Tax Authorities within a week. Within three weeks a cause–of–death statement has to be sent to SCB. At SCB, the cause–of–death statements are recorded in an annual cause–of–death register, which also includes demographic variables copied from the Register of the

Total Population (RTB). The register is used to produce the official statistical tabulations, but is also available for medical research. The register now contains information on individual deaths from 1952 to 1991.

The County Administrations register of reported death (which do not include the cause of death) is used to check the cause–of–death register for comprehensiveness. For the data of year 1991, SCB was unable to obtain death certificates in 356 cases.

The death certificates are coded at SCB. The underlying cause of death is selected manually and validated by the ACME program (supplied by the National Center for Health Statistics, North Carolina). A validity study 1986 of 5300 death certificates by an independent control coding procedure showed a coding error of 3.6 percent on the 3–digit–level and 1.4 percent on the chapter level. In 1990 the underlying cause of death was studied in 2195 certificates by independent coding: on the 4–digit–level 4.4 percent of coding errors occurred, 3.0 percent on 3–digit–level and 0.7 percent on ICD chapter level. The validity is dependent on the age and the cause of death, e.g. injury is among the more valid causes of death.

The fatal injuries are about 5,000 per year in Sweden. About 93 percents of the diagnoses are at present based on autopsy result or diagnostic procedures at hospital.

A limitation according to the injury field is that the place of injury is not registered. There are ongoing discussions within the nordic countries to add the place of occurrence and a free text description of an injury event.

"Cases of Death" Register

The Cases of Death Register is handled by Statistics Sweden and is based on a record linkage of Causes of Death 1961–70 and the Population Census (FoB) 1960. The foremost value is in the more valid occupational information.

A new record linkage has been done with the Causes of Death 1971–80 and FoB 1970. Some data from the register have been analyzed, but no report have been published so far. The general use of the cases of death register have decreased in the latest years, and the check of the civil registration numbers were time consuming. By now ad hoc record linkage is used when special questions arise and someone will pay for the analysis.

The National Hospital Discharge Register

To provide data on in–patient utilization to researchers, planners and decision makers a National Hospital Discharge was established within the National Board of Health and Welfare in 1964, with data from parts of the country. The register is based on the local County Council registers. From 1978 to 1983 data are available from 18 out of 26 County Councils (about 85 percent of the population), 1984 is lacking, but from 1985 all public hospitals in Sweden are participating.

The variables included are diagnoses, surgical procedures, external causes to injury or poisoning, date for admission and discharge. For the period 1964–83 also civil registration number. From November 1, 1993 the County Councils, according to a new legislation, are obliged to deliver data with a civil registration number. Registration numbers from the period 1985–93 may be added.

The number of discharges per year is about 1.7 million, of which 160,000 are due injuries. Missing data on discharges were estimated to 2 percent in a study 1989. A study of the 1986 year register has shown that the medical information on the detailed 5–digit–level has major classification errors, about 17 percent, but with moderate problems (7 percent) when data are grouped in DRG or when using the Nordic 99–diagnosis list [9]. The injury data, however, have less errors, about 7 percent on 5–digit–level.

The E–code on 4–digit–level show totally 22 percent errors, of which 14 percent were due to a use of a wrong E–code.

Local Trauma Registers

A few hospitals in Sweden have started trauma register, e.g., Lund University Hospital in 1993 [10]. The information is used for quality assurance and evaluation of the trauma care. The data are compiled from the ambulance and the emergency records and in–patient care.

Out–Patient Register

The Centre of Epidemiology at the National Board of Health and Welfare has initiated a National Out–patient Register with a content corresponding to the Hospital Discharge Register. The register, based on data from the local level, has gradually been established for the out–patient hospital care, with about half of the County Councils participating at present. Information from the primary health care is limited to a few County Councils. The medical information—consisting of diagnosis and external causes of injury or poisoning (E–code)—is increasing, but still insufficient. Personal identification is lacking in the central register. A complete register from the whole of Sweden would provide information of an estimated total amount of about 800,000 annual injuries in Sweden, treated by physicians and not admitted to hospitals or being lethal.

Local Surveillance Systems

Almost every County Council has registered injuries during the last decade. According to a survey in April 1993 about 50 percent had an ongoing injury surveillance system. But, these registration activities are limited in some respects. In most of the Counties not all hospitals are involved in the registration. Some registrations focus on special groups and areas, e.g. child injuries, school injuries and traffic injuries. Considering these limitations about 25 percent of the Swedish population is covered by an injury surveillance system.

The data collecting is based on the Swedish version of the NOMESCO Classification [11, 12]. This classification is multi–axial, each axis describing the site of occurrence, the mechanism of injury and the activity of the victim. There is also a possibility for a detailed free–text description of the injury event.

Besides the information about the patient (civil registration number, age, sex, place of residence, etc.) the main axes of the NOMESCO classification above are mainly on the 1–digit–level, the supplementary situation code, the date of injury and the diagnosis are to be considered as a minimum data set.

Registration of more detailed or extended variables mirrors local interests in special preventive areas. Examples of these are sport and traffic injuries, injuries among children or the elderly, at institutions etc.

The amount of missing data shows a great variation from 5 percent to 50 percent, but the most frequent amount is about 5–10 percent. No studies have been performed on the quality of the coding procedure.

Traffic Injuries

Police is required to complete a report on all road traffic accidents with personal injury. These reports are compiled and analyzed by Statistics Sweden. Police reports include comprehensive information about the conditions relevant for the cause of the accident as well as personal identification.

Different studies have shown a significant under–reporting of these data [13, 14].

Occupational Injuries

Swedish legislation requires employers to report all occupational injuries causing sick leave to the local Social Insurance Office. Copies of these reports are sent to the labor inspectorate and Swedish Occupational Injury Information System (ISA), administered by the National Board of Occupational Safety and Health. The purpose of the register is prevention of accidents. The register includes information about the injured person, the employer, the work situation, extent of the injuries, and a description of the injury event.

There is a significant under–reporting of the occupational injury data, shown in different studies [15, 16].

<u>The Insurance Companies Injury Registers</u>

The insurance companies collect different kinds of data about different types of injuries. Among others there are information related to occupational, traffic, sport and leisure–time injuries. However, the information is not stored as databases with possibility to make tabulations.

Community and National Injury Information Systems

The different sources for describing the injury problem and for evaluating the outcome of preventive activities have been presented above. The data generated by the public health care system provides the most comprehensive information on injuries because no injury type is excluded.

The focus at the national level has up to now been on fatal or in–patient hospital discharge injuries, which are the most severe. However, this gives a limited picture of the problem. Most of the injuries are treated in out–patient care with different types of injuries sustained in different sectors of the society. For example about 75 percent of the injuries occur in homes or during leisure time.

The National Injury Prevention Program in Sweden [17] starting 1986 have promoted local injury out–patient registration activities, now covering about 1/4 of the Swedish population, which could be used on the national level, compiled to a national out–patient register.

The local surveillance systems cover patients treated in emergency departments and in many cases within primary health care. This includes patients treated only in out–patient care, as well as those admitted to hospital in–patient care and those with fatal outcome. By tradition and technical reasons this information is stored and analyzed apart from the other sources of information on injuries. By linking the injury cases of the causes of death, the discharge and the local out–patient registers more comprehensive injury pattern can be described. The purpose is to validate and to add useful data. The NOMESCO classification of accident monitoring is, with almost no exception, used in the local surveillance systems—including when a registration of intentional injuries are performed—and has shown to be the most applicable data collection instrument. The classification gives possibilities to collect the information on different levels of details. For the performance and evaluation of preventive efforts on the local level the data have to be more detailed.

The first step in the process to establish a national surveillance system is to link information from the Cause of Death Register to the Hospital Discharge Register. This is possible by the civic registration numbers which are now also available in the Hospital Discharge Register. Such a performance has been initiated by the Centre for Epidemiology at the National Board of Health and Welfare.

The next step—to include data information from the local surveillance systems—needs a permission to collect personal identification data, which according to an ongoing legislative process might be possible from 1996.

This comprehensive model with general information on injuries—within the framework of a minimum data set—including data from all sectors and all types of injuries provides a useful foundation to define national policies and to measure if targets have been achieved.

The data needs of the national agencies responsible for injury prevention in different sectors (e.g., consumer, traffic, occupational, child or elderly safety) are to some extent fulfilled by the minimum data set. Detailed information have to be provided (at cost) in cooperation with a few County Councils. A possible linkage may be performed to other data sources, such as the police reported traffic injuries and the occupational injuries.

The present trends concerning the local surveillance systems are towards a continuous registration by a minimum data set. Time limited projects that focus on special areas of interest can be made by expanding to a higher level of detail or by using the supplementary parts in the NOMESCO classification, e.g., the traffic module or the external injury factor/product module. Further supplements are in progress.

The most urgent problem is to improve the validity of the local systems, with less under-coverage and misclassifications and to improve the geographical representation. The role of the Centre for Epidemiology is to facilitate that work, to collect and analyze representative national data, and to coordinate the work with the national agencies and the County Councils.

References

1. National Board of Health and Welfare. Strategies for a Safe Sweden (In Swedish. Separate summary in English). Stockholm: National Board of Health and Welfare, 1991. (Report 1991:18).

2. Callmer E, Eriksson CG, Sanderson C, Svanström L. SCPP – Evaluation group. Final report. Stockholm: Karolinska Institute, Department of Social Medicine., 1986. (Grey report 128).

3. Sanderson C, Svanström L. Contributions of Social Medicine and Systems Analysis to Formulating Objectives for Community–based Cancer Prevention Programme. Scand J Soc Med 1988;16:35–40.

4. Svanström L. Methods of evaluation of child accident prevention programmes. In: The Healthy Community. Child Safety as a part of Health Promotion Activities. Stockholm: Folksam, 1987:111–130.

5. Statistics Sweden. S:Official Statistics of Sweden Population Statistics 1992 (In Swedish Summary in English) 1993.

6. Statistics Sweden. Official Statistics of Sweden. Census statistics 1990 (In Swedish. Summary in English). Stockholm: Statistics Sweden, 1993.

7. Statistics Sweden. Official Statistics of Sweden. Living Conditions. Health and Medical care 1980–89 (In Swedish. Summary in English). Stockholm: Statistics Sweden, 1992. (Report no 76).

8. Statistics Sweden. Official Statistics of Sweden. Causes of Death 1991. Stockholm: Statistics Sweden, 1993.

9. Nilsson AC, Spetz CL, Carsjö K, Nightingale R, Smedby B. The validity of the Hospital Discharge register (In Swedish). Läkartidningen, 1994;91:598–605.

10. Lenninger K. The Trauma Registry at Lund University Hospital (In Swedish). Lund: Lund University Hospital, 1994.

11. Nordic Medico–Statistical Committee (NOMESCO). Classification for Accident Monitoring. 2nd revised edition. No 35. Copenhagen: NOMESCO, 1990.

12. Swedish National Board of Health and Welfare. Classifications of unintentional injuries 1989. Stockholm: Allmänna Förlaget, Customers Services, 1989.

13. Traffic injuries 1985 (In Swedish). Stockholm: Official Statistics of Sweden. Statistics Sweden., 1985.

14. Schelp L, Ekman R. Road Traffic Accidents in a Swedish Municipality. Public Health 1990;104:55–64.

15. Jacobsson B, Schelp L. One–year incidence of occupational injuries among teenagers in a Swedish rural municipality. Scand J Soc Med 1988;16:21–25.

16. National Board of Occupational Safety and Health. Occupational diseases and occupational accidents 1990 (In Swedish). Stockholm: Official Statistics of Sweden. Statistics Sweden, 1992.

17.   Svanström L, Schelp L, Skjönberg G. The Establishment of a National Safety Promotion Programme for Prevention of Accidents and Injuries—The first Swedish "Health for all"—programme Implemented in Practice. Health Promotion 1988;4:343–347.

Figure 1. Preventive work - level/message

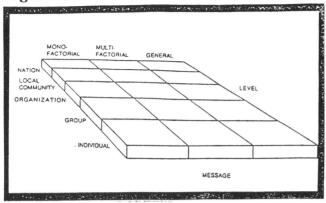

Figure 2. Intervention/level/risk/injury

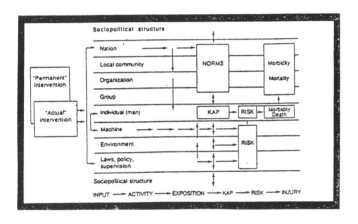

Figure 3. Possible study designs at evaluation of intervention programs.

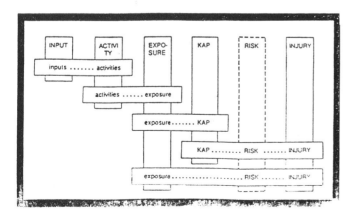

Injury Surveillance: The Role of Data Linkage

by Patricia C. Dischinger, Ph.D.

Introduction

Injury surveillance efforts have frequently been hampered by the lack of readily available information on injury cause/mechanism. Unfortunately, those sources of information with the most injury detail are usually lacking with regard to data about the mechanism of injury. Hospital discharge records, for example, frequently do not have complete E–code data. Conversely, sources of information with detail about the cause of the injury, such as police crash reports, frequently do not include much detail concerning the injuries themselves. In recent years detailed injury information has become increasingly available with the widespread use of trauma registries (1). While trauma registries are biased in that they include only those patients with the most serious injuries, (2) they do provide a comprehensive source of surveillance data, with detailed information concerning the nature and severity of the injuries (3,4). Thus, linkage of data from several sources provides information not otherwise available, allowing valuable insights into injury causation.

Injury surveillance is important in order to identify patterns and types of injuries in the population (5–7). Based on such surveillance, more in–depth epidemiologic studies of risk can be conducted. Since risk factors and patterns for fatal and non–fatal injuries frequently differ (8), both mortality and morbidity data should be included in any injury surveillance effort. By combining data from multiple sources, it is possible to examine various degrees of injury severity, and to optimize the utility of the available information. As pointed out in Injury in America, "the U.S. requires effective injury surveillance systems for gathering and integrating information from a variety of sources on which to base the planning and evaluation of control efforts. This would include...the collection of more refined data on specific types and causes of injuries and exposures to injurious environments" (9).

Maryland provides an interesting "laboratory" for injury surveillance, as there is a wealth of data systems already in place which can be used to address questions related to injury. It is one of the few states with a centralized EMS system (10) consisting of a network of trauma hospitals, with coordinated transportation and communication services (11). There is a centralized repository for ambulance/helicopter reports, a statewide trauma registry, state hospital discharge records, and a coordinated system of medical examiners, with a central location for autopsy records.

Despite the availability of these various data sources, however, there is no uniform identifier which can serve to link all the records. Each of the data sources addresses different aspects of the injury–related incident. Traffic records, for example, are routinely utilized by law enforcement agencies, highway planners, managers in departments of transportation, and researchers. They are also used by emergency medical services agencies (EMS), and injury prevention planners. However, the crash report is usually prepared by the police officer who was at the scene of the crash, from data obtained at the scene. The crash report form does not include descriptions of the injuries, rather only a crude overall injury severity code (no injury, possible injury, non–incapacitating, incapacitating, or fatal injury). Details of the injury must be obtained from hospital records, either outpatient or inpatient.

The police report does not show the history of previous infractions of the drivers involved; thus, the driver record must be obtained separately. The police report also does not give details of damage to the vehicle beyond the damage severity codes of "disabling, functional, other vehicle damage, no damage, unknown." Nor does the form indicate the response times and treatments rendered by the emergency medical system; for this the ambulance runsheet is required. Also, records of rehabilitation services provided after discharge from the hospital are not documented; hospital discharge records do, however, indicate whether the patient was discharged to an inpatient rehabilitation facility or to home.

For victims that die, death certificates are available from the Division of Vital Records of the Department of Health and Mental Hygiene; autopsy records must be obtained from the Chief Medical Examiner of the State of Maryland. Cost information is maintained by hospital billing departments, the Maryland Health Services Cost Review Commission (HSCRC) and individual insurance companies.

Thus, for an individual crash event, relevant information must be obtained from separate data sources and, if necessary, manually linked. Each of the agencies involved may have a computer database of all or parts of their data, but these are typically "sanitized" by removal of identifiers such as names and addresses, before the computer file is made available, even to another state agency. Therefore, in order to understand the pre–crash, crash, and post–crash circumstances and the consequences and costs of injuries incurred, methods to link already available computerized data, and methods of obtaining non–computerized data, must be explored.

Sources of Injury Information

The available sources of data are briefly described below:

– Police crash reports. Police crash reports document details of all injury–causing crashes occurring throughout the state. While the exact nature of the injuries is not documented, each report includes a code (the KABCO code), which is a five–point scale based on whether there was no injury, minor injury, non–incapacitating injury, incapacitating injury, or a fatal injury. There is no indication, however, of whether or not the injured person was admitted to a hospital, or the final disposition of the injury.

– Maryland Ambulance Information System. For each person transported by ground or air ambulance throughout the state, an ambulance runsheet is completed. The runsheet documents the time elapsed between the injury and field response, as well as the mechanism of the injury, and the patient's vital signs. Runsheets are optically scanned and stored centrally at the Maryland Institute for Emergency Medical Services Systems (MIEMSS).

– Trauma Registries. Information on patients treated in trauma centers is entered into the Maryland Trauma Registry. There are currently nine trauma centers located throughout the state. The trauma registry includes basic information about pre–hospital care, status of the patient on admission, diagnoses, treatment and ultimate outcome. The registry is not population–based, and therefore, unto itself does not provide adequate data to quantitate the effectiveness of various preventive measures such as seatbelt and helmet use. However, despite this limitation, in combination with other databases, the registry can provide valuable information on patients with serious injuries. Other, more detailed registries are also frequently maintained by specific trauma specialty groups, such as orthopaedics.

– Hospital Discharge Records (HSCRC). For all patients discharged from acute care hospitals throughout the state, a discharge record is generated. This record includes information on the diagnoses, acute care charges, payor type and outcome dispositions for each patient. E–codes, which document the cause or mechanism of the injury, are currently available only for approximately half of all injury discharge records.

– Medical Examiner's Records. In Maryland there is a statewide medical examiner's system, with centralized records on all deaths throughout the state. Information on the causes of the injuries is kept in a computerized registry; however, data on the injuries themselves are not currently computerized.

– Death Certificates. All death certificates for deaths occurring to Maryland residents are maintained by the State Health Department, Division of Vital Records.

– Driver's Records. Driver histories may be obtained from the Maryland Department of Motor Vehicles.

Data Linkage Methodology

From the point of view of ongoing, electronic linkage of already available data, the ideal would be to have an identified state agency authorized to receive the full confidential files from each data owner, with names and other private information, within approximately three months of the injury–causing event. The data could then be linked and the individual identifier information removed before public release and after analysis by the different agencies for their own system evaluation and/or prevention activities. It may be that state legislation would be necessary in order to require all of the groups involved to augment their present computer information systems to include the necessary additional confidential information and to submit it to the designated central state agency.

Nevertheless, given current concerns about the confidentiality of data included in these various data sources, other means are currently required to accomplish these linkages. The two main strategies for data linkage are summarized below, followed by examples of studies using each method:

(1) A **sequential linkage method** requires identification of cases from a central source, and subsequent linkage of that information with other databases. For example, as discussed below in the Motorcycle Study, all injured motorcyclists were identified using police crash reports. Then, based on information from the crash report, it was possible to obtain enough information to link with ambulance runsheet, hospital discharge, and other databases. If this linkage process were successful, it would be possible to relate every police report to a list of injuries, if any, which resulted from the crash. This level of detail would allow for sensitive, and long–awaited, measures of system effectiveness and provide a basis for the monitoring of injury prevention efforts.

(2) A **probabilistic linkage** is based on collections of various variables, not unique, which in combination provide the best linkage between two different databases. Such a linkage does not require the use of confidential data. The success of such a linkage, however, is highly dependent upon the quality and completeness of this select set of variables.

In many instances, electronic linkage of data from multiple sources can be accomplished using several key indicators. Some key indicators include: date of the injury, date of birth of the injured, gender, and place of injury occurrence. Usually, the name of the victim is not accessible using available data sources. With the increasing availability of geographic information systems, another key variable in the future may be the longitude/latitude of the injury–related incident.

Table 1 shows the key variables of the various databases, with the most useful linkage variables highlighted.

Examples of Surveillance Studies Using Data Linkage

Several examples of injury surveillance studies which have resulted from linkage of two or more already existing databases are described below. The first, the Motorcycle Study (12) is an example of the sequential data linkage type.

The Motorcycle Study

Although there are many opportunities for such data linkages, these efforts are frequently manpower intensive, as there is no single identifier which can be used in an automatic linkage. In a surveillance study of motorcyclists conducted in Maryland, data from the following sources were linked: police crash reports, ambulance runsheets, EDs, trauma registries, hospital discharge records, driving records, and autopsy reports. In order to carry out this study, injured motorcyclists were identified from police crash reports. From the crash report, it was possible to ascertain the hospital, if any, to which the injured cyclist was taken. A data collection form was then sent to each hospital, requesting information on the diagnoses for each individual and whether the cyclist had been treated and released, admitted, or died in the emergency room. For those admitted to hospitals, the hospital record number was used to access the hospital discharge database. From this database, information on discharge diagnoses and hospital costs (charges) was obtained. If the motorcyclist died, autopsy reports were identified and abstracted at the Medical Examiner's Office. Driver histories were also requested for each of the motorcyclists included in the study.

Figure 1 illustrates the final, linked database, with the diagram of the motorcycle representing the police crash report, which was the starting point for case identification. The linkage success rate is illustrated in Table 2. During the one–year study period, there were 1882 police–reported motorcycle crashes, involving 1900 motorcycle drivers, 362 motorcycle passengers, and 40 pedestrians struck by motorcycles. Of the 1900 drivers, 1360 (72 percent) were transported to hospitals. Of this group, outcome data were available for 911 motorcyclists; 39 percent were either admitted or transferred, 54 percent were treated and released, and 5 percent died. The remaining 2 percent left the emergency department against medical advice.

Based on the findings from this study, several recommendations were made regarding data linkage. First, it was recommended that the police crash form be modified so that it would be possible, in the event of multiple persons injured, to determine which person was transported to which hospital.

Secondly, the recommendation was made that the ambulance runsheet have a "tearsheet" at the bottom, stamped with the same number, which would be filled out by the hospital ED staff. The tearsheet would
indicate the disposition of the patient (treated and released, transferred, admitted, or died). It would then be returned to a central data repository where the data would be entered. With these two modifications, then, it would be possible, at least for vehicular injuries, to effect a linkage between police reports, ambulance records, and hospital discharge records. After a one–year trial of the tearsheet, however, it is apparent that compliance is not good, primarily because of the manpower required to complete the paperwork in the ED (13). Meanwhile, the Health Services Cost Review Commission (HSCRC) has agreed to add the ambulance runsheet number to its computerized records. While this assumes that the runsheet is legible, and that it will be put into the medical record, this development means that, at least for hospitalized cases, there can be an ongoing linkage between the crash, ambulance, and hospital records.

The following studies are examples of studies conducted using probabilistic data linkage:

Linkage of Trauma Registry and Hospital Discharge Records

To address the question of what proportion of injured patients admitted to hospitals are treated by trauma teams, a linkage between HSCRC and trauma registry data was attempted for those hospital discharges occurring in calendar year 1988. Using the HSCRC tape, all patients with a discharge diagnosis which included an ICD–9 code between 800.00 and 959.99 were selected (N=38,692). Of this group, 16,368 (42.3 percent) were admitted to trauma hospitals, with the remainder admitted to community hospitals. Included in the registry were 7,534 of these patients. For this subgroup admitted to trauma hospitals, an electronic linkage between trauma registry and HSCRC data was achieved for 74.3 percent. Of those unmatched, a large proportion were found to have been hospitalized for 24 hours or less or to have had an ISS of less than 13. Data from this linkage have been used in a study of the costs of intentional injury in Maryland (14). Using the trauma registry, patients admitted as a result of gunshot wounds, stabbings, or beatings were identified; cost information was then obtained through a linkage with the hospital discharge tapes.

Linkage of Trauma Registry and Police Crash Report Databases

–   Study of the Pattern of Injuries in Lateral vs. Frontal Collisions

In this study, clinical data on the nature and severity of injuries was linked with data from police crash reports for 3675 car/truck drivers admitted to trauma centers (15). From the computerized vehicle diagram on the police crash report, it was possible to distinguish between crashes with primarily frontal vs. left lateral impacts. Different patterns of injuries were noted for drivers in these two types of collisions (see Table 3). Injuries to the face and lower extremities were significantly greater in frontal collisions; thorax, abdominal and pelvic injuries were significantly greater in lateral collisions.

In addition, drivers in lateral collisions were found to have significantly more multiple injuries to the abdomen and thorax. This information has potential use for clinical decision making, since drivers admitted to trauma centers following left lateral collisions have a higher incidence of occult abdominal and thoracic injuries.

Linkage of Trauma Registry, Police Report, and Toxicology Databases

–   Study of Alcohol Use Among Injured Sets of Drivers and Passengers

Crash report and blood alcohol concentration (BAC) data were linked for 109 injured driver/passenger pairs admitted to a Level I trauma center and identified using the trauma registry (16). Among those occupants, 47 drivers (43 percent) (mean BAC, 147 mg/dl) and 45 passengers (41 percent) (mean BAC, 127 mg/dl) were BAC+. No occupant was BAC+ in 57 crashes (52 percent); both were BAC+ in 40 (37 percent); and only one was BAC+ in 12 (11 percent). When both occupants were BAC+, the driver had the higher BAC in 68 percent of cases, and when one was BAC+, it was the driver 58 percent of the time. In six additional alcohol–related crashes with one driver and two passengers, the "wrong" occupant was driving on five occasions. Hence, in the 58 crashes involving BAC+ occupants, the least appropriate occupant was driving 67 percent of the time.

From this data it is not appropriate to conclude that "designated driver" initiatives are ineffective. This study is based on a select group of individuals admitted to a trauma center, i.e., "numerator" data. However, the findings from this study seem to indicate a need for educational efforts that are directed not only toward encouraging drivers not to drink, but also toward discouraging passengers from traveling with drinking drivers. To fully assess the need for such educational endeavors, studies of driver/passenger BAC+ status among the non–injured motoring population are needed.

Summary

Linkage of already available sources of data provides an effective way of conducting injury surveillance. Although most of these injury sources are not population–based, they provide data which allow for generation of hypotheses for further epidemiologic study. Even without unique identifiers, an acceptable data linkage success rate can be attained using probablistic linkage techniques. Meanwhile, new techniques should be explored to find ways to effect an ongoing linkage of injury data sources.

In–depth studies may require even more detail concerning the mechanism of injury. In such instances, already available data may be augmented for the purposes of the study. For example, in an ongoing study of lower extremity injuries to motor vehicle occupants, crash reconstruction data are being obtained for the crashes which resulted in these injuries (17). By correlating the detailed findings about the crash with information about the specific nature and severity of the injury, it is possible to postulate the actual mechanism (e.g., dorsiflexion, inversion, eversion, axial load) which caused the injury. Such information, when combined with observations from the less detailed surveillance data, and with experimental research, can provide specific suggestions for injury mitigation.

References

1.   Report from the 1988 Trauma Registry Workshop, Including Recommendations for Hospital–based Trauma Registries. J Trauma 29(6):827–834, 1989.

2.   Payne SR, Waller JA: Trauma registry and trauma center biases in injury research. J Trauma 29(4):424–429, 1989.

3.   Pollock DA, McClain PW: Trauma registries: current status and future prospects. JAMA 262(16):2280–2283, 1989.

4.   Lloyd LE, Graitcer PL: The potential for using a trauma registry for injury surveillance and prevention. Am J Prev Med 5:34–37, 1989.

Table 2 – Results of Sequential Record Linkage

File	Drivers %	Passengers %	Pedestrians %
Past driving history of motorcycle drivers licensed in Maryland	83	–	–
Pre–hospital care of those transported by Maryland ambulances or helicopters (two counties were not reporting)	71	64	29
Emergency Department reports of treatments of crash victims transported to identified Maryland hospitals (five civilian hospitals plus clinics and federal hospitals did not take part in this study)	79	72	82
Emergency Department reports of treatments of crash victims transported to the 45 cooperating hospitals	92	92	92
Hospital discharge reports of crash victims identified as admitted to the participating Maryland hospitals	91	83	100
Trauma centers trauma registry data of crash victims identified as transported to Maryland trauma centers	77	72	29
Autopsy records of those identified as motorcyclists or struck pedestrians killed in motorcycle crashes in Maryland	98	100	100

Table 3 – Incidence of Specific Organ/Skeletal Injuries by Direction of Impact

Injury	Number (%) in Frontal Crashes (n=2804)	Number (%) in Left Lateral Crashes (n=376)	p Value
Head/neck	1531 (54.6)	187 (49.7)	0.08
Brain	488 (17.4)	68 (18.1)	NS
AIS 4+	149 (5.3)	25 (6.7)	NS
Skull	420 (15.0)	35 (9.3)	<0.003
Face	1268 (45.2)	102 (27.1)	<0.0001
Thorax	680 (24.3)	137 (36.4)	<0.0001
Chest Wall	354 (12.6)	101 (26.9)	<0.0001
Lung	131 (4.7)	27 (7.2)	0.036
Diaphragm	7 (0.3)	10 (2.7)	<0.0001
Abdomen	693 (21.2)	138 (28.7)	<0.001
Liver	77 (2.8)	16 (4.3)	NS
Spleen	72 (2.6)	30 (8.0)	<0.0001
Kidney	50 (1.8)	10 (2.7)	NS
Intestine	44 (1.6)	3 (0.8)	NS
Bladder	5 (0.2)	13 (3.5)	<0.0001
Pelvis	154 (5.5)	75 (20.0)	<0.0001
Lower Ext.	508 (18.1)	26 (6.9)	<0.0001
Femur	208 (7.4)	17 (4.5)	0.04
Patella	84 (3.0)	1 (0.3)	<0.002
Tibia/fib.	127 (4.5)	4 (1.1)	<0.001
Ankle/foot	138 (4.9)	4 (1.1)	<0.001
Tarsal	113 (4.0)	1 (0.3)	<0.0001

Figure 1 - Motorcycle Study Linked Database

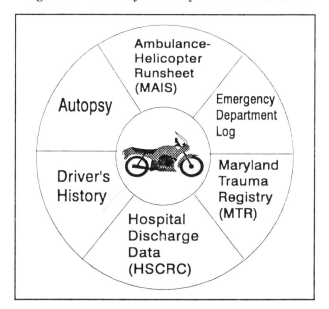

Coding Issues

E–Coding of Morbidity Data

by David H Stone, M.D. and Kevin McGeechan, B.Sc.

Background

The population of Scotland suffers a relatively high risk of injury in comparison with other parts of the United Kingdom for reasons which are unclear. Some claim that the inclement weather is to blame, others that the defiant personality of the Scots leads to risk–taking behaviour. A more plausible explanation is the extremely high level of poverty which casts a long shadow over Scottish society. This manifests itself not only in the economic deprivation of many individuals and families but in poor housing design and other environmental hazards to safety which are especially prevalent in the densely populated urban areas of the central belt.

Injury prevention in Scotland has received a major boost from a governmental policy statement contained in a document entitled "Scotland's Health—A challenge To Us All." This was issued at about the same time as its English counterpart "The Health of the Nation." These may be regarded as ideological descendants of the 1978 Alma Ata Declaration which led to the World Health Organisation's Health for All Strategy and its accompanying targets for health promotion. Both highlighted accidents as one of a handful of key areas requiring urgent attention by government departments.

Probably the most serious obstacle to the development of a comprehensive injury prevention strategy is the lack of appropriate data for injury surveillance—a sine qua non for planning and evaluating interventions. Of those data which do exist, mortality statistics are the most widely quoted, partly because the recording and classification of injury deaths generally adopts the format of the International Classification of Disease and is therefore often accompanied by some basic causal descriptors in the form of so–called E (External Cause) codes. This dependence on mortality data distorts the totality of the injury picture since deaths constitute less than one per cent of all injuries presenting to health services. In particular, there is a worrying deficiency of injury morbidity data which fulfil three important criteria of public health information: their routine availability, their population–based orientation and their inclusion of causal variables. Scotland, however, is almost unique in having an database which meets all three criteria. It is known as the Scottish Morbidity Record (SMR) system.

The SMR system is a routine hospital activity monitoring scheme dating back to 1961. It is operated by the Information and Statistics Division of the Common Services Agency of the Scottish Health Service. A computer–coded form (SMR 1) is completed on the discharge, death or transfer of every non–obstetric and non–psychiatric in–patient or day case from any Scottish hospital. The form records a range of administrative and clinical data, including ICD 9 diagnostic and E–codes, which are abstracted from the case record by trained clerical staff.

Relatively little use has been made of the SMR system for injury research or prevention. We therefore decided, on the gentle prompting of the organisers of this ICE, to explore the possibilities further. We set out to try to answer the following question: what is the potential of E–coded Scottish hospitalisation data for injury surveillance? Specifically, we wanted to know the completeness of E–coding of SMR data, and the epidemiological and preventive potential of the database.

Materials and Methods

All hospitalisation episodes arising from injury or poison diagnoses recorded on the SMR1 database were analysed using a linked file for the period 1984–91 for Scottish residents. The linkage enabled us to generate data on continuous inpatient stays (i.e., excluding transfers or re–admissions within 24 hours of the initial discharge) rather than episodes of hospitalisation.

We used two ICD 9 dimensions to tabulate the data: injury and poisoning diagnoses (ICD codes 800–999) and E–codes (ICD codes E800–E999). We then computed annual injury and external cause rates by relating the SMR1 data to age–specific population denominators derived from mid–year population estimates of the Registrar General for Scotland for the years 1984–91. We also cross–tabulated the injury diagnoses with E–codes to obtain bi–directional frequency distributions. Age standardisation was achieved by the direct method using the 1986 population as the standard.

The data were presented as diagrammatic and graphic displays using Harvard Graphics for Windows.

Results

A total of 713,398 hospitalisation episodes were analysed. Of these, 701,580 (98.3 percent) had an E–code recorded.

Table 1 shows the annual proportions of records of continuous inpatient stays (CIS) with an E–code recorded over the period 1984–91. These are consistently high, ranging from 96.9 percent to 100 percent.

We were able to generate an enormous number of tabulations, charts and graphs based on these E–coded injury hospitalisations. The following examples have been selected to illustrate the potential of the database for descriptive and monitoring purposes rather than as an exhaustive account of the wide range of its analytical possibilities.

Motor vehicle traffic accidents (MVTA) are one of the largest contributors to injury morbidity and are denoted by the codes E810–E819. Being a heterogeneous group of phenomena, data relating to MVTAs are of limited preventive value unless the role of the victim (as driver, passenger or other) is identified. The fourth digit extension to the code enables this to be analysed. Figure 1 is a pie chart showing the proportions of MVTA victims who were drivers, passengers, motor cyclists, pedal cyclists, pedestrians or others for the year 1991. The three largest categories were drivers (25 percent), pedestrians (24 percent) and passengers (13 percent).

Similarly, falls (E880–E888) represent a large but uninformative category. A fifth digit extension provides an opportunity to code place of occurrence of the fall. Figure 2 illustrates a recurring problem with the use of many of the E–codes—incompleteness of coding. While 25 percent of female fall victims hospitalised in 1991 are recorded as having experienced their injury in the home, in almost two–thirds of cases the place of occurrence was not specified. Whether this was due to deficiencies in the clinical recording of the circumstances of the falls or to a systematic failure to assign the appropriate codes cannot be determined from these data.

By relating the hospitalisation numerators to population denominators, age standardised annual injury hospitalisation rates can be derived. Figure 3 shows the temporal trend in discharge rates for falls for the whole of Scotland. Based on crosstabulations of falls against the resultant injuries, the graphs in Figure 4 provide a more revealing insight into the pattern of interaction between injury causes and outcomes over time. Falls are associated with head injuries more frequently in males than in females, who suffer more often from lower limb dislocations or fractures. In both sexes, however, fall–related head injuries are declining while lower limb injuries are increasing in frequency.

At times, the distinction between the cause and outcome of an injury appears to become blurred and it is therefore important for the investigator to include both dimensions while retaining an open mind about which is which. Figure 5 depicts the upward trend in suicide (E950–E959) as a cause of injury in females, the largest component "injury" being poisoning. In this case, the E–code (suicide) is more appropriately described as the outcome while the injury diagnosis (poisoning) is the cause. On the other hand, there is little ambiguity about assault (E960–E969) as the cause of a rising rate of male admissions and the various associated injuries (notably to the head) as the result (Figure 6), or traffic accidents (E810–E819) as the cause of a declining rate of hospitalisations and a range of injuries (mainly of the head and limbs) as their result (Figure 7).

All of the above examples have illustrated the analytical approach which takes the injury cause (as reflected by the E–code) as the starting point. This may seem logical when planning preventive measures. In some ways, however, the injury itself may be more important—if, for example, the resource implications for hospital specialties are being considered. To this end, the analysis can be reversed and the injury used as the starting point, and the contrast with the causally based approach can yield surprises. Figure 8, for example, suggests that the discharge rate for head injuries has barely changed despite an apparently declining causal contribution from MVTAs. Yet the previous illustration (Figure 7) seemed to indicate that both MVTAs and head injuries were declining in frequency. This latter conclusion would be erroneous since it fails to take account of the changing pattern of causes of head injuries, at least in males, which are increasingly associated with assaults and decreasingly with MVTAs. Thus an injury oriented analysis is as important—and should be complementary to—a causally oriented one.

Discussion

This rapid and relatively superficial overview of the potential of the SMR system for injury analysis scarcely does justice to the complexities and possibilities of the data. Our intention is to carry this work forward by extending and refining the types of analyses we have presented here, and to encourage our international colleagues to contrast their own injury morbidity experience with ours.

At the same time, we recognise that progress is likely to be hampered by the methodological constraints inherent in any hospitalisation based injury morbidity database as well as in the well–documented limitations of the ICD E–codes themselves. In particular, there are three worrying—and to date unanswered—questions to which we must find answers urgently.

First, how valid are the injury diagnoses—and the E–codes assigned to them—as recorded in routine hospitalisation morbidity systems?

Second, how useful in practice are hospitalisation morbidity systems for local injury surveillance and prevention?

Third, how confident are we that E–coded injury data are comparable both within and between countries?

Our provisional conclusions about the potential role of E–coded injury morbidity data in injury investigation, surveillance and prevention may be summarised as follows.

1.   The systematic E–coding of routine hospitalisation data is eminently feasible: in Scotland, it approaches 100 percent. Further work is necessary to establish the local, national and international validity and comparability of both the principal injury diagnoses and their assigned E–codes.

2.   E coded hospitalisation data offer valuable insights into the causes and epidemiological patterns (including secular trends) of injuries, although the practical utility for prevention of such analyses remains unclear.

3.   The crosstabulation of injury types against their causes illuminates the nature of the injury hospitalisation phenomenon in ways which are more relevant to prevention than unidimensional analysis.

4.   Routine hospitalisation data (such as those collected by the SMR system) can play an important role in the epidemiological investigation of injuries provided that the inherent theoretical and practical limitations of using hospitalisations—and E–codes—to measure injury morbidity are recognised.

5.   Given the current paucity of causal information on injury morbidity world–wide, the routine use of E–coding of hospitalisation data should be placed high on the agenda of international initiatives such as this ICE and EURORISC (see Appendix).

Appendix

A brief word about EURORISC. The acronym stands for European Review of Research on Injury Surveillance and Control. The idea grew out of a growing realisation that re–inventing the wheel was a tremendously wasteful activity and that one could learn a great deal from colleagues working on injury surveillance in various parts of Europe. A grant application was therefore submitted to the Biomed programme of the European Commission in 1993. As yet, no outright rejection has been received but nor has any funding materialised.

The aim of EURORISC is to investigate the feasibility of establishing a transnational collaborative network of injury surveillance and control researchers in countries of the European Union.

Its three specific objectives are: to establish a central clearing house for information exchange, to initiate collaborative projects with particular emphasis on the evaluation of interventions and to accelerate progress towards the harmonisation of injury surveillance and control methods in Europe.

So far, eight potential participants have been identified in six countries (United Kingdom, Sweden, France, Netherlands, Italy and Greece). Since the future of the embryonic project is uncertain, and it may be logical to integrate it with existing global efforts such as those initiated by the World Health Organisation and the US National Center for Health Statistics.

References

1.   Kohli HS, Knill–Jones RP. How accurate are SMR 1 (Scottish Morbidity Record 1) data? Health Bulletin (Edinburgh). 50, 14–23. 1992.

2.   Ribbeck BM, Runge JW, Thomason MH, Baker JW. Injury surveillance: a method for recording E–codes for injured emergency department patients. Annals of Emergency Medicine, 21, 37–46. 1992.

3.   Smith GS, Langlois JA, Buechner JS. Methodological issues in using hospital discharge data to determine the incidence of hospitalized injuries. American Journal of Epidemiology, 134, 1146–58. 1991.

4.   Smith T. Accidents, poisoning and violence as a cause of hospital admissions in children. Health Bulletin (Edinburgh), 49, 237–44. 1991.

5.   Tursz A, Crost M, Lelong N. Basic principles of epidemiology applied to accident research. In: Rogmans W, Schuurman M (eds), Proceedings of International Seminar on Accident Data, Baden, Austria. 1989.

Table 1 - % of Injury (ICD 800-999) CIS Discharges with an E Code Recorded

Year	No. of CIS discharges	With E code recorded
1984	76103	100.0%
1985	75875	100.0%
1986	74494	96.9%
1987	76077	98.7%
1988	78257	99.5%
1989	78011	98.5%
1990	81871	98.7%
1991	85911	99.7%

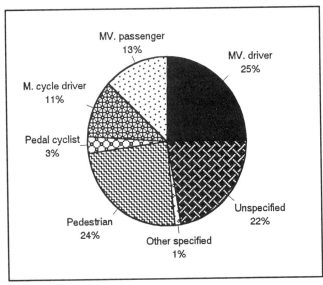

Figure 1. Fourth digit classification for MVTA (ICD E810-819), males discharged from Scottish hospitals, 1991

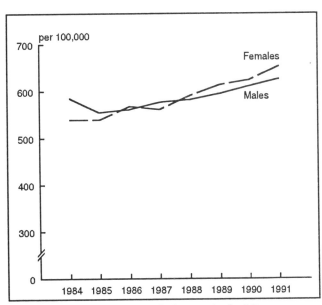

Figure 3. Age standardised CIS discharge rates for falls (ICD E880-888), Scotland 1984-91

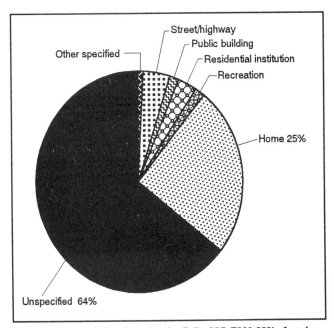

Figure 2. Fifth digit classification for Falls (ICD E880-888), females discharged from Scottish hospitals 1991

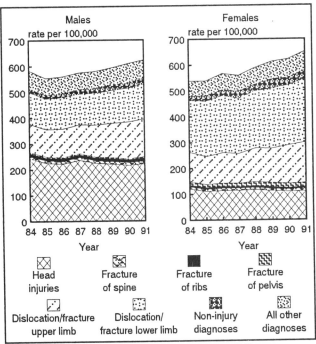

Figure 4. Age standardised CIS discharge rate for Falls (ICD E880-888), Scotland 1984-91

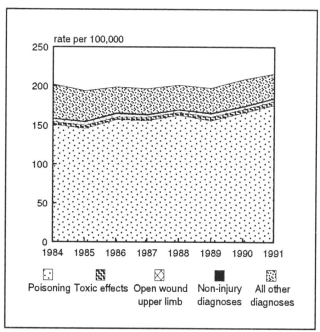

Figure 5. Age standardised CIS discharge rate for Suicide (ICD E950-959), females Scotland 1984-91

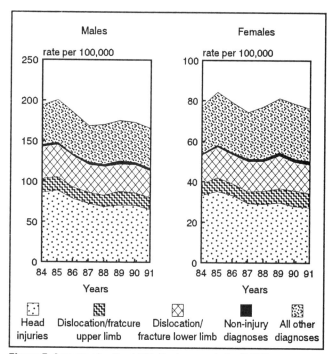

Figure 7. Age standardised CIS discharge rate for MVTA (ICD E810-819), Scotland 1984-91

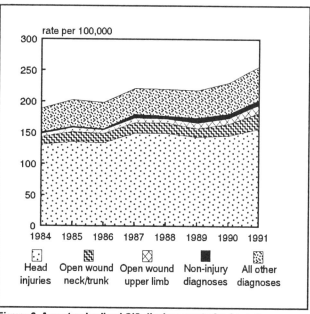

Figure 6. Age standardised CIS discharge rate for Assault (ICD E960-969), males Scotland 1984-91

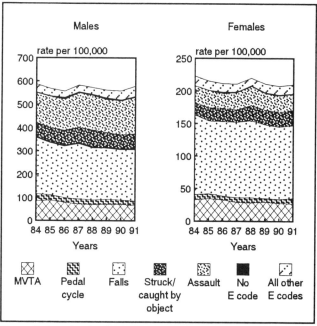

Figure 8. Age standardised CIS discharge rate for Head Injuries, Scotland 1984-91

The ICD–10 Classifications of Injuries
and External Causes

by A.C.P. L'Hours

Introduction

The Tenth Revision of the ICD[1] published in 1992 is the most radical since the Sixth Revision in 1948 and in many respects represents a new classification rather than an updating of the previous revision that has been in use since 1977.

The adoption of an alphanumeric coding scheme of one letter and two numbers at the three–character level with decimal subdivisions at the fourth character has almost doubled the size of the coding frame as compared to ICD–9. This has enabled new categories to be created for a number of entities with the fourth character being used for enhanced clinical and other detail.

Chapters XIX, Injury, poisoning and certain other consequences of external causes (using the letters S and T) and XX, External causes of morbidity and mortality (using the letters V, W, X and Y) have perhaps undergone the most change of all the 21 chapters of ICD–10 and both bring new taxonomic approaches that will result in easier and more accurate coding as well as facilitating the analysis and interpretation of the coded data.

In drafting these two chapters, a conscious effort was made to maintain a clear distinction between the event itself (the external cause) and the effect on the individual (the injury or other consequence). This was achieved by avoiding terminology related to the trauma in the external cause chapter and descriptions of the event in the injury chapter. There are however terms, such as drowning and electrocution, that are used to describe the cause as well as effect and these are used in both chapters.

The expression <u>certain</u> other consequences of external causes has been used in the title of chapter XIX. Some other consequences such as drug–induced and radiation–related disorders are included in other chapters, while other longer term consequences are better classified by the International Classification of Impairments, Disabilities, and Handicaps (ICIDH).[2]

The view has been expressed that these two chapters could usefully serve as the basis for the development of an adaptation of ICD–10 for injury prevention.

The Revision Process

The broad lines of the Tenth Revision of the ICD were set at the Preparatory Meeting on ICD–10 held at the Headquarters of the World Health Organization (WHO) in Geneva, Switzerland from 12 to 16 September 1983.[3]

The meeting recommended an alphanumeric coding scheme for ICD–10 of one letter and two numbers at the three–character level with numeric subdivisions where necessary to form the fourth–character level. The full range of codes therefore runs from A00.0 to Z99.9.

The first Expert Committee on ICD–10[4] met in San Francisco in June 1984 and the first draft proposal for ICD–10[5] containing only the three–character codes and titles was circulated to WHO Member States, Nongovernmental Organizations in official relations with WHO, WHO Collaborating Centres for Classification of Diseases, and other interested groups and individuals in August 1984. Comments were requested by the end of January 1985.

The second draft proposal for ICD–10[6] containing both the three– and four–character codes and titles was circulated, on the same basis as the first draft, in August 1986 and comments were requested by 15 January 1987.

The chapter on External causes of morbidity and mortality[7] however was not circulated until September 1986 and comments were requested by 15 March 1987.

At the Second Expert Committee on ICD–10[8] held in Geneva in November 1987, a full draft proposal containing three– and four–character titles with inclusion and exclusion terms was presented for the first time.

Throughout the revision process, WHO received valuable advice and guidance from the annual meetings of the Heads of WHO Collaborating Centers for Classification of Diseases. The Centers are located in institutions in Canberra, Australia; Sao Paulo, Brazil; Beijing, China; London, England; Le Vésinet, France; Moscow, Russian Federation; Uppsala, Sweden; Hyattsville, USA; and Caracas, Venezuela. At their annual meetings, the Centre Heads are also joined by representatives of the Dutch National Committee for Classification and Coding and the Office of the ICD, Japan.

The International Conference for the Tenth Revision of the International Classification of Diseases,[9] attended by delegates from 43 Member States, was held in Geneva from 26 September to 2 October 1989. Following approval by the WHO Executive Board and the World Health Assembly in 1990, Volume 1 of ICD–10 was published in 1992 and the classification came into use in two countries in 1994. Several other countries will adopt it in 1995.

Chapter XIX: Injury, Poisoning and Certain Other Consequences of External Causes

At the meeting of Heads of WHO Collaborating Centers for Classification of Diseases held in San Francisco from 29 May to 4 June 1984, two separate proposals for the revision of the chapter related to injuries were presented.

One, prepared by the WHO Unit responsible for coordinating the periodic revision of the ICD,[10] followed the traditional approach of using the type of injury as the main axis of classification at the level of the blocks of categories with the site of involvement being identified at the three and four–character levels. The other, undertaken by the Accident Analysis Group of Odense University Hospital, Denmark,[11] took into account suggestions made by the WHO Joint EURO/Global Steering Committee on the Development of Indicators for Accidents.

The proposal was incompletely elaborated in that it covered only injuries in its biaxial classification using body region and type of injury with no provision being made for injuries of unspecified site. Also the proposal had not been discussed with the Nordic Medico Statistical Committee (NOMESCO) and it was thought that some Scandinavian countries would have preferred the traditional approach.

The Centre Heads recommended[12] that the proposal following the traditional approach, which had changed little over successive revisions, should form the basis for the injury chapter in the first formal draft proposal for ICD–10.[5] This recommendation was endorsed by the First Expert Committee on ICD–10.[4]

At their meeting in Sao Paulo, Brazil in April 1985, the Centre Heads heard that, at its meeting in Reykjavik in August 1984, the WHO Joint EURO/Global Steering Committee on the Development of Indicators for Accidents had requested that the Centre Heads reconsider the rejection by both their group and the Expert Committee of the draft chapter on Injury and Poisoning.

The Committee on the Development of Indicators for Accidents were of the view that an arrangement of injuries according to topography would be easier to apply and suitable for use by health workers at all levels. The accuracy of coding would also be enhanced by this approach.

The Centre Heads therefore rediscussed this issue and concluded that this approach should be tested before a final decision could be taken.[13]

Prior to the meeting of the Centre Heads held in Tokyo in April 1986, the proposed version of chapter XIX was reviewed at a NOMESCO Seminar at Hesselet, Denmark from 14 to 16 January 1986. For this review, a limited number of hospital cases and death certificates were used. The Seminar gave rise to a number of recommendations which were subsequently incorporated in a revised draft that formed the basis of the second draft proposal for ICD–10 circulated in August 1986.[6]

Field testing was carried out by the Department of Health Economics and Public Health, Odense University, Denmark using 700 consecutive emergency room contacts during 1 to 15 December 1986 and 245 acute trauma–related admissions randomly sampled over the period 1 January to 31 May 1986. The results were reported to the Centre Heads at their meeting in June 1987.[14]

On the basis of comments received and the results of the field trials that had been carried out, the chapter was further revised and another version was presented to the Centre Heads when they met in Paris in March 1989. The primary axis of classification of body region however still did not allow for the assignment of imprecise descriptions of injuries that related only to the trunk, upper limbs, lower limbs or unspecified limb.

Three possible solutions were proposed to this problem. One (option A) which required minimum rearrangement of the systematic structure of the chapter and provided a new block of categories for injuries to broader body regions, one (option B) which required greater rearrangement and condensation of the effects of foreign bodies into a single three–character code, and a third solution (option C) which involved reducing the amount of space available for detail by creating body regions for upper limb, lower limb and a trunk. After detailed discussion, the Centre Heads requested the secretariat to proceed with a further revision of this chapter on the basis of option A.

A revised version was prepared in time for the Revision Conference that was held in September/October 1989 and subsequently approved by WHO Executive Board and the World Health Assembly in 1990.

The "S" series of codes (S00–S99) is used to classify injuries related to single "body regions". The 10 body regions are the following:

S00–S09	Head
S10–S19	Neck
S20–S29	Thorax
S30–S39	Abdomen, lower back, lumbar spine and pelvis
S40–S49	Shoulder and upper arm
S50–S59	Elbow and forearm
S60–S69	Wrist and hand
S70–S79	Hip and thigh
S80–S89	Knee and lower leg
S90–S99	Ankle and foot

Within each block of 10 three–character categories, specific injury types are identified at the three–character level:

Superficial injury
Open wound
Fracture
Dislocation, sprain and strain
Injury to nerves and spinal cord
Injury to blood vessels
Injury to muscle and tendon
Crushing injury
Traumatic amputation
Injury to internal organs
Other and unspecified injuries

The same injury type usually has the same third character in the code but there are some exceptions made necessary by the importance of certain injuries, so that:

S05	which, in the matrix approach, would normally mean Injury to blood vessels of head has been used to identify Injuries of eye and orbit
S06	(Injury to muscle and tendon of head) relates to Intracranial injury
S26	(Injury to muscle and tendon of thorax) relates to Injury of heart
S27	(Crushing injury of thorax) relates to Injury of other and unspecified intrathoracic organs
S28	(Traumatic amputation of part of thorax) groups both crushing injury and traumatic amputation
S36	(Injury to muscle and tendon of abdomen, etc.) is used to identify Injury of intra–abdominal organs
S37	(Crushing injury of abdomen, etc.) relates to Injury of pelvic organs
S38	(Traumatic amputation of abdomen, etc.) groups both crushing injury and traumatic amputation.

In each case where there is a deviation from the matrix meaning of the code, the injury type is assigned a fourth–character subcategory at SX9:

S090	Injury of blood vessels of head
S091	Injury of muscle and tendon of head
S290	Injury of muscle and tendon at thorax level
S390	Injury of muscle and tendon of abdomen, etc.

The "T" series of codes (T00–T98)

Injuries involving multiple body regions are assigned to T00–T07. The three–character categories identify the main injury types:

T00	Superficial injuries
T01	Open wounds
T02	Fractures
T03	Dislocations, sprains and strains
T04	Crushing injuries
T05	Traumatic amputations

Category T06 covers other injuries involving multiple body regions and is subdivided as follows:

T06.0	Brain and cranial nerves with nerves and spinal cord at neck level
T06.1	Nerves and spinal cord involving other multiple body regions
T06.2	Nerves involving multiple body regions
T06.3	Blood vessels involving multiple body regions
T06.4	Muscles and tendons involving multiple body regions
T06.5	Intrathoracic organs with intra–abdominal and pelvic organs
T06.6	Other specified injuries involving multiple body regions

Injuries that are unspecified as to the body region involved are assigned to T08–T14:

T08	Fracture of spine, level unspecified
T09	Other injuries of spine and trunk, level unspecified
T10	Fracture of upper limb, level unspecified
T11	Other injuries of upper limb, level unspecified

T12   Fracture of lower limb, level unspecified
T13   Other injuries of lower limb, level unspecified
T14   Injury of unspecified body region

Categories T08, T10 and T12 are unsubdivided as they relate specifically to fractures, while T09, T11, T13 and T14 are subdivided according to the broad injury types.

Foreign bodies which were attributed 10 three–digit categories in ICD–9 are accommodated in only five categories in ICD–10. This has been achieved by using broader anatomical groups at the category level. The only ICD–9 site that can no longer be specifically coded is the lacrimal punctum while the nasal sinus, nostril, small intestine, colon, urethra and bladder are now separately identifiable.

Burns and corrosions (T20–T32)

The ten categories assigned to these injuries in ICD–9 are increased to 13 in ICD–10. Apart from burns confined to the eye and adnexa, ICD–9 did not distinguish between thermal and chemical burns. In ICD–10, fourth–character subdivisions are used both to distinguish between burns and corrosions and whether first, second, third or unspecified degree. The three additional categories are used to identify burn and corrosion of ankle and foot (T25), burn and corrosion of respiratory tract (T27) and corrosions according to extent of body surface involved (T32).

Frostbite was classified within four fourth–digit subcategories of category 991 of ICD–9 (Effects of reduced temperature). In ICD–10, three three–character categories (T33–T35) are used to classify superficial frostbite, frostbite with tissue necrosis and frostbite involving multiple body regions or of unspecified degree. The fourth–character subcategories identify the site of involvement.

The remaining categories in this chapter are grouped as follows:

T36–T40   Poisoning by drugs, medicaments and biological substances
T51–T65   Toxic effects of substances chiefly nonmedicinal as to source
T66–T78   Other and unspecified effects of external causes
T79   Certain early complications of trauma
T80–T88   Complications of surgical and medical care, not elsewhere classified
T90–T98   Sequelae of injuries, of poisoning and of other consequences of external causes

There has been some concern expressed regarding comparability of injury data between ICD–9 and ICD–10. Annex A shows the ICD–9 groups of injuries with the equivalent ICD–10 codes. Although it is necessary to group dislocations with sprains and strains and superficial injuries with contusions, it is possible to approximate the ICD–9 groupings. The only problem area relates to traumatic amputation (classified as an open wound in ICD–9) and crushing injury of unspecified body region that are both assigned to T14.7 in ICD–10. Annex B groups ICD–10 injury types from the different body regions. Again, the only difficulty relates to T14.7.

Chapter XX: External Causes of Morbidity and Mortality

The traditional ICD approach to the classification of external causes, while perhaps relevant to mortality uses was, in many respects, considered to be inadequate for the needs of injury prevention programmes and policies. Several groups had been working on alternative methods of classification and at the first Expert Committee on ICD–10 in 1984, two multi–axial approaches were presented—one by the WHO Joint Euro/Global Steering Committee on the Development of Indicators for Accidents[15] and the other by NOMESCO.[16] Both classifications were, however, incompletely elaborated as they placed the emphasis on accidents and it was also doubtful whether a departure from the basic principle of the ICD as a single–variable axis classification could be accepted for one chapter. The first draft proposal for ICD–10 that was circulated in August 1984[5] therefore followed the traditional approach for this chapter.

At the meeting of Heads of WHO Collaborating Centers for Classification of Diseases in 1985, two further proposals were submitted. A NOMESCO document showing a multi-axial approach for accident monitoring[17] and a proposal from the Centers for Disease Control(CDC)/Consumer Product Safety Commission (CPSC) in the United States[18] which took a more traditional approach but reallocated space in accordance with their concept of the needs of prevention programmes. The Centre Heads appreciated the work of the two groups but felt that such proposals might more appropriately be considered in the context of a specialty–based application of the ICD for injury prevention.

In 1986, the Centre Heads reviewed another two proposals, one prepared by a WHO Working Party, which occupied 400 three–character categories and was strongly influenced by the systematic approach of the NOMESCO classification. The other, drawn up by CDC and CPSC in the USA was constructed within the 200 three–character categories that were available in the ICD–9. These two draft proposals were contained in a single document.[19] After considering the two proposals, the Center Heads recommended that the best aspects of the two drafts should be merged into a revision proposal that would utilize only three alphabetical characters but that would be completed down to the fourth–character level.

Representatives of the two groups and of WHO met in Odense from 19 to 22 August 1986 under the auspices of NOMESCO and with the generous support of the administration of the Odense Sygehus, to produce a draft proposal on the basis of the recommendations of the Centre Heads. The draft prepared by the working group was circulated to WHO Member States, and other interested groups and individuals as a part of the second formal draft proposal for ICD–10[7] in September 1986. Comments were requested by 15 March 1987. The comments received were discussed at a meeting held in Atlanta, USA in March 1987 by representatives from the United States, NOMESCO and WHO.

A further revision was prepared and submitted to the Centre Heads in June 1987.[20] The Centre Heads identified a number of deficiencies and as a result the Centre for North America offered to prepare a revised proposal.[21] Subsequently, the WHO Secretariat proceeded with a further elaboration[22] in which the order of sections was changed to permit a more efficient use of the available space and to reflect comments that had been received too late for consideration by the Atlanta meeting. Unfortunately the timetable for revision did not allow for the two groups to collaborate in the preparation of the drafts so that two different versions were put before the second Expert Committee on ICD–10 in November 1987.

The Expert Committee found advantages and disadvantages in both the draft proposals. In addition to a number of specific comments, it recommended that WHO and the North American Center proceed with a synthesis of the two drafts, that the resulting classification should be tested by one or more collaborating centers and the results presented to the 1988 meeting of Heads of WHO Collaborating Centers for the Classification of Diseases.

Representatives of WHO, the North American Center and NOMESCO came together from 3 to 5 February 1988 at the National Center for Health Statistics, Hyattsville, Maryland, USA and prepared the revised draft proposal using the order of categories contained in the WHO proposal. The revised draft proposal[23] was sent to WHO Collaborating Centers for field testing and at their 1988 meeting, the Centre Heads heard results of testing carried out in Brazil,[24] Denmark,[25] England,[26] Finland,[27] Sweden,[28] the United States[29] and Venezuela.[30] The detailed findings were referred to the secretariat for development of the draft proposal to be submitted to the Revision Conference.

Some further refinements were made to the draft that was submitted to the Centre Heads at their 1989 meeting and the resultant classification was submitted to the International Conference for the Tenth Revision of the ICD held in Geneva from 26 September to 2 October 1989.

It should be noted that this chapter forms an integral part of ICD–10. The ICD–9 designation of this classification as being supplementary has been discontinued in an effort to encourage its use for both ambulatory and in–patient morbidity systems.

The proposal as presented to the Revision Conference and included in the published ICD–10 uses the code range V01–Y99.

The letter V is used for transport accidents. The first eight blocks of 10 categories identify the victim's mode of transport at the second character level:

V0   Pedestrian
V1   Pedal cyclist
V2   Motorcycle rider
V3   Occupant of three–wheeled motor vehicle
V4   Car occupant
V5   Occupant of pick–up truck or van
V6   Occupant of heavy transport vehicle
V7   Bus occupant

The third character identifies the victim's counterpart or the circumstances of the accident:

VX0   Collision with pedestrian or animal
VX1   Collision with pedal cyclist
VX2   Collision with two– or three–wheeled motor vehicle
VX3   Collision with car, pick–up truck or van
VX4   Collision with heavy transport vehicle or bus
VX5   Collision with railway train or railway vehicle
VX6   Collision with other non motor vehicle
VX7   Collision with fixed or stationary object
VX8   Noncollision transport accident
VX9   Other and unspecified transport accident

This matrix approach is shown in more detail at Annex C. It should be noted that code V00 is not used as in the matrix this would relate to a collision between a pedestrian and another pedestrian. Such events are classified to W51.

The fourth–character is used to identify both the activity of the victim and whether the event was a traffic or a nontraffic accident:

VXX.0   Driver, nontraffic
VXX.1   Passenger, nontraffic
VXX.2   Person on outside of vehicle, nontraffic
VXX.3   Unspecified occupant, nontraffic
VXX.4   Person boarding or alighting
VXX.5   Driver, traffic
VXX.6   Passenger, traffic
VXX.7   Person on outside of vehicle traffic
VXX.9   Unspecified occupant, traffic

The remainder of land transport accidents are covered by categories V80–V89:

V80   Animal–rider or occupant of animal–drawn vehicle
V81   Occupant of railway train or railway vehicle
V82   Occupant of streetcar
V83   Occupant of special vehicle mainly used on industrial premises
V84   Occupant of special vehicle mainly used in agriculture
V85   Occupant of special construction vehicle
V86   Occupant of special all–terrain or other motor vehicle designed primarily for off–road use
V87   Traffic accident of special type but victim's mode of transport unknown
V88   Nontraffic accident of specified type but victim's mode of transport unknown
V89   Motor– or nonmotor–vehicle accident, type of vehicle unspecified

V80–V86   show the victim's mode of transport while the fourth–character subdivisions relate to the circumstances of the accident.

V87–V88   are used for accidents where information is available regarding the vehicles involved or the circumstances of the accident but the victim's mode of transport is unknown.

V89   covers those circumstances where the only available information relates to that unspecified motor–vehicle or non motor vehicle was involved and whether the event was a traffic accident or a nontraffic accident.

Apart from transport accidents, the remainder of the categories are only shown at the three–character level as there are standard fourth–character subcategories for W00–Y34 (except Y06 and Y07, maltreatment syndromes) to identify the place of occurrence of the external cause.

Place of occurrence:

.0   Home
.1   Residential institution
.2   School, other institution and public administrative area
.3   Sports and athletics area
.4   Street and highway
.5   Trade and service area
.6   Industrial and construction area
.7   Farm
.8   Other specified places
.9   Unspecified place

As the place of occurrence is not relevant to legal intervention (Y35), operations of war (Y36) and complications of medical and surgical care (Y40–Y84), the fourth character is used to provide more detail about the nature of the event or, in the case of adverse effects of drugs, the type of substance involved.

In addition to the fourth characters for place of occurrence, a further subclassification is provided for optional use in a supplementary character position (i.e., the fifth character or beyond according to the structure of the data system) to indicate the activity of the injured person at the time the event occurred. These activity codes are intended to be used with all categories including those where the place of occurrence codes do not apply:

0   While engaged in sports activity
1   While engaged in leisure activity
2   While working for income
3   While engaged in other types of work
4   While resting, sleeping, eating or engaging in other vital activities
8   While engaged in other specified activities
9   During unspecified activities

Falls have been moved to the beginning of the W series of codes at W00–W19 and new groupings have been created at:

W20–W49	Exposure to inanimate mechanical forces
W50–W64	Exposure to animate mechanical forces
W65–W74	Accidental drowning and submersion
W75–W84	Other accidental threats to breathing
W85–W99	Exposure to electric current, radiation and extreme ambient air temperature or pressure
X00–X09	Exposure to smoke, fire and flames
X10–X19	Contact with heat and hot substances
X20–X29	Contact with venomous plants and animals

X30–X39	Exposure to forces of nature
X40–X49	Accidental poisoning and exposure to noxious substances
X50–X57	Overexertion, travel and privation
X58,X59	Exposure to other and unspecified accidental factors

The last category in the group of accidents X59, Exposure to unspecified factors includes Fracture not otherwise specified, which was previously classified in the section on Falls.

The ICD–9 section of Suicide and Self–inflicted injury is redesignated as Intentional self–harm and appears at X60–X84.

Assault, including neglect and abandonment and other maltreatment syndromes which are subdivided to identify the perpetrator, is shown at X85–Y09.

The ICD–9 section of injury undetermined whether accidentally or purposely inflicted is now designated Event of undetermined intent at Y10–Y34.

Legal intervention and Operations of war which each occupied ten three–digit categories in ICD–9 are both given a single three–character category at Y35 and Y36.

Complications of medical care are brought together in contiguous blocks of categories within Y40–Y84. This includes a new group at Y70–Y82 for Medical devices associated with adverse incidents in diagnostic and therapeutic use.

Sequelae of external causes which were included at the end of the relevant sections of accident, suicide, undetermined, etc. in ICD–9 have been brought together at Y85–Y89.

Finally, the last section in this chapter concerns supplementary factors related to causes of morbidity and mortality classified elsewhere. This includes two categories to identify the involvement of alcohol, one subdivided by blood alcohol content and the other identifying alcohol intoxication as mild, moderate, severe and very severe on the basis of assessment of behaviour, functions and responses. The other categories in the group may be used as additional codes to identify conditions as nosocomial, work–related, environmental–pollution related, and life–style related.

An overview of the blocks of categories in this chapter is given at Annex D.

References

1. International Classification of Diseases and Related Health Problems. Tenth Revision. Vol 1: Tabular List. Geneva, World Health Organization, 1992.

2. International Classification of Impairments, Disabilities, and Handicaps. Geneva, World Health Organization, 1980.

3. Report of the Preparatory Meeting on ICD–10. Geneva, World Health Organization, 1983 (unpublished document DES/ICD–10/83.19).

4. Report of the Expert Committee on the International Classification of Diseases. First meeting on the Tenth Revision. Geneva, World Health Organization, 1984 (unpublished document DES/ICD–10/84.34).

5. Circulation of First Draft Proposal for the Tenth Revision of the International Classification of Diseases. Geneva, World Health Organization, 1984 (unpublished document ICD/I/1984).

6. Circulation of the Second Draft Proposal for the Tenth Revision of the International Classification of Diseases. Geneva, World Health Organization, 1986 (unpublished document WHO/DES/ICD/II/1986).

7. Circulation of the Second Draft Proposal for the Tenth Revision of the International Classification of Diseases (ICD–10). Draft Chapter XX: External Causes of Morbidity and Mortality. Geneva, World Health Organization, 1986 (unpublished document WHO/DES/ICD/II/1986 Annex 2).

8. Report of the Expert Committee on the International Classification of Diseases. Second Meeting on the Tenth Revision. Geneva, World Health Organization, 1987 (unpublished document WHO/DES/EC/87.38).

9. Report of the International Conference for the Tenth Revision of the International Classification of Diseases. Geneva, World Health Organization, 1989 (unpublished document WHO/ICD10/REV.CONF/89.9/Rev.1).

10. Alphanumeric approach to the Tenth Revision of the International Classification of Diseases. Geneva, World Health Organization, 1984 (unpublished document DES/ICD/C/84.5).

11. Kruse T and Frandsen PA. Tenth Revision of the ICD, Draft Chapter XVII: Injury and Poisoning, Proposal for Revision of Categories and Subcategories. Geneva, World Health Organization, 1984 (unpublished document DES/ICD/C/84.22).

12. Report of the Meeting of Heads of WHO Collaborating Centres for Classification of Diseases. Geneva, World Health Organization, 1984 (unpublished document DES/ICD/C/84.48).

13. Report of the Meeting of Heads of WHO Collaborating Centres for Classification of Diseases. Geneva, World Health Organization, 1985 (unpublished document DES/ICD/C/85.27).

14. Kruse T, Frandsen PA, Röck ND. Injury, poisoning and other consequences of external causes: field testing of chapter XIX, ICD–10 (second draft). Odense, Odense University, 1987 (Background document No. 2 for Meeting of Heads of Collaborating Centres for Classification of Diseases, Leningrad, USSR, 1987).

15. Kruse T. Tenth Revision of the ICD, Draft Chapter XXI: External Cause of Injury and Poisoning, Proposal for Revision. Geneva, World Health Organization, 1984 (unpublished document DES/ICD/C/84.26).

16. Development of a Nordic Classification for Accident Monitoring by the Nordic Medico–Statistical Committee (NOMESCO). Geneva, World Health Organization, 1984 (unpublished document DES/ICD/C/84.47).

17. Nordic Medico–Statistical Committee. Nordic Classification of Accident Monitoring: Codes and Manuals. Geneva, World Health Organization, 1985 (unpublished document DES/ICD/C/85.21).

18. Centers for Disease Control/Consumer Product Safety Commission Work Group to revise ICD–10 Injury Codes. Proposed Modification of ICD–10 Chapter on External Causes of Morbidity and Mortality. Geneva, World Health Organization, 1985 (unpublished document DES/ICD/C/85.9)

19. Tenth Revision of the ICD, Draft Chapter XX: External Causes of Morbidity and Mortality. Proposal for Revision of ICD Categories. Geneva, World Health Organization, 1986 (unpublished document WHO/DES/ICD/C/86.020).

20. Draft Chapter XX: External Causes of Morbidity and Mortality. Geneva, World Health Organization, 1987 (unpublished document DES/ICD/C/87.20).

21. WHO Collaborating Center for Classification of Diseases for North America. Modification to the ICD–10 Third Draft Proposal for Chapter XX: External Causes of Morbidity and Mortality. Geneva, World Health Organization, 1987 (unpublished document WHO/DES/EC/ICD–10/87.22).

22. Draft Chapter XX: External Causes of Morbidity and Mortality. Geneva, World Health Organization, 1987 (unpublished document WHO/DES/EC/ICD–10/87.20).

23. Field Trial Version of the Chapter on External Causes of Morbidity and Mortality. Geneva, World Health Organization, 1988 (unpublished document DES/ICD/C/88.17).

24. Laurenti R and Jorge MHPM. Field Trial of Chapter XX (External Causes of Morbidity and Mortality). Geneva, World Health Organization, 1988 (unpublished document DES/ICD/C/88.19).

25. Kruse T and Röck ND. Preliminary Report of Field Trial of ICD–10, Draft Chapter XX, Based on Morbidity Data. Geneva, World Health Organization, 1988 (unpublished document DES/ICD/C/88.24).

26. Comments of the Chapter of External Causes of Morbidity and Mortality by the WHO Centre, London. Geneva, World Health Organization, 1988 (unpublished document DES/ICD/C/88.29).

27. Karkola K. Comments on the Field Trial Version of the Chapter on External Causes of Morbidity and Mortality from Finland. Geneva, World Health Organization, 1988 (unpublished document DES/ICD/C/88.25).

28. Smedby B. Comments on the Field Trial Version of the Chapter of External Causes of Morbidity and Mortality from Sweden. Geneva, World Health Organization, 1988 (unpublished document DES/ICD/C/88.26)

29. WHO Collaborating Center for Classification of Diseases for North America. Results of a Test of Adequacy of Draft of ICD–10 Chapter XX. Geneva, World Health Organization, 1988 (unpublished document DES/ICD/C/88.7).

30. Bridge Study ICD–9/10, Venezuela. Preliminary Report. Geneva, World Health Organization, 1988 (unpublished document DES/ICD/C/88.35).

Annex A

ICD–9 Groups of Injuries with Equivalent ICD–10 Codes

Fractures (800–829)

S02, S07.0, S07, S12, S22, S32, S42, S52, S62, S72, S82, S92, T02, T08, T10, T12, T14.2

Dislocation (830–839)
Sprains and strains (840–848)

S03, S13, S23, S33, S43, S53, S63, S73, S83, S93, T03, T09.2, T11.2, T13.2, T14.3

Intracranial injury (850–854)

S06, T06.0

Internal injury of chest, abdomen and pelvis (860–869)

S26, S27, S36, S37, S39.6, T06.5

Open wounds (870–897)

S01, S05.2,–S05.7, S08, S09.2, S11, S18, S21, S28.1, S31, S38.2, S38.3, S41, S48, S51, S58, S61, S68, S71, S78, S81, S88, S91, S98, T01, T05, T09.1, T09.6, T11.1, T11.6, T13.1, T13.6, T14.1, T14.7 part

Injury to blood vessels (900–904)

S09.0, S15, S25, S35, S45, S55, S65, S75, S85, S95, T06.3, T11.4, T13.4, T14.5

Late effects (905–909)

T90–T98

Superficial injury (910–919)
Contusion with intact skin surface (920–924)

S00, S05.0, S05.1, S05.8, S05.9, S10, S20, S30, S40, S50, S60, S70, S80, S90, T00, T09.0, T11.0, T13.0, T14.0

Crushing injury (925–929)

S17, S28.0, S38.0, S38.1, S47, S57, S67, S77, S87, S97, T04, T14.7 part

Effects of foreign body entering through orifice (930–939)

T15–T19

Burns (940–949)

T20–T32

Injury to nerves and spinal cord (950–957)

S04, S14, S24, S34, S44, S54, S64, S74, S84, S94, T06.1, T06.2, T09.3, T09.4, T11.3, T13.3, T14,4

Certain traumatic complications (958)

T79

Injury, other and unspecified (959)

S05, S09.7, S09.8, S09.9, S19, S29.7, S29.8, S29.9, S39.7, S39.8, S39.9, S49.7, S49.8, S49.9, S59.7, S59.8, S59.9, S69.7, S69.8, S69.9, S79.7, S79.8, S79.9, S89.7, S89.8, S89.9, S99.7, S99.8, S99.9, T06.8, T07, T09.8, T09.9, T11.8, T11.9, T13.8, T13.9, T14.8, T14.9

Poisoning by drugs, medicaments and biological substances (960–979)

T36–T50

Toxic effects of substances chiefly nonmedicinal as to source (980–989)

T51–T65

Other and unspecified effects of external causes (990–995)

T33–T35, T66–T78

Complications of surgical and medical cause not elsewhere classified (996–999)

T80–T88

Annex B

ICD–10 Injury Types Grouped by Codes from the Different Body Regions

Superficial injury (including contusions)

S00, S10, S20, S30, S40, S50, S60, S70, S80, S90, T00, T09.0, T11.0, T13.0, T14.0

Open wound

S01, S11, S21, S31, S51, S61, S71, S81, S91, T01, T09.1, T09.6, T11.1, T13.1, T14.1

Fracture

S02, S12, S22, S32, S42, S52, S62, S72, S82, S92, T02, T08, T10, T12, T14.2

Dislocation, sprain and strain

S03, S13, S23, S33, S43, S53, S63, S73, S83, S93, T03, T09.2, T11.2, T13.2, T14.3

Injury to nerves and spinal cord

S04, S14, S24, S34, S44, S54, S64, S74, S84, S94, T06.1, T06.2, T09.3, T09.4, T11.3, T13.3, T14.4

Injury to blood vessels

S09.0, S15, S25, S35, S45, S55, S65, S75, S85, S95, T06.3, T11.4, T13.4, T14.5

Injury to muscle and tendon

S09.1, S16, S29.0, S39.0, S46, S56, S66, S76, S86, S96, T06.4, T09.5, T11.5, T13.5, T14.6

Crushing injury

S07.0, S07.8, S17, S28.0, S38.0, S38.1, S47, S57, S67, S77, S87, S97, T04, T14.7 part

Traumatic amputation

S08, S18, S28.1, S38.2, S38.3, S48, S58, S68, S78, S88, S98, T05, T09.6, T11.6, T13.6, T14.7 part

Injury to internal organs

S06, S26, S27, S36, S37, S39.6, T06.5

Other and unspecified injuries

S05, S09.2, S09.7, S09.8, S09.9, S19, S29.7, S29.8, S29.9, S39.7, S39.8, S39.9, S49.7, S49.8, S49.9, S59.7, S59.8, S59.9, S69.7, S69.8, S69.9, S79.7, S79.8, S79.9, S89.7, S89.8, S89.9, S99.7, S99.8, S99.9, T06.0, T06.8, T07, T09.8, T09.9, T11.8, T11.9, T13.8, T13.9, T14.8, T14.9

Annex C
Table of land transport accidents
In collision with or involved in:

Victim and mode of transport	Pedestrian or animal	Pedal cycle	Two- or three-wheel motor vehicle	Car (automobile) pick-up truck or van	Heavy transport vehicle or bus (coach)	Other motor vehicle	Railway train or vehicle	Other nonmotor vehicle including animal-drawn vehicle	Collision with fixed or stationary object	Noncollision transport accident	Other or unspecified transport accident
Pedestrian	(W51.-)	V01.-	V02.-	V03.-	V04.-	V09.-	V05.-	V06.-	(W22.5)	-	V09
Pedal cycle	V10.-	V11.-	V12.-	V13.-	V14.-	V19.-	V15.-	V16.-	V17.-	V18.-	V19.-
Motorcycle rider	V20.-	V21.-	V22.-	V23.-	V24.-	V29.-	V25.-	V26.-	V27.-	V28.-	V29.-
Occupant of:											
—three-wheeled motor vehicle	V30.-	V31.-	V32.-	V33.-	V34.-	V39.-	V35.-	V36.-	V37.-	V38.-	V39.-
—car (automobile)	V40.-	V41.-	V42.-	V43.-	V44.-	V49.-	V45.-	V46.-	V47.-	V48.-	V49.-
—pick up truck or van	V50.-	V51.-	V52.-	V53.-	V54.-	V59.-	V55.-	V56.-	V57.-	V58.-	V59.-
—heavy transport vehicle	V60.-	V61.-	V62.-	V63.-	V64.-	V69.-	V65.-	V66.-	V67.-	V68.-	V69.-
—bus (coach)	V70.-	V71.-	V72.-	V73.-	V74.-	V79.-	V75.-	V76.-	V77.-	V78.-	V79.-
—animal-drawn vehicle (or animal rider)	V80.1	V80.2	V80.3	V80.4	V80.4	V80.5	V80.6	V80.7	V80.8	V80.0	V80.9

CHAPTER XX
External causes of morbidity and mortality
(V01–Y98)

V01–X59	Accidents	
	V01–V99	Transport accidents
	V01–V09	Pedestrian injured in transport accident
	V10–V19	Pedal cyclist injured in transport accident
	V20–V29	Motorcycle rider injured in transport accident
	V30–V39	Occupant of three–wheeled motor vehicle injured in transport accident
	V40–V49	Car occupant injured in transport accident
	V50–V59	Occupant of pick–up truck or van injured in transport accident
	V60–V69	Occupant of heavy transport vehicle injured in transport accident
	V70–V79	Bus occupant injured in transport accident
	V80–V89	Other land transport accidents
	V90–V94	Water transport accidents
	V95–V97	Air and space transport accidents
	V98–V99	Other and unspecified transport accidents

W00–X59	Other external causes of accidental injury	
	W00–W19	Falls
	W20–W49	Exposure to inanimate mechanical forces
	W50–W64	Exposure to animate mechanical forces
	W65–W74	Accidental drowning and submersion
	W75–W84	Other accidental threats to breathing
	W85–W99	Exposure to electric current, radiation and extreme ambient air temperature and pressure
	X00–X09	Exposure to smoke, fire and flames
	X10–X19	Contact with heat and hot substances
	X20–X29	Contact with venomous animals and plants
	X30–X39	Exposure to forces of nature
	X40–X49	Accidental poisoning by and exposure to noxious substances
	X50–X57	Overexertion, travel and privation
	X58–X59	Accidental exposure to other and unspecified factors

X60–X84	Intentional self–harm

X85–Y09	Assault

Y10–Y34	Event of undetermined intent

Y35–Y36	Legal intervention and operations of war

Y40–Y84	Complications of medical and surgical care	
	Y40–Y59	Drugs, medicaments and biological substances causing adverse effects in therapeutic use
	Y60–Y69	Misadventures to patients during surgical and medical care
	Y70–Y82	Medical devices associated with adverse incidents in diagnostic and therapeutic use
	Y83–Y84	Surgical and other medical procedures as the cause of abnormal reaction of the patient, or of later complication, without mention of misadventure at the time of the procedure

Y85–Y89	Sequelae of external causes of morbidity and mortality

Y90–Y98	Supplementary factors related to causes of morbidity and mortality classified elsewhere

Data Needs for Planning
and Monitoring Accident and Injury Prevention

A comparison of the ICD– and the NOMESCO classification systems

by H. Bay–Nielsen, M.D. and B. Frimodt–Møller, M.D.

We are very pleased to have this opportunity to present an overview of the most important differences between accident registration systems based on the ICD–10 Classification and the NOMESCO Classification. We consider it as very important to stress: A classification is designed for a certain purpose _and_ misuse of the classification for other purposes may obstruct cognition and the scientific process.

ICD–10 and earlier revisions are structured for stratification of fatal accidents, but the stratification of injured treated in hospitals and emergency departments is insufficient. Figure 1 demonstrates that the structure of ICD corresponds to the distribution of E–codes in fatalities, but not in admissions—and it differs substantially from the injured visiting emergency rooms. This reflects the fact that the panel of main contributors in the development of ICD–10 was representatives from central statistical bureaus with responsibility for the important mortality statistics.

It is our allegation that the ICD Classification is primarily structured for fatalities and as a basis for a classical, simple reporting system, i.e., sequential list useful in simple tabulations with subdivision in age and sex (c.f., Figure 2). Coding for place of occurrence and activity is optional. The place of occurrence classification is at a high hierarchical level and is too crude to be useful in injury prevention. Information on occupational accidents can only be obtained if you use the optional activity code. Sports injuries are not specified at all.

Furthermore, the lack of hierarchical structure in ICD inhibits processing on databases constructed on the ICD classification. As an example, traffic accidents are only defined at 4th digit level and in different positions throughout the transport section. Retrieval of traffic accident data demands complicated and time consuming programming and processing.

When considering accident prevention it is important to take a quantitative aspect into account. Figure 3 shows the dimensions of the injured as known to the hospital sector. For every fatal accident we have 40 admitted to a hospital and 300 victims treated at emergency rooms. For those sectors in society which are responsible for injury prevention and accident registration, systems based on fatal accidents are insufficient.

The NOMESCO classification was developed on _initiative_ by those sectors in society which are responsible for injury prevention. The ICD based injury classification systems could not fulfil their demands for data on the circumstances of injury. NOMESCO (Nordic Medico–Statistical Committee) set up a specific working group which produced and published a "Classification for Accident Monitoring" in 1989 and a second edition in 1990.

These sectors (c.f., Figure 4) expressed the following list of the most important information needed for injury prevention in ranked order:

- Place of occurrence as specified as possible
- Type of activity of the victim
- Injury mechanism
- Product involved in the accident
- Free text describing the circumstances of the event

These variables have therefore been included in the NOMESCO classification. The classification is developed for use in the emergency rooms, bearing in mind that the emergency rooms are the "gateway" to the hospitals and that you can obtain the most precise information on the circumstances of the accidents in emergency rooms.

We aimed at a multiaxial and hierarchical classification which could facilitate data processing including systematic data retrieval, analyses etc. The classification is contained in the folder which will be distributed at this meeting; the ICD was acknowledged as the instrument for classifying fatal accidents.

Figure 5 demonstrates the reason for contact code, which sorts out diseases from accidents, violence and self harm. Each of these 3 categories of injured are coded separately following the classification's basic module:

- Place of occurrence
- Activity of the victim
- Injury mechanism

Figure 6 demonstrates the classification system. Occupational accidents are coded following the industrial module worked out in collaboration with Nordic occupational health agencies. Traffic accidents are coded following the vehicle module worked out in collaboration with the Nordic Committee on Road Accident Research. Sports codes describe sports accidents by the type of sports. All types of injury may be coded for the product involved in the event. This product classification comprising all types of products was worked out by a Nordic group representing the Nordic Consumers' Agencies.

The increasing interest concerning violence in our countries was followed up by another NOMESCO initiative. Recently, we held a seminar with representatives of police, researchers on violence, criminologists, and forensic medicine. At this seminar we produced a supplementary module for violence aiming at classifying the most important information about circumstances of violence. This information is needed for planning prevention of violence.

The following examples (c.f., Figure 7–9) show the use of the NOMESCO Classification.

The Activity code elicits three major categories of accidents: The place of occurrence code gives further specification of home and leisure accidents among children; use of the vehicle accident module traffic accidents may be further specified for mode of transport. These examples have illustrated the data needed for targeted prevention. As a final example, Figure 10 shows the coding of a case story illustrating the differences between the ICD–10 and NOMESCO with regard to the information kept in the database.

All major injury registration systems in Europe use multiaxial injury classifications: PORS (Netherlands), HASS (U.K.), EHLASS (European Home and Leisure Accident Surveillance System) and they are all compatible with the NOMESCO system. These classifications have proved their efficiency in rendering the information demanded by the sectors responsible for prevention. They are designed for this purpose.

We propose a collaborative effort on developing an *international classification of external causes of injuries* for use in emergency departments.

References

1.   International Statistical Classification of Diseases and Related Health Problems. Tenth Revision. WHO Geneva 1992.

2.   Classification for Accident Monitoring. 2nd revised edition. Nordic Medico–Statistical Committee (NOMESCO). Copenhagen 1990.

3.   Classification of External Causes of Injuries in the Arctic. Trial version. NOMESCO 1993.

4.   Surveillance Systems on Home and Leisure Accidents in Europe. Consumer Safety Institute. Amsterdam 1992.

5.   The Role of Accident Data. In designing, monitoring and evaluating measures aiming at improving consumer safety in Europe. European Consumer Safety Association (ECOSA). Amsterdam 1993.

6.   Prevention of Accidents. A Basic Data Set and guidelines for its use. WHO/Regional Office for Europe. EUR/ICP/APR 113. Copenhagen.

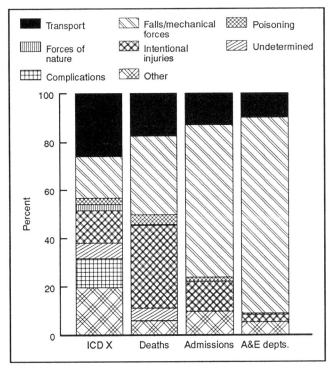

Figure 1. Use and misue of the ICD

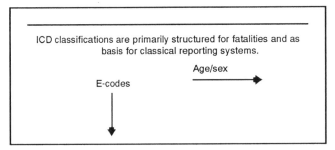

Figure 2.

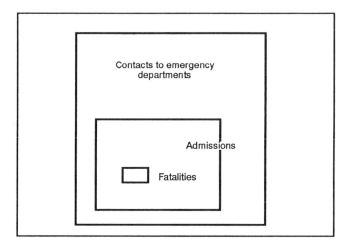

Figure 3. Casualties known to the hospital sector

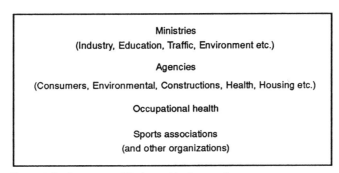

Figure 4. Sectors responsible for accident prevention

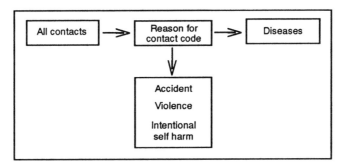

Figure 5. NOMESCO reason for contact code

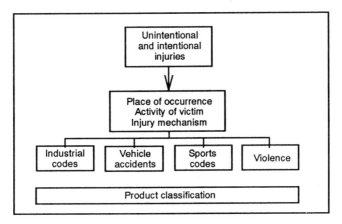

Figure 6. NOMESCO: the structure of the classification

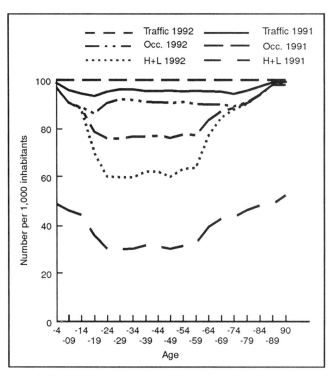

Figure 7. Emergency room contacts activity code 1991 and 1992

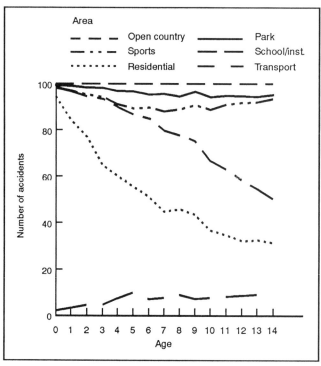

Figure 8. Home and leisure accidents children 0-14 years place of occurrence

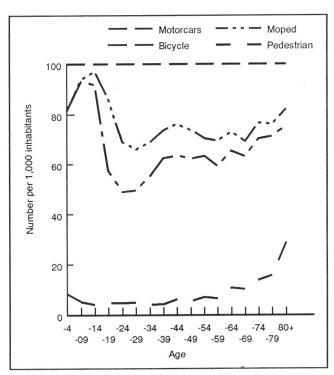

Figure 9. Emergency room contacts vehicle accidents

	ICD-10	NOMESCO
	Girl, 3 years, *fell* off mother's *bicycle* or *path* in *residential area*	
V18	Pedal cyclist injured in noncollision transport accident	Residential area (path – nontraffic)
V18.1	Passenger injured in nontraffic accident	Fall Bicycle Single accident Passenger

Figure 10. Case story

Use of Narrative Text Fields in Occupational Injury Data

by Nancy Stout, Ed.D. and E. Lynn Jenkins, M.A.

Surveillance data on occupational injuries and deaths are frequently analyzed in order to identify high–risk worker populations, characterize injury circumstances, and determine potential risk factors. Results drive injury prevention efforts at the national, state and local levels, and impact legislation and regulatory policy. The inclusion of narrative fields in injury surveillance data allow for identification of specific hazards and injury incidents. NIOSH maintains several surveillance systems that include narrative fields.

Analyses of these narrative entries, through computerized key–word searches and manual review, has allowed us to go beyond the limits of coded data to better understand specific circumstances and risks.
NIOSH's primary system for surveillance of fatal occupational injuries is the National Traumatic Occupational Fatalities System, or NTOF. NTOF is comprised of information from death certificates for people who die from injuries at work. Death certificates are provided by all 50 states for cases that meet these criteria: age 16 years or older, external cause of death (E800–E999), and a positive response to the "injury at work?" item. The NTOF database contains data on fatal occupational injuries since 1980.

We recently released a publication: "Fatal Injuries to Workers in the United States, 1980–1989: A Decade of Surveillance", that Dr. Satcher described, which provides an overview of the NTOF surveillance system and contains both national and state–specific analyses of worker deaths for the decade of the 1980s.

We frequently use NTOF data to respond to requests for information, from within CDC as well as from other federal organizations, states, and the public. In the U.S. there are two agencies that share responsibility for occupational safety and health: NIOSH is a research organization that conducts research, assesses risk, and develops prevention efforts, while the Occupational Safety and Health Administration, or OSHA, is a regulatory agency that develops and enforces occupational safety and health regulations. NIOSH frequently provides data and testimony to OSHA when they are proposing new rulemaking for occupational safety. This is important to us because this is one of the most effective ways we can implement our findings to shape national policy to prevent occupational injuries.

One reason NTOF is so useful is that it contains narrative data that allow us to examine detail that is not typically available, because most databases consist solely of coded data. NTOF contains narrative entries for industry, occupation, an injury description, and immediate, underlying and contributory causes of death. To demonstrate the value of these narrative data, I would like to describe some examples of analyses of narrative injury data that have impacted national programs or policies.

First, OSHA requested data pertaining to their proposed rule for confined space entry. Deaths in confined spaces are not limited to an industry or occupation group, nor are they specific to one cause of death, so they are difficult to identify in any surveillance data, and impossible if the data are all coded.

With NTOF, we were able to first select E–Codes that could potentially be confined space–related deaths (e.g., suffocation, poisoning). This narrowed the data to about 2000 cases for a 6–year period. Then we reviewed the injury description narratives to confirm deaths in confined spaces (758 cases for 1980–1985). The narrative information is not always detailed or specific enough to identify all such deaths, but we were able to determine that at least 126 deaths a year occurred in confined spaces, and were able to further analyze this subset to identify characteristics of these victims. For example, they were most frequently employed in construction or mining, and the leading causes of death were mechanical suffocation, poisoning by gas, explosion, and drowning. OSHA used these data to help justify the need for and determine the specifications for the recently enacted OSHA confined space safe–entry procedures.

In developing the Agricultural Initiative in 1989, the U.S. Congress requested data illustrating the major occupational safety hazards related to agricultural machinery. We knew from previous narrative data analysis that tractors were the leading cause of death, and we knew from literature and from working with the data that tractor roll–overs were a major problem, but that had not been documented or quantified at the national level. Again we turned to the narrative data.

We first selected cases with E–codes for agricultural machines, then we did a keyword search for the word "tractor" (which is not a unique E–code). Finally, we manually reviewed the injury descriptions. We were able to document that tractors accounted for 69 percent of all agricultural machinery–related deaths (1523 cases), and that 52 percent of these resulted from roll–overs and 16 percent were run–overs. Funding was allocated for several injury prevention programs as a result of these findings.

Incidentally, in another analysis of narrative data we discovered that many tractor incidents are missed by limiting analysis to the E–code for agricultural machines, because according to ICD–9 rules, tractors are correctly coded as motor vehicles if they are on a public roadway under their own power.

Another example is an OSHA request for data on fatalities to line clearance tree trimmers for testimony pertaining to standards for protective equipment for the electrical power industry. Tree trimmers can be coded into a number of different occupation categories (linemen, gardeners, laborer, etc.) so they cannot be identified by occupation codes. To identify tree trimmers in NTOF, we did a keyword search of the occupation, industry, and injury description fields for terms such as tree trimmer, arborist, and tree surgeon. We found 127 cases for 1980–1985. We were able to document that at least 21 tree trimmers were killed on the job each year, and that 41 percent were electrocutions, and 33 percent were fatal falls. Also, all but one were males and two–thirds were less than 35 years old. Again, these findings helped shape national occupational safety regulatory policy that recently went into effect. NIOSH also published an Alert on this topic to warn workers of the magnitude of this problem and the hazards they face from electrocution as well as from falls.

A few years ago, several deaths were brought to our attention of farmers who had entered their manure pits and been overcome and died from methane gas asphyxia. Tragically, other family members and co–workers also died in rescue attempts. We realized that we needed to alert the public of deaths due to methane asphyxia in manure pits on farms. Although we had investigated a few cases, we wanted to try to determine the national magnitude of this problem. So we subset potential cases from the NTOF data by appropriate E–codes, such as suffocation and poisoning, which narrowed us to 2000 cases, then we manually reviewed the injury descriptions to confirm cases that occurred in manure pits.

Although death certificates do not always contain enough detail to identify all cases, we did find that at least 16 people died from asphyxia in manure pits, and that 5 episodes resulted in multiple deaths from rescue attempts. We published an MMWR article on this and issued an Alert. Incidentally, we recently got a phone call from a farmer who was getting ready to go into his manure pit to fix something and he remembered seeing our publication. He called us to ask what he should do to stay alive when he went into his pit. We were able to appropriately advise him, and were pleased that our information is reaching those at risk.

Another OSHA request for information on hazards in the logging industry resulted in this analysis of narrative data. We selected cases coded as logging industry and examined the distribution of cause of death. After finding that a large proportion of cases were due to machines, we selected cases coded to the machinery E–code and reviewed the injury descriptions to better understand the circumstances of these deaths. We found that almost half of the machinery–related deaths in logging were the result of roll–overs. We had previously determined that the leading cause of death in this industry—struck by falling objects—was largely due to falling trees and logs. While that is not so surprising, we also found that of ALL worker deaths E–coded as being struck by falling objects, in all industries, 30 percent are from trees alone. Again, we could not have learned any of this from coded data. Without the narrative data, we would not have a clue as to what falling objects were killing workers or how we could attempt to prevent these deaths.

We also used narrative data to identify and understand worker deaths caused by falls from suspension scaffolds, to examine deaths from trench cave–ins, from falls through skylights and roof openings, deaths from forklift trucks, from electrocutions during work with scaffolds near overhead power lines, from entanglements with hay bailers that resulted in scalpings, and from homicides of convenience store workers. We published Alerts on many of these topics, using these NTOF analyses in support of other data and information, to request assistance in preventing these deaths.

These are just a few examples of the uses and value of narrative data. None of these analyses would have been possible with coded data, as none of these cases are identifiable through E–codes or other coded data alone. The narrative information, particularly injury description, allow us to go beyond the limits of coded data to drive NIOSH research and initiatives as well as national regulatory policy, to prevent worker deaths.

We also want to emphasize the value of E–codes in addition to narrative data. In many of these examples the E–codes allowed us to subset a large database to a manageable number of cases for manual review or to determine which words to use in keyword searches. Without this ability, many cases may be missed. Also, to determine overall distributions of cases, such as identifying the leading causes of death or conducting international comparisons, coded data are essential. Unfortunately, this may be why databases that lack E–codes are under–utilized. Both coded and narrative data are valuable in injury surveillance efforts.

Another value of narrative data is the ability to code or recode variables to alternative coding schemes. For example, there are three US standard coding schemes for occupation, two for industry, and three for injury circumstances, as well as numerous schemes unique to agencies or other nations. Most schemes are not comparable, and data coded to one cannot be directly converted to another. This prohibits comparisons between databases, particularly international comparisons. It also often prevents the computation of rates, if denominator and numerator databases are coded to different schemes (which is frequently the case in the U.S.).

Coding schemes also change periodically. U.S. employment codes generally change every decade, and even internationally standardized codes such as the ICD are periodically modified. When surveillance systems convert to a new code structure, the ability to monitor trends over time is often lost. Narrative data can be recoded to provide comparability of data between systems, years, and countries.

There have been a number of efforts in recent years to develop software that automatically codes narrative data into numeric codes. Dr. Rosenberg described NCHS efforts in developing and improving software that codes cause of death. There is currently a collaborative effort underway in the U.S., between NIOSH, NCHS, and several other organizations, to develop intelligent software that will automatically code occupation and industry narratives into standard numeric codes. Similar efforts have also taken place in other countries and have been applied to other variables. Information about various coding software has not been assimilated, to my knowledge, and this may be another area for this International Collaborative Effort to address. It would certainly be valuable to coordinate and integrate these coding programs. Automated coding software makes it easier, less expensive, and more reliable to automate narrative data than to code variables prior to automation. Narrative data not only provide valuable detail, but also provide the flexibility to adapt existing data to changes and future needs.

References

1. Castillo, DN, Landen, DD, Layne, LA. 1994. Occupational Injury Deaths of 16– and 17–year–olds in the United States. American Journal of Public Health, 1994:84.

2. Etherton, JR, Myers, JR. 1990. The use of rollover protection on farm tractors in West Virginia. B.Das ed., Advances in Industrial Ergonomics and Safety II, Taylor and Francis, Philadelphia, PA. pp. 819–825.

3. Etherton, JR, Myers, JR, Jensen, RC, Russell. JC, Braddee, RW. 1991. Agricultural machine–related deaths. Amer. Jour. Pub. Hlth. 81(6):766–768.

4. Fosbroke, DE, Myers, JR. 1994. Logging fatalities in the United States by region, cause of death, and other factors—1980 through 1988. Journal of Safety Research, 25(2).

5. Jenkins, EL, Hard, DL. 1992. Implications for the use of E–codes of the International Classification of Diseases and narrative data in identifying tractor–related deaths in agriculture, United States, 1980—1986. Scand J Work Environ Health, 92(18) Suppl 2:49—50.

6. Myers, JR, Casini, VJ. 1989. Fatalities attributed to methane asphyxia in manure pits—Ohio,Michigan, 1989. Centers for Disease Control. Mortality and Morbidity Weekly, 38(33):583–586.

7. Myers, JR, Fosbroke, DE. Logging fatalities in the United States by region, cause of death, and other factors—1980 through 1988. Accepted for publication by the Journal of Safety Research, November 2, 1993.

8. Roerig, S, Melius, J, Casini, VJ, Myers, JR, Snyder, KA. 1992. Scalping incidents involving hale balers – New York. Centers for Disease Control. Mortality and Morbidity Weekly Report, 41:27:489–491.

9. Snyder, KA, Bobick, TG, Hanz, JL, and Myers, JR. 1992. Grain–handling fatalities in production agriculture, 1985–1989. In: American Society of Agricultural Engineers 1992 International Winter Meeting. December 15–18, 1992, Nashville, TN. Paper No. 92–5509.

10. Stout, N, Frommer, MS, Harrison, J. 1990. Comparison of work–related fatality surveillance in the U.S.A. and Australia. Journal of Occupational Accidents, 90(13):195–211.

11. Stout–Wiegand, N. 1987. Characteristics of Work–related Injuries Involving Forklift Trucks. Journal of Safety Research, 87(18):179–190.

12. U.S. Department of Health and Human Services. 1989. NIOSH Alert: Preventing Worker Deaths and Injuries from Falls through Skylights and Roof Openings. DHHS (NIOSH) Publication No. 90–100.

13. U.S. Department of Health and Human Services. 1990. NIOSH Alert: Request for Assistance in Preventing Deaths of Farm Workers in Manure Pits. DHHS (NIOSH) Publication No. 90–103.

14. U.S. Department of Health and Human Services. 1992. NIOSH Alert: Request for Assistance in Preventing Falls and Electrocutions During Tree Trimming. DHHS (NIOSH) Publication No. 92–106.

15. U.S. Department of Health and Human Services. 1992. NIOSH Alert: Request for Assistance in Preventing Worker Injuries and Deaths Caused by Falls From Suspension Scaffolds. DHHS (NIOSH) publication No. 92–108.

16. U.S. Department of Health and Human Services. 1994. Worker Deaths in Confined Spaces: A Summary of NIOSH Surveillance and Investigative Findings. DHHS (NIOSH) Publication No. 94–103.

17. U.S. Department of Health and Human Services. 1993. NIOSH Alert: Request for Assistance in Preventing Homicide in the Workplace. DHHS (NIOSH) Publication No. 93–109.

Assessing and Improving the Quality of Data From Medical Examiners and Coroners

by Gib Parrish, M.D.

Background

Medical examiners and coroners (ME/C) investigate and certify approximately 400,000 (20 percent) of the two million deaths that occur annually in the United States, including virtually all homicides and suicides and most deaths related to unintentional injuries (Table 1).[1] To gather information about the cause, manner, and circumstances of investigated deaths, ME/Cs conduct scene investigations, autopsies, and toxicological tests in many, though not all, of these investigations (Table 2). As a result, data collected by ME/Cs are a valuable source of information on deaths due to injuries. They are used by researchers to conduct epidemiologic studies of these deaths and by government agencies, including the U.S. Departments of Health and Human Services, Labor, and Transportation, to monitor trends and patterns of injury–related mortality (Table 3). Because of the usefulness of data collected by ME/Cs, considerable recent effort has been expended to assess and, when necessary, to improve the quality of these data. This effort has addressed three aspects of the quality of ME/C data: 1) the completeness of reporting to ME/Cs of deaths that fall under their legal jurisdiction; 2) the quality of the investigation of reported deaths; and 3) the quality, completeness, and usefulness of the data recorded–either manually or electronically–about investigated deaths.

Completeness of Reporting

Most studies of the completeness of reporting of injury–related deaths to ME/Cs have relied on linking computerized state or federal vital records data files with ME/C data files and subsequently assessing the overlap of the two data sources for specific causes of death. Recent studies of this type have addressed head and neck injury,[2] occupational injury,[2,3] disaster–related injury, child abuse, and carbon monoxide poisoning. Some of these studies have also assessed the availability and comparability of information contained in ME/C records with that contained in automated vital records files. One recent study in Iowa by Dijkhuis et al., linked ME/C records with vital records for all injury–related deaths and found that age, cause, manner, and county of death were strong predictors of whether a particular death was reported to and investigated by a ME in Iowa.[2] The 1993 National Mortality Follow–back Survey currently being conducted by the National Center for Health Statistics will assess the completeness of the reporting of deaths to ME/Cs, as well as the comparability of ME/C data with the data contained on the death certificate, for a nationally representative sample of injury–related and non–injury–related deaths.

Quality of Investigations

Wide variation exists in the quality and extent of the investigation of deaths reported to ME/Cs (Table 4). This variation is partly due to the existence of approximately 2,200 separate death investigation jurisdictions in the United States.[1] The lack of standardized methods for investigating deaths, the lack of adequate training for many ME/Cs and other death investigators, and the lack of adequate resources for conducting investigations add further to this variation.[2] Assessments of the quality and extent of investigations have primarily relied on process measures, such as the autopsy rates in different jurisdictions. For example, Pollock et al., found that autopsy rates in 1989 for deaths due to nonhomicidal blunt and penetrating trauma–deaths typically investigated by ME/Cs–ranged from 10 percent in Oklahoma to 95 percent in Hawaii and were higher in metropolitan (58.2 percent) than in nonmetropolitan (29.9 percent) counties. Furthermore, rates for blunt and penetrating trauma (homicidal and nonhomicidal combined) were higher in jurisdictions served by medical examiners (63.9 percent) than in those served by coroners (52.3 percent).[3]

To improve the quality of death investigations, the American Academy of Forensic Sciences has developed model guidelines for investigating deaths;[4] the National Association of Medical Examiners has developed an inspection and accreditation program for ME/C offices;[5] seven states now require specific training for their coroners;[1,6] several states have developed training materials, including investigation manuals, to aid their ME/Cs; and at least five academic centers offer short–term, continuing education courses in death investigation.[3] Other efforts to improve the quality of death investigation, including the passage of legislation in almost half of the states to establish programs to review childhood fatalities due to injuries and other causes, are currently being planned or implemented.[7]

Quality and Usefulness of Data

The quality and completeness of the data recorded–either manually or electronically–for investigated deaths has also received attention (Table 5). Two recent surveys of ME/C offices have assessed the extent and nature of the automation of their death investigation and administrative data.[8,9] These surveys found that data collection and storage methods vary tremendously for different ME/C jurisdictions. Some jurisdictions lack any record–keeping system, whereas others have detailed, computerized, high–quality records that are maintained by staff specifically hired to manage their jurisdiction's information system. For those offices that have computerized their records, the amount of data on each case varies widely, from offices that automate only basic demographic and cause–of–death information to those with extensive information on each case, including a detailed, narrative description of the circumstances of death and the quantitative results of post–mortem toxicological tests. In most states, the lack of centralized data collection and storage hampers wider use of ME/C data.

To assist in the effort to improve the quality, completeness, and use of data collected by ME/C offices, the Centers for Disease Control and Prevention established the Medical Examiner/Coroner Information Sharing Program (MECISP) in 1987. MECISP has 1) developed guidelines for collecting data, including model death investigation forms and a model data set–the Death Investigation Data Set or "DIDS";[4] 2) provided on–site consultation on information management to more than 20 large ME/C offices; 3) provided financial resources to assist offices in upgrading their information management systems; and 4) facilitated the analysis and use of data from 16 ME/C offices.

Conclusions and Recommendations

The investigations performed by medical examiners and coroners are potentially the best source of data on injury–related mortality, and most other sources of data on injury–related mortality are based on information obtained during these investigations. Nevertheless, major logistical and resource barriers to improved quality and optimal use of data from ME/C offices remain. To overcome these barriers, the public and those responsible for making public health and public safety policy at the local, state, and federal levels need to recognize the importance of high–quality death investigations and the data derived from them and to provide the resources necessary to continue and expand efforts at improving the completeness of reporting, the quality of investigation, and the quality of data (Table 6). Federal programs that work with ME/C offices or that use their data need better coordination to ensure that available federal resources produce the greatest benefit. Since resources are limited, initial federal efforts should focus on statewide medical examiner systems and on populous metropolitan counties in order to maximize population coverage and to minimize administrative and other program costs. States without statewide death investigation systems can increase the usefulness of ME/C from their county–based jurisdictions by centrally collecting data from these jurisdictions. Local, state, and federal programs that monitor or study injury–related mortality should consider the benefits of placing staff and resources directly in ME/C offices, where the investigations are conducted and the data collected. Finally, since any source of data has both its strengths and weaknesses, ME/C data should be used in conjunction with other data sources, such as vital records, to provide the most complete and accurate picture of injury–related mortality.

Table 1. Deaths Investigated by Medical Examiners and Coroners

- Homicides
- Suicides
- Accidental traumatic deaths (e.g., falls, burns, drownings)
- Deaths caused by drugs or toxic agents
- Deaths caused by agents that threaten public health
- Deaths that occur during employment
- Deaths that occur while a person is in custody or confinement
- Sudden, unexplained deaths

Table 2. Components of Death Investigation

- Report of death to ME/C
- Determination of circumstances of death
- Scene investigation
- Post–mortem examination
    - external exam
    - autopsy
    - laboratory tests (e.g., the presence of alcohol, drugs)
- Certification of cause and manner of death
- Report of findings to interested parties
- Medicolegal testimony

Table 3. Examples of the Use of Data from Death Investigations

To monitor trends and patterns of injury–related mortality:

- State and local injury control programs
- Fatal Accident Reporting System for motor vehicle–related deaths
- Drug Abuse Warning Network for substance abuse–related deaths
- Medical Examiner Coroner Alert Project for consumer product–related deaths
- Census of Fatal Occupational Injuries for work–related deaths
- Violent Criminal Apprehension Program for serial homicides

To conduct epidemiologic studies of specific causes of death:

- Hypo– and hyperthermia
- Substance abuse
- Motor vehicle crashes

- Carbon monoxide poisoning
- Drowning
- Firearms
- Injuries while at work

Table 4. Quality of Death Investigations–Issues

- 2,200 separate death investigation jurisdictions in the United States
- Variety of organizational locations (e.g., law enforcement agencies, health departments)
- Lack of standardized methods for investigating deaths
- Lack of standardized definitions (e.g., manner, cause of death)
- Inadequate training for many ME/Cs and other death investigators
- Inadequate resources for conducting investigations

Table 5. Barriers to Quality and Completeness of Death Investigation Data

- Variety of data collection and management methods
  - Most ME/C offices not fully computerized
  - Variety of hardware and software systems
- Inadequate budget for information management
- Lack of staff trained in information management and analysis
- Records not centralized in many states
- Lack of coordinated data collection by federal agencies

Table 6. Recommendations

- Increase recognition of importance of high–quality death investigations and data
- Provide resources at local, state, and federal levels for improvements
- Improve coordination of federal programs to provide greatest benefit
- Focus efforts on statewide ME systems and large urban counties
- Encourage states to coordinate investigations and data collection
- Base surveillance and studies of injury–related mortality in ME/C offices
- Use ME/C data in conjunction with other sources of data

References

1. Combs DL, Parrish RG, Ing R. *Death investigation in the United States and Canada, 1992.* Atlanta: Centers for Disease Control, 1992.

2. Nelson DE, Sacks JJ, Sosin DM, McFeeley P, Smith SM. Sensitivity of multiple–cause mortality data for surveillance of deaths associated with head or neck injuries. *MMWR* 1993;42(SS–5):29–35.

3. Stout N, Bell C. Effectiveness of source documents for identifying fatal occupational injuries: a synthesis of studies. *Am J Public Health* 1991;81(6):725–728.

4. Bureau of Labor Statistics. *Fatal workplace injuries in 1991: a collection of data and analysis.* DL Report 845. Washington: Bureau of Labor Statistics, 1993:83.

5. Dijkhuis H, Zwerling C, Parrish G, Bennett, Kemper HCG. Medical examiner data in injury surveillance: a comparison with death certificates. *Am J Epidemiology* 1994;139(6):637–643.

6. Hanzlick R, Combs D, Parrish RG, Ing RT. Death investigation in the United States, 1990: A survey of statutes, systems, and educational requirements. *J Forensic Sci* 1993;38(3):628–632.

7. Pollock DA, O'Neil JM, Parrish RG, Combs DL, Annest JL. Temporal and geographic trends in the autopsy frequency of blunt and penetrating trauma deaths in the United States. *JAMA* 1993;269(12):1525–1531.

8. Lipskin BA, Field KS, editors. *Death investigation and examination: medicolegal guidelines and checklists.* Colorado Springs, CO: Forensic Sciences Foundation Press, 1984.

9. Bell JS, editor. *Standards for inspection and accreditation of a modern medicolegal investigative system.* St. Louis, MO: National Association of Medical Examiners, 1980.

10. American Academy of Forensic Sciences. *Academy News.* Colorado Springs: American Academy of Forensic Sciences, 1994 May;24(3).

11. Durfee M, Gellert GA, Tilton–Durfee D. Origins and clinical relevance of child death review teams. *JAMA* 1992;267(23):3172–3175.

12. Hanzlick RL. Automation of medical examiner offices. *Am J Forensic Med Pathol* 1993;14(1):34–38.

13. Parrish RG, Maes EF, Ing RT. Computerization of medical examiner and coroner offices: a national survey [Abstract]. In: *American Academy of Forensic Sciences Program, 1992 Annual Meeting.* Colorado Springs: American Academy of Forensic Sciences, 1992:152.

14. Hanzlick RL, Parrish RG. Death investigation report forms (DIRFs): Generic forms for investigators (IDIRFs) and certifiers (CDIRFs). *J Forensic Sci* 1994;39(3):629–636.

15. Baron RC, Thacker SB, Gorelkin L, Vernon AA, Taylor WR, Choi K. Sudden death among Southeast Asian refugees: an unexplained nocturnal phenomenon. *JAMA* 1983;250:2947–2951.

16. Berkelman RL, Herndon JL, Callaway JL, et al. Fatal injuries and alcohol. *Am J Prev Med* 1985;1(6):21–28.

17. Bern C, Lew J, McFeeley P, Ing D, Ing RT, Glass RI. Diarrheal deaths in children living in New Mexico: toward a strategy of preventive interventions. *Journal of Pediatrics.* 1993;122(6):920–922.

18. Blaser MJ, Jason JM, Weniger BG, Elsea WR, Finton RJ, Hanson RA, Feldman RA. Epidemiologic analysis of a cluster of homicides of children in Atlanta. *JAMA* 1984;251:3255–3258.

19. Brison RJ, Wicklund K, Mueller BA. Fatal pedestrian injuries to young children: a different pattern of injury. *Am J Public Health* 1988;78(7):793–795.

20. Bureau of Labor Statistics. *Fatal workplace injuries in 1991: a collection of data and analysis.* DL Report 845. Washington: Bureau of Labor Statistics, 1993.

21. Campbell S, Hood I, Ryan D, et al. Death as a result of asthma in Wayne County medical examiner cases, 1975–1987. *J Forensic Sci* 1990;35(2):356–364.

22. Centers for Disease Control. Sudden unexpected, nocturnal deaths among Southeast Asian refugees. *MMWR* 1981;30(47):581–584.

23. Centers for Disease Control. Sudden unexplained death syndrome in Southeast Asian refugees: a review of CDC surveillance. *MMWR* 1987;36(1SS):43SS–53SS.

24. Centers for Disease Control. Update: sudden unexplained death syndrome among Southeast Asian refugees – United States. *MMWR* 1988;37(37):568–570.

25. Centers for Disease Control. Earthquake–associated deaths – California. *MMWR* 1989;38:767–770.

26. Centers for Disease Control. Cyanide poisoning associated with over–the–counter medication – Washington State, 1991. *MMWR* 1991;40:161–168.

27. Centers for Disease Control. Preliminary report: medical examiner reports of deaths associated with hurricane Andrew—Florida, August 1992. *MMWR* 1992;41:641–644.

28. Centers for Disease Control. Outbreak of an acute illness—Southwestern United States, 1993. *MMWR* 1993;42:421–424.

29. Copeland AR. Suicide by jumping from buildings. *Am J Forensic Med Pathol* 1989;10(4):295–298.

30. Emerick SJ, Foster LR, Campbell DT. Risk factors for traumatic infant death in Oregon, 1973 to 1982. *Pediatrics* 1986;77(4):518–522.

31. Goodman RA, Mercy JA, Loya F, et al. Alcohol use and interpersonal violence: alcohol detected in homicide victims. *Am J Public Health* 1986;76(2):144–149.

32.   Goodman RA, Mercy JA, Rosenberg ML. Drug use and interpersonal violence. Barbiturates detected in homicide victims. *Am J Epidemiol* 1986;124(5):851–855.

33.   Hanzlick R, Parrish RG. Deaths among the homeless in Fulton County, Georgia, 1988–90. *Public Health Reports* 1993;108(4):488–491.

34.   Jones ST, Liang AP, Kilbourne EM, et al. Morbidity and mortality associated with the July 1980 heat wave in St. Louis and Kansas City, MO. *JAMA* 1982;247:3327–3331.

35.   Kellerman AL, Reay DT. Protection or peril? An analysis of firearm–related deaths in the home. *N Engl J Med* 1986;314(24):1557–1560.

36.   Kellerman AL, Rivara FP, Rushforth NB, et al. Gun ownership as a risk factor for homicide in the home. *N Engl J Med* 1993;329:1084–1091.

37.   Kellerman AL, Rivara FP, Somes G, et al. Suicide in the home in relation to gun ownership. *N Engl J Med* 1992;327:467–72.

38.   Kirschner RH, Eckner FAO, Baron RC. The cardiac pathology of sudden, unexplained nocturnal death in Southeast Asian refugees. *JAMA* 1986;256:2700–2705.

39.   MayoSmith MF, Hirsch PJ, Wodzinski SF, Schiffman FJ. Acute epiglottitis in adults. An eight–year experience in the state of Rhode Island. *N Engl J Med* 1986;314(18):1133–1139.

40.   Patetta MJ, Cole TB. A population–based descriptive study of housefire deaths in North Carolina. *Am J Public Health* 1990;80(9):1116–1117.

41.   Philen RM, Combs DL, Miller L, Sanderson LM, Parrish RG, Ing R. Hurricane Hugo–related deaths: South Carolina and Puerto Rico, 1989. *Disasters* 1992;16(1):53–59.

42.   Quan L, Gore EJ, Wentz K, et al. Ten–year study of pediatric drownings and near–drownings in King County, Washington: lessons in injury prevention. *Pediatrics* 1989;83(6):1035–1040.

43.   Robinson CC, Kuller LH, Perper J. An epidemiologic study of sudden death at work in an industrial county, 1979–1982. *Am J Epidemiology* 1988;128(4):806–820.

44.   Ruttenber JA, Luke JL. Heroin–related deaths: new epidemiologic insights. *Science* 1984;226:14–20.

45.   Schierer CL, Hood IC, Mirchandani HG. Atherosclerotic cardiovascular disease and sudden deaths among young adults in Wayne County. *Am J Forensic Med Pathol* 1990;11(3):198–201.

46.   Smith SM, Middaugh J. Injuries associated with three–wheeled all–terrain vehicles—Alaska, 1983–84. *JAMA* 1986;255:2454–2458.

47.   Sniezek JE, Horiagon TM. Medical–examiner–reported fatal occupational injuries, North Carolina, 1978–1984. *Am J Ind Med* 1989;15:669–678.

48.   Substance Abuse and Mental Health Services Administration. *Annual medical examiner data 1992*. DHHS Publication No. (SMA) 94–2081. Rockville: Substance Abuse and Mental Health Services Administration, 1994.

49.   University of California at Los Angeles, Centers for Disease Control*: The epidemiology of homicide in the city of Los Angeles, 1970–79*. DHHS, PHS, CDC, August 1985.

50.   Wintemute GJ, Kraus JF, Teret SP, et al. Ten–year study of pediatric drownings and near–drownings in King County, Washington: lessons in injury prevention. *Pediatrics* 1989;83(6):1035–1040.

51.   Bureau of Labor Statistics. *Fatal workplace injuries in 1992: a collection of data and analysis*. Washington, DC. 1994 U.S. Department of Labor, Report 870: page 83.

52.   Centers for Disease Control. Enumerating deaths among homeless persons: a comparison of medical examiner and shelter records. *MMWR* 1993;42(37):719–726.

53.   Conroy C, Russell JC. Medical examiner/coroner records: uses and limitations in occupational injury epidemiologic research. *J Forensic Sci* 1990;35(4):932–937.

54.   Cragle D, Fletcher A. Risk factors associated with the classification of unspecified and/or unexplained causes of death in an occupational cohort. *Am J Public Health* 1992;82:455–457.

55.   Dijkhuis H, Zwerling C, Parrish G, Bennett, Kemper HCG. Medical examiner data in injury surveillance: a comparison with death certificates. *Am J Epidemiology* 1994;139(6):637–643.

56.   Forensic Sciences Foundation (Lipskin BA, Field KS, editors). *Death investigation and examination: Medicolegal guidelines and checklists*. Colorado Springs, CO: Forensic Sciences Foundation Press; 1984.

57.   Goodman RA, Herndon JL, Istre GR, et al. Fatal injuries in Oklahoma: descriptive epidemiology using medical examiner data. *South Med J* 1989;82(9):1128–1134.

58.   Goodman RA, Istre GR, Jordan FB, Herndon JL, Kelaghan J. Alcohol and fatal injuries in Oklahoma. *Journal of Studies on Alcohol* 1991;52:156–161.

59.   Graitcer PL, Williams WW, Finton RJ, Goodman RA, Thacker SB, Hanzlick R. An evaluation of the use of medical examiner data for epidemiologic surveillance. *Am J Public Health* 1987;77(9):1212–1214.

60.   Hanzlick RL. BLURBs. A coding scheme for toxicologic data. *Am J Forensic Med Pathol* 1993;14(1):31–33.

61.   Hanzlick R. Survey of medical examiner office computerization. *Am J Forensic Med and Path* 1994;15(2):110–117.

62.   Hanzlick RL, Parrish RG. Death investigation report forms (DIRFs): Generic forms for investigators (IDIRFs) and certifiers (CDIRFs). *J Forensic Sci* 1994;39(3):629–636.

63. Hanzlick RL, Parrish RG, Ing R. Features of commercial computer software systems for medical examiners and coroners. *Am J Forensic Med and Path* 1993;14(4):334–339.

64. Jobes DA, Berman AL, Josselson AR. The impact of psychological autopsies on medical examiners' determination of manner of death. *J Forensic Sci* 1986;31(1):177–189.

65. National Association of Medical Examiners (Bell JS, editor). *Standards for inspection and accreditation of a modern medicolegal investigative system.* St. Louis, MO: National Association of Medical Examiners; 1980.

66. Nelson DE, Sacks JJ, Sosin DM, McFeeley P, Smith SM. Sensitivity of multiple–cause mortality data for surveillance of deaths associated with head or neck injuries. *MMWR* 1993;42(SS–5):29–35.

67. Smith SM, Goodman RA, Thacker SB, et al. Alcohol and fatal injuries: temporal patterns. *Am J Prev Med* 1989; 5(5):296–302.

68. Smith SM, Middaugh J. An assessment of potential injury surveillance data sources in Alaska using an emerging problem: all–terrain vehicle associated injuries. *Public Health Reports* 1989;104:493–498.

69. Soslow AR, Woolf AD. Reliability of data sources for poisoning deaths in Massachusetts. *Am J Emerg Med* 1992;10:124–127.

70. Stout N, Bell C. Effectiveness of source documents for identifying fatal occupational injuries: a synthesis of studies. *Am J Public Health* 1991;81(6):725–728.

71. Centers for Disease Control. Autopsy frequency – United States, 1980–1985. MMWR 1988;37(12):191–194.

72. Centers for Disease Control. Death investigation – United States, 1987. *MMWR* 1988;38(1):1–4.

73. Combs DL, Parrish RG, Ing R. *Death investigation in the United States and Canada, 1992.* Atlanta: Centers for Disease Control, 1992.

74. Durfee M, Gellert GA, Tilton–Durfee D. Origins and clinical relevance of child death review teams. *JAMA* 1992;267(23):3172–3175.

75. Hanzlick RL. Automation of medical examiner offices. *Am J Forensic Med Pathol* 1993;14(1):34–38.

76. Hanzlick R, Parrish RG. The failure of death certificates to record the performance of autopsies [Letter]. *JAMA* 1993;269(1):47.

77. Hanzlick R, Combs D, Parrish RG, Ing RT. Death investigation in the United States, 1990: A survey of statutes, systems, and educational requirements. *J Forensic Sci* 1993;38(3):628–632.

73. Hanzlick RL, Parrish RG, Combs DL. Standard language in death investigation laws. *J Forensic Sci* 1994;39(3):637–643.

74.   Pollock DA, O'Neil JM, Parrish RG, Combs DL, Annest JL. Temporal and geographic trends in the autopsy frequency of blunt and penetrating trauma deaths in the United States. *JAMA* 1993;269(12):1525–1531.

Suicide Misclassification in an International Context

by Ian R.H. Rockett, Ph.D. and Gordon S. Smith, M.B., Ch.B., M.P.H.

Within the context of international research, data misclassification has been a persistent and contentious topic in the suicide literature.[1-8] Guiding this paper is the central question of whether official national suicide data are sufficiently reliable and valid to scientifically justify their use in international comparative studies. Are real differences and similarities in cross–national suicide rates obscured by artifactual differences? The paper moves from consideration of general potential sources of suicide misclassification to the presentation of techniques and data deemed useful in assessing the severity of the problem.

Manner of Death and Medicolegal Decision–Making

When an individual dies, the primary classification decision concerns whether manner of death can be appropriately attributed to **natural causes, accident, homicide** or **suicide**.* The great preponderance of deaths are attributed to natural causes, whether due to chronic or communicable disease. Natural causes accounted for between 85 and 97 percent of reported deaths in the 28 countries whose 1990 mortality data were accessible to the authors through the *World Health Statistics Annual* published by the World Health Organization (WHO) (Table 1).** With important implications for quality of cause–of–death reporting, this helps explain relatively low autopsy rates in many countries. The mean autopsy rate was 21 percent among 25 countries reporting this information to WHO, with a range of 4 to 49 percent.[9] All other things being equal, a low autopsy rate increases the likelihood that some suicides are misclassified under natural causes.

Results of a 1971 WHO survey provide insight into the process of suicide case ascertainment.[10] Normally, the train of decision–making concerning manner of death begins with a proximate physician. But when a suicide (or other unnatural death) is suspected, police are often the first authorities called to the scene. They play a key role in questioning relatives, nonrelative witnesses, as well as physicians connected to the case, and in locating notes or observing aspects of the scene indicative of suicide. Sometimes police are assisted directly in their interrogations by a coroner, medical examiner or ancillary personnel.

The WHO research indicates that practicing physicians involved in a possible suicide case rarely possess sole responsibility for ruling on manner of death. In fact, this decision is usually in the province of the public authorities: coroner, medical examiner, police or judiciary. A majority of countries responding to the survey possessed a coroner or medical examiner system or equivalent. While medical examiners are medically qualified, coroners may have law degrees, medical degrees or both. The decision to autopsy is usually made by a coroner or other legal representative of the State, but this may rest with police or local physicians. Autopsies are mostly performed by qualified pathologists. Suspected poisonings require a toxicological examination, which is often, but not invariably conducted in a dedicated forensic laboratory. Forensic medical training appears prominently featured in the qualifications of those charged with making a ruling, or contributing directly to a ruling, on possible suicides.

The WHO survey reveals that the level of appointment of persons serving as a coroner or medical examiner varies from the national through the state or provincial level to the local level. Those in the office may be full–time or

---

*Injury epidemiologists increasingly prefer to substitute the rubric **unintentional injury** for **accident** in order to nullify connotations of fatalism and implied unavoidability. But since **accident** is routinely used in classifying manner of death, and coding external cause of injury mortality under the *International Classification of Diseases* (ICD), it is retained for use in this paper. It seems noteworthy that the rubric **natural causes** also is routinely used in classifying manner of death, and that this use might well be counterproductive with regard to case ascertainment and prevention of premature mortality.

**For comparative purposes, the United States was added as the twenty-ninth country. The U.S. data pertain to 1989.

part–time, and supervised or unsupervised. In some countries, decisions concerning suicide can be amended on the death certificate in light of subsequent evidence. Some countries also reported probable suicides within their official national suicide statistics, while others did not or might not. This issue has since been resolved in ICD–8 with inclusion of injury codes for undetermined intent.

Determining the correct manner of death harbors important implications with respect to criminal liability, insurance payments, quality of mortality statistics, and the emotional well–being of survivors.[11] Deficient empirical evidence and the burden of proof appear to impel medicolegal authorities towards ruling an equivocal injury death an accident rather than as a suicide or homicide,[10] although the undetermined injury intent category would be the appropriate place for such a death. But burden of proof is more important in shaping the decision–making of coroners than that of medical examiners. The latter are more guided by the balance of probabilities, and hence are likely to be less conservative in their judgments. To illustrate these system differences, the procedure used in many states of the United States is contrasted with that of England. In American states with a medical examiner system, the medical examiner possesses sole authority to rule a death a suicide or not, based on the accessible evidence. In England, a formal judicial coroner's court makes the final determination based on testimony from a variety of sources, including forensic experts.

Impairing generalizability, responses to the WHO survey were received on behalf of only 26 countries. Nevertheless, this research does reveal diversity in medicolegal procedures and decision–making, which could be expected to generate artifactual cross–national variation in suicide reporting.

Complications of Method and Duration

Ability to detect suicide varies with the method used, and there is considerable international variation in terms of the distribution of methods among reported suicides.[12–14] In the absence of other evidence, violent methods of the order of hanging, shooting and stabbing make detection easier for medicolegal authorities than so–called nonviolent methods like drowning, poisoning and gassing.[7,15–18] These last three methods have been labeled equivocal, along with some others such as jumping from a height, lone driver vehicular crashes, and one form of shooting, Russian roulette.

Among suicides in which a rapidly lethal method was used, those by drowning seem most difficult to correctly discern, especially without witnesses. Toxicological evidence of a lethal overdose in an adult is suggestive of a suicidal poisoning, especially when the substances involved are not associated with abuse. This suggestion is based on the notion that an adult who overdoses, does so wittingly. However, the co–presence of alcohol and/or some other highly addictive psychoactive drug, when not the lethal agent, can cast doubts about intent. For drugs of abuse, it is especially difficult to determine intent because of the unknown and variable strength of many "street" drugs. Some adults also may truly be ignorant about the demarcation line between a safe dose and an overdose.

Slow suicides, those whose duration extends over several months or even years, seem rarely likely to be registered as suicides in any country.[19] Whether common or not, a suicidal decision by some individuals may lead to a protracted, tortuous and lethal trail of excessive use of alcohol and/or other psychoactive drugs, malnutrition or undernutrition, or some combination of wilful destructive behaviors. A more obvious, but probably still grossly underreported kind of slow suicide, is one that commences with an attempt, and ends months later in death from medical complications.

Individual Sociodemographic Characteristics

Heterogeneity across populations could have implications for artifactual differences in international suicide rates. Sociodemographic characteristics of suicide victims, for example, all possess potential for differential misclassification. This issue is illustrated here by reference to three such characteristics: age, sex and race.

With respect to age, elderly deaths are less thoroughly investigated than deaths in younger people. Older people are more likely to die from natural causes than younger people, which helps account for their lower autopsy rates.[9] Also, they are believed to be more prone to choose nonviolent methods of suicide, and slow methods like starvation or deliberate neglect of necessary personal medical attention and treatment.[19,20] In concert, these factors promote the expectation that the accuracy and completeness of suicide certification is less for the elderly than for their younger counterparts.

Recent data confirm the frequently reported finding that male suicide rates exceed corresponding female rates (Table 2). While this situation may well accurately portray the direction of observed national sex differences in suicide rates, differential misclassification may ensue from females being more inclined to choose nonviolent methods than are males.[12,13]

Warranting more intensive and extensive investigation is the relationship between race, ethnicity and differential suicide misclassification. Predictably, research conducted in the United States provides evidence of their connection.[21-23] In one example, a New York study, which focused on race and misclassification, published Health Department records of suicides were compared with the suicide records of the Medical Examiner (ME).[22] The ME records on suicides, serving as the gold standard in this study, included in addition to cases signed out to the Health Department, cases medically considered suicide, but not attaining the legal status, and cases overlooked by the Health Department because final disposition was not requested. Following the introduction of the injury with undetermined intent codes under ICD–8, black suicide cases were almost twice as likely to be underenumerated in Health Department records as white cases. One major explanation was the relatively high use by blacks of an equivocal suicide method, jumping. But in addition, case histories for blacks were less complete than those for whites. Unknown is whether racism and racial socioeconomic differences influenced the history taking.

While sociodemographic characteristics differentially relate to suicide underenumeration within a country, it seems probable that these differentials are less pronounced in some countries than others. Thus, adjusting international suicide rates for population composition may or may not ease problems with their use.

Sociocultural Milieu

The search for the meaning of suicides must extend beyond purely individual characteristics and circumstances to the sociocultural milieu in which these events occur. But like sociodemographic heterogeneity, sociocultural heterogeneity can be a source of artifactual differences in international suicide rates.

Religion is a sociocultural variable, which has received serious attention from suicidologists dating back to the work of the French sociologist, Emile Durkheim, in the nineteenth century.[24] A famous Durkheimian hypothesis is that adherents of religions or religious denominations, which foster a high degree of social integration, are less prone to suicide than counterparts whose religious affiliation encourages or is permissive towards individualism or the pursuit of free inquiry. The social integration argument was used by Durkheim to explain a lower reported suicide rate in Roman Catholic countries than in Protestant countries.

A plausible alternative explanation to that of Durkheim in accounting for international suicide rate differences, such as those still frequently reported between predominantly Roman Catholic and Protestant countries, is that these differences really reflect variation in the social condemnation of suicide and the reluctance of physicians to certify a death a suicide.[25] Proponents argue that suicide rates are actually socially constructed, and that the greater the social condemnation of suicide the more deficient the reporting. Whether the source is related to religion and/or other factors, social condemnation may induce suicide victims to disguise the intent of their acts. Moreover, it may similarly function to encourage family and friends, and sometimes even medicolegal authorities themselves, to withhold or suppress crucial evidence like a suicide note, or knowledge of behavior or conversation consistent with suicide ideation.

Assessing Reliability

Three empirical approaches are identified here, which have been employed by epidemiologists, to assess the reliability or precision of international suicide statistics. The first, labeled the experimental approach, is aimed at determining whether medicolegal officials differ in assigning manner of death in a common set of cases. In a blinded study, in which Danish and English officials made such assignments for a sample of each other's cases, differentials in reported suicide rates were attributed to variation in ascertainment procedures.[26] However, this finding was contradicted in a second study involving English and Scottish officials.[27] The discrepant results might be explained by the fact that in the latter study, cases being reviewed were not restricted to equivocal ones.

A second approach to the reliability question compares rankings of suicide rates of immigrants in a particular country with rate rankings in the countries of origin. Two studies, conducted in Australia (n=17)[28] (see, for example, Table 3) and the United States (n=11),[29] respectively, demonstrated a high degree of consistency between rankings. Rank–order correlation coefficients ranged between 0.8 and 0.9. Their findings induced the authors of both studies to conclude that cross–national differences in reported suicide rates were real, and not artifacts of variable case ascertainment procedures. These procedures were assumed to be consistent within countries; a weak assumption. All Australian states and territories possess a coroner system, but national reporting of suicide does not invariably depend upon it.[30] The medicolegal system in the United States is diverse and highly decentralized.[10] Immigrants in neither country are uniformly distributed geographically by ethnicity. In addition, there are examples of inconsistency in the rankings in the two studies, and the magnitude of rate differences may be affected by ascertainment procedures. These concerns have generated a third approach for addressing the reliability issue, known as rate reformulation.

With rate reformulation, cross–national comparisons are conducted using reported suicide rates, and rates combining suicide with other mortality categories thought prone to contain hidden suicides. A 22 nation mortality study, which involved a comparison of suicide rates with combined rates for suicide and injury of undetermined intent, produced a rank–order correlation coefficient of 0.89 ($p < .001$).[31] This coefficient rose to 0.95 with the removal of a single outlier, Chile. A second study, based on 19 European countries, adopted the same technique, excepting that accidental poisonings also were added to suicides and injury deaths of undetermined intent (Table 4).[6] The correlation coefficient of 0.96 ($p < 0.001$) reflected highly congruent rankings. Thus, expanding the suicide category to allow for possible misclassification under other injury categories did not appreciably alter the rankings reported for the suicide rates alone.

Besides epidemiologists, sociologists are the other main utilizers of international suicide statistics for research purposes. Sociological interest is driven primarily by the quest for understanding social causation; by the search for macro–explanations of cross–national rate variation, such as the roles of industrialization, urbanization, and religion.[32] The groundwork for a fourth approach for assessing the reliability of international suicide data is evident in an innovative sociological study.[33] Taking official county–level suicide rates as the dependent variable, its authors performed a two–step multivariate analysis using both putative social causation factors, and a set of social construction factors as predictors. The latter variables are explicitly incorporated into their model in order to determine if systematic misreporting renders official suicide data useless for testing social causation theories. These variables are the type of system charged with classifying manner of death, procedures for selecting medicolegal officials, and nature of facilities accessible to these officials over the course of an investigation. The authors conclude that while systematic misreporting occurs, it exerts a minor impact on the "explanatory" power of social construction predictors of suicide rates. Their study was limited to a single country, albeit an extremely diverse one, the United States. It has been criticized for a number of deficiencies, including the omission of age as a covariate, and the failure to examine differences between suicide certifications made by coroners and medical examiners, respectively.[17] But despite deficiencies, there is a need to apply its research question and methodology to the international arena.

On balance, to the extent that they are representative, the findings reported from the preceding studies give reason for confidence that international suicide data are adequate for scientific purposes from the standpoint of spatial reliability. Temporal reliability does not appear problematic either. The introduction of the undetermined injury intent category under ICD–8 had potentially important implications for allocating equivocal injury deaths. But research conducted in the United States and Australia suggests that any associated artifactual suicide rate changes at the national level are small.[34,35] However, as the ensuing sections demonstrate, the validity of international suicide data is much more difficult to dismiss as a scientific concern.

Assessing Validity

Borrowing from the language of disease screening, the validity of suicide data can be examined from the complementary perspectives of sensitivity and specificity. Sensitivity measures the degree to which suicides are correctly certified. Specificity is the equivalent measure for nonsuicides. Since suicide tends not to be overenumerated, the specificity of suicide certification should not be problematic for international research. Specificity is inferred to reach or approach 100 percent.[36]

With considerable cross–national variation, the sensitivity of suicide certification falls well short of the high standard established for specificity. This is due to the interplay of forces already identified, such as sociodemographic characteristics of suicide victims, choice of method and duration of event, prevailing sociocultural milieu, and nature and training of medicolegal decision–makers and auxiliary staff. A range for sensitivity estimates has been reported of 26 percent and 83 percent, with estimates concentrating between 56 percent and 71 percent.[36] However, these figures are probably inflated due to the difficulty in obtaining a suitable gold standard, such as ME/coroner records which incorporate psychological autopsies. Moreover, the more developed countries predominate among countries upon whose data these estimates derive. Primarily due to a lack of economic resources and appropriately trained personnel, sensitivity estimates for the less developed countries should be closer to the lower end of the specified sensitivity range than to the upper limit.

Three external cause categories are considered prime contenders for containing misclassified suicides. They are accidental poisoning (ICD–9 E850–869), accidental drowning (E910), and injury of undetermined intent (E980–989). The mortality ratio of the combined death rate for these combined categories to the suicide rate is a guide in estimating theoretical upper limits for various national suicide rates. Figure 1 draws attention to this potential in 29 countries whose mortality data were accessed for this paper. The degree of potential suicide misclassification varies directly with the magnitude of the ratio. Other violence (E980–999), which includes war–related injury, is used for computing the ratio in lieu of being able to extricate injury of undetermined intent. However, the former is generally believed to have been of no or minor consequence for mortality in the reporting countries in the observation year.

The ratio of the rates for the selected combined injury categories to suicide reveal a range extending from 0.1 for Austria to 4.1 for Mexico. Thus, in the implausible scenario that all of the combined injury deaths are misclassified suicides, reclassification would only increase the Austrian suicide rate by 10 percent. At the other extreme, the Mexican rate would increase more than four–fold. Other nations exhibiting potential for a high degree of suicide misclassification include Malta, Portugal and a number of Eastern European countries. Examining potential misclassification by suicide method for these countries would be interesting, but is not possible on the basis of the published WHO mortality data.

Figure 2 displays a second set of ratios, which provide for highly liberal upper limits for suicide rates. These ratios incorporate another possible source of misclassified suicides, the residual natural cause mortality category of symptoms, signs and ill–defined conditions (ICD–9 780–799).[37] In this instance, the range extends from 0.2 for Austria and Hungary to 16.8 for Greece.

Computing and examining ratios of the type presented above would be useful in selecting countries for an international suicide study, in a way which would minimize concerns with validity and be consistent with the need for fair comparisons. Artifactual differences in cross–national suicide rates will not necessarily invalidate conclusions based on observed trends. But the selection process should make allowance for major differentials in potential suicide misclassification.

Drowning and Elderly Japanese Females[***]

Through reference to routinely published WHO mortality data, the preceding section illustrates the potential, in gross terms, for undercounting suicide in 29 selected countries. As previously stated, WHO does not report suicide data disaggregated by method. Yet the distribution of suicide methods varies cross–nationally, and this has important implications for differential misclassification. A case for this being a viable issue is proposed by means of a hypothesis concerning one nonviolent and equivocal method of suicide in one sub–population, elderly Japanese females. The method is drowning, which like **harikari** or self–disembowelment, has attained major symbolic importance in Japan.[38] Elderly are operationalized here as persons 65 years and older, and the observation period is the 1979–81 triennium.

Elderly Japanese of both sexes register comparatively high suicide rates within and across populations, and the male rates exceed those of females.[39] In a comparison involving the populations of Japan and seven other countries, all known for ease of water access, elderly Japanese also manifested a clear excess risk of accidental drowning (Table 5). Whereas only one in 24 Japanese male suicides was attributed to drowning, the proportion among female suicides was one in eight (Table 6). In the adjacent age groups, 65–74 years and 75 and older, female drowning suicide rates were two–and–a–half times those of corresponding male rates (Figure 3).

It is hypothesized that suicide of elderly females is relatively underenumerated due to misclassification of suicidal drowning as accidental drowning. At the core of this hypothesis is the finding that between ages 25–34 and 75 and older, the ratio of drowning suicides to accidental drownings declined by 81 percent for females as compared with only 49 percent for males (Figure 4). Moreover, the ratio was 5:1 at ages 25–34, while always below parity for males. The differential ratio decline might simply result from age–sex variation in exposure to, and proficiency in water. This does not seem particularly plausible, and has not been demonstrated. A Japanese national study found that less than 10 percent of elderly accidental drownings had witnesses.[40] By contrast, one–third of those in the 15–64 age group was witnessed.

Two arguments are proposed, in addition to the nature of the ratio shift, which reinforce the drowning suicide misclassification hypothesis. First, Japanese females hold a six year advantage over males in life expectancy at birth, and are at much greater risk of being widowed, and living alone.[41] These differences reduce the likelihood that older female victims of suicide, irrespective of method, will have survivors well situated to assist medicolegal authorities in their investigation and deliberations. In 1985, for example, 70 percent of 75–79 year old females were widowed as compared with 20 percent of corresponding males. Furthermore, between 1970 and 1985 the percentage of females from the 1900–04 birth cohort, living separately from their families, rose from 9.6 to 19.3. Further emphasizing this trend of increasing isolation are results from surveys of wives of childbearing age conducted by the *Mainichi Shimbun*, a leading Japanese newspaper.[41] In 1950, 55 percent of responders planned to be dependent upon their children in old age. This percentage decreased to 18 in 1988. With similar implications for the living arrangements of the elderly, 75 percent of responders in 1963 regarded personal care of aged parents as normal, compared with 63 percent in 1988.

The second argument for suspecting relative underenumeration of elderly female suicide in Japan revolves around persisting sex roles and changing attitudes to suicide in the social, cultural, political and economic metamorphosis characterizing the post–World War II era. Traditionally an acceptable, and even honorable manner of death,[2,24] suicide is much less so in contemporary Japan.[42] But the formative years of Japanese, designated elderly in the period 1979–81, preceded both the United States' occupation and the revolution in global communications. Therefore, this sub–population might well have retained a traditional view of suicide being an appropriate means for terminating life. However, since Japan has remained a male–dominated society,[41,43,44] elderly females may be more inclined than elderly males to disguise their suicides in order to protect their families against social stigmatization.

[***]The material presented in this section is drawn from a previously published source: Rockett IRH, Smith GS. Covert suicide among elderly Japanese females: questioning unintentional drownings. *Social Science and Medicine* 36(11); 1993: 1467-1472.

Japan has the longest population life expectancy at birth in the world, among the highest living standards, historically positive attitudes towards suicide, and a relatively ethnically and racially homogeneous population. These factors are all conducive to comprehensive and accurate suicide registration. But the evidence presented here, as a rationale for the drowning suicide hypothesis, suggests that Japan is not immune to problems with the sensitivity of suicide certification; at least among the group at highest reported risk of suicide, the elderly. The drowning suicide misclassification hypothesis needs testing at the level of prefectures, the local level. If substantiated, it further underscores the caution that researchers should exercise, if tempted to uncritically accept as valid the magnitude, and even the existence and direction, of observed age– and sex–specific differentials in cross–national suicide rates.

Conclusion

Unless specifically addressing issues of data quality, international suicide studies typically use underlying cause–of–death data emanating from national death certificates. For the more developed countries, the evidence presented here indicates that such national data achieve acceptable standards of reliability. The validity of suicide certification, or more precisely the sensitivity, poses greater problems for scientific users.

Epidemiologists, who are interested in official international suicide data for comparative descriptive purposes, should exercise restraint in selecting countries and drawing conclusions. Whether these data are suitable for what sociologists refer to as social causation studies, and epidemiologists call correlational or ecological studies, requires further investigation. Generally, the quality of suicide data for the less developed countries is likely to be grossly deficient. Without adjustment, the use of such data is highly questionable.

Suicide is widely acknowledged as a public–health problem, although an underenumerated one. Identifying high–risk groups, understanding etiology, and designing and implementing effective prevention programs are ultimately contingent upon obtaining an accurate and detailed description of its magnitude. There is a serious need to improve the sensitivity of suicide certification in most countries. To this end, and to enhance data comparability, there would be great value in WHO creating a global working group to standardize criteria for defining suicide and ascertaining cases, along the lines of a recent collaborative multi–disciplinary and multi–organizational effort in the United States coordinated by the Centers for Disease Control and Prevention (CDC). A comprehensive update of the 1971 WHO survey, too, would aid in the formation of the group, and in specifying its responsibilities.

Finally, while not necessarily the panacea for suicide data problems, greater international use should be made of the psychological autopsy.[46–49] This approach involves followback interviews with family, friends and acquaintances of a decedent to specifically look for possible antecedents of his or her possible suicide. If psychological autopsies were implemented in all or a random sample of equivocal fatal injury cases, this would assist in computing correction factors to refine estimates of true suicide rates. Benefits would also accrue with regard to etiologic understanding and to prevention.

References

1.	Zilboorg G. Suicide among civilized and primitive races. *American Journal of Psychiatry* 92; 1936: 1347–1369.

2.	Dublin LI. *Suicide: A Sociological and Statistical Study.* New York: Ronald Press, 1963.

3.	Douglas JD. *The Social Meaning of Suicide.* Princeton University Press, 1967.

4.	McCarthy PD, Walsh D. Suicide in Dublin, I. The under–reporting of suicide and the consequences for national statistics. *British Journal of Psychiatry* 126; 1975: 301–308.

5.	Halbwachs M. *The Causes of Suicide.* London: Routledge and Kegan Paul, 1978.

6. Sainsbury P, Jenkins JS. The accuracy of officially reported suicide statistics for purposes of epidemiological research. *Journal of Epidemiology and Community Health* 36; 1982: 43–48.

7. Kleck G. Miscounting suicides. *Suicide and Life–Threatening Behavior* 18; 1988: 219–235.

8. Speechley M, Stavraky KM. The adequacy of suicide statistics for use in epidemiology and public health. *Canadian Journal of Public Health* 82; 1991: 38–42.

9. World Health Organization. *World Health Statistics Annual.* Geneva: WHO, 1993.

10. Brooke E. (Ed.). *Suicide and Attempted Suicide.* Public Health Papers 58. Geneva: World Health Organization, 1974.

11. Litman RE, Curphy T, Schneidman ES, Farberow NL, Tobachnick N. Investigations of equivocal suicides. *Journal of the American Medical Association* 184; 1963: 924–929.

12. Monk M. Suicide. Pp. 1385–1397 in *Public Health and Preventive Medicine*, 12th ed. (Edited by Last JM). Norwalk, CT: Appleton–Century Crofts, 1986.

13. Kolmos L, Bach E. Sources of error in registering suicide. *Acta Psychiatrica Scandinavica.* Supplement 336 76; 1987: 22–41.

14. Rockett IRH, Smith GS. Covert suicide among elderly Japanese females: questioning unintentional drownings. *Social Science and Medicine* 36; 1993: 1467–1472.

15. Holding TA, Barraclough BM. Psychiatric morbidity in a sample of a London coroners' open verdicts. *British Journal of Psychiatry* 127; 1975: 133–143.

16. Holding TA, Barraclough BM. Psychiatric morbidity in a sample of accidents. *British Journal of Psychiatry* 130; 1977: 244–252.

17. Jobes DA, Berman AL, Josselson AR. Improving the validity and reliability of medical–legal certifications of suicide. *Suicide and Life–Threatening Behavior* 17; 1987: 310–325.

18. Guidotti TL. Mortality of urban transit workers: indications of an excess of deaths by suicide using gas. *Occupational Medicine* 42; 1992: 125–128.

19. McIntosh JL, Hubbard RW. Indirect self–destructive behavior among the elderly: a review with case examples. *Journal of Gerontological Social Work* 13; 1988: 37–48.

20. Miller M. *Suicide After Sixty: The Final Alternative.* New York: Springer, 1979.

21. Andress, VR. Ethnic/racial misidentification in death: a problem which might distort suicide statistics. *Forensic Science* 9; 177: 179–183.

22. Warshauer ME, Monk M. Problems in suicide statistics for whites and blacks. *American Journal of Public Health* 68; 1978: 383–388.

23. Hlady GW, Middaugh JP. The under–recording of suicides in state and national records, Alaska, 1983–1984. *Suicide and Life Threatening Behavior* 18; 1988: 237–244.

24. Durkheim E. *Suicide: A Study in Sociology.* New York: Free Press, 1951.

25. Gibbs J. Suicide. Pp. 281–321 in *Contemporary Social Problems.* (Edited by Merton RK, Nisbet R). New York: Harcourt, Brace and World, 1961.

26.   Atkinson MW, Kessel N, Dalgaard JB. The comparability of suicide rates. *British Journal of Psychiatry* 127; 1975: 247–256.

27.   Ross O, Kreitman N. A further investigation of differences in the suicide rates of England and Wales and Scotland. *British Journal of Psychiatry* 127; 1975: 575–582.

28.   Whitlock FA. Migration and suicide. *Medical Journal of Australia* 2; 1971: 840–848.

29.   Sainsbury P, Barraclough BM. Differences between suicide rates. *Nature* 220; 1968: 1252.

30.   Cantor CH, Dunne MP. Australian suicide data and the use of "undetermined" death category (1968–1985). *Australian and New Zealand Journal of Psychiatry* 24; 1990: 381–384.

31.   Barraclough BM. Differences between national suicide rates. *British Journal of Psychiatry* 122; 1973: 95–96.

32.   Stack S. The effect of religious commitment on suicide: a cross–national analysis. *Journal of Health and Social Behavior* 24; 1983: 362–374.

33.   Pescosolido BA, Mendelsohn R. Social causation or social construction of suicide? An investigation into the social organization of official rates. *American Sociological Review* 51; 1986: 80–100.

34.   National Center for Health Statistics. Provisional estimates of selected comparability ratios based on dual coding of 1966 death certificates by the seventh and eighth revisions of the International Classification of Diseases. *Monthly Vital Statistics Report* 17; 1968: 8.

35.   Burvill PW, McCall MG, Stenhouse NS, Woodings TL. The relationship between suicide, undetermined deaths and accidental deaths in the Australian born and migrants in Australia. *Australian and New Zealand Journal of Psychiatry* 16; 1982: 179–184.

36.   O'Carroll PWA. A consideration of the validity and reliability of suicide mortality data. *Suicide and Life–Threatening Behavior* 19; 1989: 1–16.

37.   Johnson HRM. The incidence of unnatural deaths which have been presumed to be natural in coroner's autopsies. *Medicine, Science and the Law* 9; 1969: 102–106.

38.   Iga M, Yamamoto J, Noguchi T, Koshinga J. Suicide in Japan. *Social Science and Medicine* 12A; 1978:507–516.

39.   Rockett IRH, Smith GS. Homicide, suicide, motor vehicle crash and fall mortality: United States' experience in comparative perspective. *American Journal of Public Health* 79; 1989: 1396–1400.

40.   Statistics and Information Department (Minister's Secretariat). *Economic and Social Aspects of Accidental Deaths, Except Traffic Accidents* (in Japanese). Japanese Ministry of Health and Welfare, Tokyo, 1979.

41.   Martin LG. The graying of Japan. *Population Bulletin* 44, 1989.

42.   Iga, M, Tatai K. Characteristics of suicides and attitudes toward suicide in Japan. Pp. 255–280 in *Suicide in Different Cultures* (Edited by Farberow NL). Baltimore: University Park Press, 1975.

43.   Samuma K. The Japanese family in relation to people's health. *Social Science and Medicine* 12A: 1978: 469–478.

44.   Preston, SH, Kono S. Trends in well–being of children and the elderly in Japan. Pp. 277–307 in *The Vulnerable* (Edited by Palmer JL **et al**.). Washington, DC: Urban Institute, 1988.

45. Rosenberg ML, Davidson LE, Smith JC, Berman AL, Buzbee H, Gantner G, Gay GA, Moore–Lewis B, Harper Mills D, Murray D, O'Carroll PW, Jobes D. Operational criteria for the determination of suicide. *Journal of Forensic Sciences* 33; 1988: 1445–1456.

46. Rudestam KE. Some notes on conducting a psychological autopsy. *Suicide and Life–Threatening Behavior* 9; 1979: 141–144.

47. Schneidman ES. The psychological autopsy. *Suicide and Life–Threatening Behavior* 11; 1981: 325–340.

48. Litman RE. 500 psychological autopsies. *Journal of Forensic Sciences, JFSCA,* 34; 1989: 638–646.

49. Beskow J, Runeson B, Asgard U. Psychological autopsies: Methods and ethics. *Suicide and Life–Threatening Behavior* 20; 1990: 307–323.

Table 1. Percentage of Deaths Attributed to Natural Causes* by Country, 1990

Country	%	Country	%
Austria	97.4	Mauritius	92.8
Bulgaria	94.9	Mexico	85.5
Canada	93.2	Netherlands	95.9
Czechoslovakia	92.9	Norway	94.2
Denmark	93.3	Poland	92.3
Germany	95.0	Portugal	93.5
Finland	90.6	Romania	92.8
France	90.8	Singapore	92.7
Greece	97.4	Switzerland	91.2
Hungary	90.9	United Kingdom	96.7
Iceland	92.6	United States**	93.0
Ireland	95.3	Uruguay	93.7
Japan	93.2	USSR	89.1
Luxembourg	94.0	Yugoslavia	93.4
Malta	96.3		

*Chronic or communicable diseases.
**Data for 1989.

Sources: Adapted from World Health Organization, *World Health Statistics Annual*, 1991 and 1992. Geneva: WHO, 1992 and 1993.

Table 2. Suicide Rates by Sex and Country, 1990

| Country | Rate* | | Ratio |
	Male	Female	M:F
Austria	34.8	13.4	2.6
Bulgaria	20.7	8.8	2.4
Canada	20.4	5.2	3.9
Czechoslovakia	27.3	8.9	3.1
Denmark**	32.2	16.3	2.0
Germany	24.9	10.7	2.3
Finland	49.3	12.4	4.0
France	29.6	11.1	2.7
Greece	5.5	1.5	3.7
Hungary	59.9	21.4	2.8
Iceland	27.4	3.9	7.0
Japan	20.4	12.4	1.6
Ireland	14.4	4.7	3.1
Luxembourg	25.2	10.8	2.3
Malta	4.6	0	***
Mauritius	17.6	10.8	1.6
Mexico	3.9	0.7	5.6
Netherlands	12.3	7.2	1.7
Norway	23.3	8	2.9
Poland	22	4.5	4.9
Portugal	13.5	4.5	3.0
Romania	13.3	4.7	2.8
Singapore	14.7	11.5	1.3
Switzerland**	31.5	12.7	2.5
United Kingdom	12.6	3.9	3.5
United States†	19.9	4.8	4.1
Uruguay	16.6	4.2	3.9
USSR	37.4	9.1	4.1
Yugoslavia	21.6	9.2	2.3

*Suicide coded according to ICD–9, except for Denmark and Switzerland (ICD–8).
**Rates per 100,000 population.
***Ratio not calculated due to zero cell.
†Data for 1989.

Sources: World Health Organization. *World Health Statistics Annual*, 1991 and 1992. Geneva: WHO, 1992 and 1993.

Table 3. Suicide Rates per 100,000: Australian Immigrants and Countries of Birth

	Male Suicide Rates				Female Suicide Rates			
Hungary	57.7	40.3	1	1	34.6	17.3	3	1
Poland	56.6	14.3	2	7	28.8	3.3	4	11
Yugoslavia	38.6	17.8	3	5	16.2	7.7	7	6
Czechoslovakia	38.5	30.4	4	3	45.7	12.3	1	4
New Zealand	33.1	11.4	5	9	19.0	6.4	5	8
Austria	33.0	32.4	6	2	44.6	13.9	2	2
Germany	32.8	26.7	7	4	14.5	13.6	9	3
Ireland	30.5	5.3	8	14	10.8	2.3	11	14
Scotland	30.3	10.0	9	10	17.7	6.6	6	7
USA	29.5	16.3	10	6	13.8	5.8	10	9
England and Wales	25.3	13.7	11	8	15.3	9.6	8	5
Spain	15.9	7.6	12	12	7.1	2.5	12	13
Netherlands	12.7	8.2	13	11	6.8	4.9	13	10
Malta	10.7	1.4	14	16	1.4	0.2	16	16
Italy	10.4	7.6	15	12	3.4	3.2	14	12
Greece	6.8	4.7	16	15	3.0	2.2	15	15
Australia	16.1				10.0			
			$r_s = 0.78*$				$r_s = 0.79*$	

*Spearman's rank correlation coefficient.

Source: Whitlock FA. Migration and suicide. *Medical Journal of Australia* II; 1971:840–848.

Table 4. Comparison of the Rank Orders of Suicide Rates and Suicide,
Undetermined and Accidental Poisoning Death Rates in 19 Countries in 1970–73

Country	Suicide and self–inflicted injury	Rank order	Suicide and self–inflicted injury and injury undetermined whether purposely or accidentally inflicted and accidental poisoning	Rank order
Austria	30.4	4	33.0	6
Bulgaria	15.1	11	19.0	11
Czechoslovakia	31.0	2	39.8	3
Denmark	30.6	3	36.4	4
Finland	29.7	5	40.8	2
France	20.4	9	25.1	9
Germany	26.8	6	29.6	7
Greece	4.1	19	7.1	18
Hungary	45.2	1	48.5	1
Italy	7.6	16	9.2	17
Netherlands	11.3	13	12.9	15
Norway	11.4	12	14.2	14
Poland	15.5	10	23.1	10
Spain	5.9	17	6.8	19
Switzerland	24.6	8	27.2	8
England and Wales	10.3	15	15.5	13
Northern Ireland	5.4	18	11.0	16
Scotland	10.6	14	17.6	12
Sweden	26.4	7	36.0	5

Spearman's rank correlation coefficient = 0.9596 n = 19 p <0.001

Source: Sainsbury P and Jenkins JS. The accuracy of officially reported suicide statistics for purposes of epidemiologic research. *Journal of Epidemiology and Community Health* 36; 1982:43–48.

Table 5. Annualized Accidental Drowning Rates by Age, Sex and Country, 1979–81*

	Age (years)											
	15–24		25–34		35–44		45–54		55–64		65–74	
	M	F	M	F	M	F	M	F	M	F	M	F
Japan	2.9	0.2	2.5	0.3	2.5	0.3	3.5	0.6	4.5	1.1	7.9	3.8
Australia	3.3	0.4	3.1	0.3	3.2	0.4	3.9	0.8	3.6	0.6	3.2	1.0
France	3.5	0.4	3.2	0.4	3.2	0.6	3.3	0.6	3.7	0.9	4.2	1.6
New Zealand	4.8	0.6	3.4	0.3	1.8	1.1	2.8	1.3	2.8	1.2	1.9	1.9
Norway	3.5	0.3	4.2	0.3	4.3	0.1	5.3	0.6	4.5	0.5	4.2	1.7
Sweden	1.5	0.2	2.6	0.3	2.3	0.7	2.4	0.6	3.1	0.7	4.3	1.0
United	1.5	0.2	1.2	0.2	1.0	0.2	0.9	0.4	1.1	0.4	1.1	0.6
Kingdom**	7.2	0.8	4.2	0.6	2.9	0.5	2.4	0.5	2.3	0.5	2.5	0.7
United States												

*Rates expressed per 100,000 population.
**Accidental drowning deaths for Northern Ireland in 1981 were not reported by WHO. For these calculations, they are estimated as the annual average for 1979 and 1980.

Source: Rockett IRH, Smith GS. Covert suicide among elderly Japanese females: questioning unintentional drownings. *Social Science and Medicine* 36(11); 1993:1467–1472.

Table 6. Percentage Drowning as Method of Suicide by Age and Sex, Japan: 1979–81

Age (years)	Male	Female	Both Sexes
15–24	3.3	5.8	4.1
25–34	4.4	10.1	6.2
35–44	3.9	11.1	6.1
45–54	3.4	12.0	6.1
55–64	4.3	13.1	8.0
65–74	4.8	14.5	9.8
75+	5.7	17.4	12.2
Total	4.1	12.5	7.3

Source: Rockett IRH, Smith GS. Covert suicide among elderly Japanese females: questioning unintentional drownings. *Social Science and Medicine* 36(11); 1993:1467–1472.

The authors wish to thank Billy M. Thomas for his assistance with data compilation.

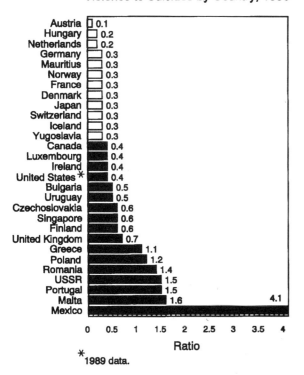

Figure 1 Ratio of Combined Deaths from Accidental Drowning, Accidental Poisoning, and Other Violence to Suicides by Country, 1990

* 1989 data.

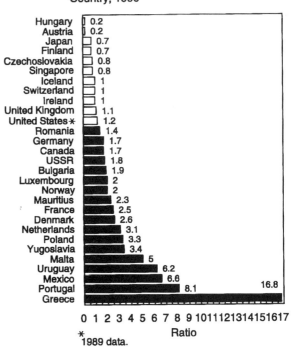

Figure 2 Ratio of Combined Deaths from Accidental Drowning, Accidental Poisoning, Other Violence, and Symptoms, Signs, and Ill-Defined Conditions to Suicides by Country, 1990

* 1989 data.

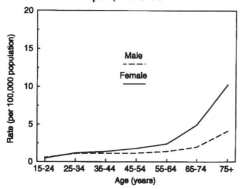

Figure 3 Annual average drowning suicide rates by age and sex: Japan, 1979-81

Source: Rockett IRH, Smith GS. Covert suicide among elderly Japanese females: questioning unintentional drownings. **Social Science and Medicine** 36(11);1993:1467-1472.

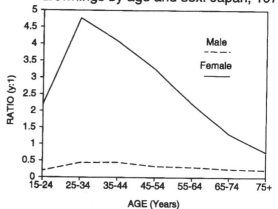

Figure 4 Ratio of drowning suicides to unintentional drownings by age and sex: Japan, 1979-81

Source: Rockett IRH, Smith GS. Covert suicide among elderly Japanese females: questioning unintentional drownings. **Social Science and Medicine** 36(11);1993:1467-1472.

Workshops

Mortality

Co-chairs: Mike Hayes, Ph.D. and Harry Rosenberg, Ph.D.

Aim – to understand why there are differences in mortality rates in different countries, and in particular to consider whether these differences are real or are related to the reporting systems, or are a mixture of both.

We considered the opportunities for errors through the various stages in the reporting system, starting with the certification of a death, working through the practices for investigating and determining the nature of the injuries and the circumstances of the event, to the reporting of these findings to the national vital statistics agency, the subsequent coding of the information, and finally its dissemination and use (figure 1). We tried to get a handle on the scale and significance of any problems that we identified and considered how matters could be improved, and by whom.

To understand a country's mortality data, we felt it essential to know the nature of their reporting system. For example, is it compulsory to report a death? Are all age groups captured equally? Even with apparently high capture rates, are all conditions reported to same level? For international comparisons to be meaningful, we need to know the ins and outs of other systems or at least to have confidence in them. It is, therefore, essential to **report on the completeness and quality of data**.

A couple of general points that do not fit comfortably on figure 1:

1 – need to be aware of the "real" data collection systems in different countries. Not the official systems, but what actually happens.

2 – need to be sensitive to the effect of language. Anne Tursz mentioned the use of the "term" accident in France.

3 – need to be sensitive to cultural issues which lead to different national practices e.g., religious blocks on Post Mortems

What is influence on statistics?

A long discussion took place on the question of identifying injury–related deaths. This is important, as it triggers the investigation and reporting system. Doctors regard completing death certificate as a chore.

– need to understand why they are being asked what they are

– need to understand their public health role

– need to understand that they are contributing to policy development

Education Needed

– initial training

– during professional examinations

– reinforcement through querying system for vital stats agency

Role of WHO

- instructions on handbooks on completing death certificates.

Quality of investigations of external cause of death and injuries (Gib Parrish's presentation)

Need to Raise Standards Among MEs and Coroners (Internationally?)

- may not get everyone to "gold" standard, but should seek uniformly good data

- further data from follow up studies and sampling

- islands of excellence, supplementing routing national data, and contributing to quality assessment.

MEs and Coroners Need to Be Working to Same Standards Internationally

- model guidelines for MEs and Coroners

- Education of MEs and Coroners on their public health role

On Medical Front

- need to be aware of what may be meant by term "autopsy"; is it verbal, or a full physical examination?

- "multiple" injuries unacceptable – poor medical description; improve through querying system.

Coding of External Causes and Injuries

Amendment of records issues

- can account for significant variations

- after legal proceedings

- need to know if amendments are included and whether on a timely basis

- may not affect all groups equally, may be a particular problem in area of homicide

- may render different countries' statistics incompatible in certain areas

- national legal frameworks may be the cause of the failure to amend databases.

Need for International Coding Trial to Examine Differences

- good model in field of diabetes

- circulate scenarios to difference countries' for coding

- be aware of translation problems

Ad Hoc National Coding Rules

–   exchange via WHO

Automated coding will help, but there is still need for manual validation and quality control

Quality Assessments of National Data

–   need to know the completeness of your own data to allow meaningful international comparisons

–   can be done by using multiple sources of data and follow back studies, and cross–linking data as in the Oxford record linkage study

–   note completeness of coverage in published statistics

Recommendations for the I.C.E.

Education

–   of doctors on death certification

–   of medical examiners and coroners on their public health role

International projects

–   descriptions of "real" systems

–   comparative coding of external cause

–   exchange of ad hoc, national coding rules

–   development of model guidelines for MEs and Coroners

Figure 1. Stages of the Reporting System and Related Issues:
Injury data from the death certificate

Death

Registration
- Coverage
- Capture rates

Injury related death?
- Education of doctors

Investigation of cause of injuries
- Raising standards
- International guidelines
- Education of ME/C
- Definition of an autopsy
- "Multiple" injuries

Coding of external cause and injuries
- Amendment of records
- International coding trials
- Exchange of ad hoc coding rules

Collation and publication of national data
- Quality assessment

Morbidity

Co-Chairs: Herbert G. Garrison, M.D., M.P.H. and George Rutherford, M.S.

The variety of terms speakers at the International Collaborative Effort on Injury Statistics Symposium used to describe injury morbidity illustrates the problem the injury morbidity workshop participants faced in their deliberations (Table 1). At the end of the first workshop session, the participants concluded that stating simply what injury morbidity is constitutes quite a challenge.

As discussed at the first workshop session, there are many reasons for the difficulty in precisely defining injury morbidity. First, there is a lack of general agreement on the answer to the question: What is an injury? For example, is an injury always an exchange or absorption of energy or can it be the subjective sense that I am or may be injured? Another reason for why it is difficult to define injury morbidity is that the various parts of medical care systems are not common to all countries. Variation in medical care systems makes using service utilization as a surrogate for injury morbidity very tricky. A final important reason involves the number of potential manifestations or degrees of injury morbidity. In contrast to injury mortality, the many manifestations of injury morbidity makes the task of trying to account for them all nearly impossible.

Despite these "nearly impossible" odds, participants in the first workshop session attempted to define injury morbidity by filling in blanks on the so-called injury pyramid. The workshop participants started from the bottom of an "injury morbidity pyramid" (Figure 1) with the following injury morbidity indicators:

- An injury to an individual that was recorded or reported (including those sensed subjectively)
- An injury that resulted in contact with a health care provider
- An injury that resulted in a visit to any health care facility
- An injury that resulted in a visit to an emergency care facility open 24 hours a day
- Disability that requires an individual to reside in an extended care facility

The workgroup did not have a chance to complete the obvious vacuum between the top injury morbidity indicator which, like the universal measure death, focuses on outcome and the other indicators in the injury morbidity pyramid which are mainly associated with health care resource utilization There was agreement that comparability will be better with outcome indicators. In addition, it was suggested that the use of coded incidence data of specific, targeted injuries would be a good way to account for morbidity.

Participants in the second workshop session discussed specific topics. The first discussion was about issues that affect the international comparability of injury morbidity data. The issues discussed included:

- How injury morbidity is defined
- The magnitude of injury morbidity which may range from none to permanent disability
- Coding
- Economics
- Differences in health seeking behavior
- Insurance practices
- The lack of standard or uniform case definitions

The quality of available injury morbidity data was another topic discussed. Many participants commented on the need for general norms for hospitalization that could be used for corrections when comparing length of stay. This is a significant problem since answers to the questions What is a hospital? What is a hospital stay? and What is a hospital day? will vary depending on the country. Another quality of morbidity data issue discussed were potential problems with the denominators used for evaluating the impact of injury morbidity. Concern was expressed specifically over inter-country differences in measuring and collecting census data.

The workgroup also discussed potential users of injury morbidity data. These include health care administrators, grant writers, injury control professionals, vital statistics agencies, acute care professionals and other health care providers, outcomes researchers, policy makers, hospitals, insurance companies, and those who have commercial needs such as for market research.

There was a discussion about how the personnel collecting injury data (e.g., health care providers) are usually not the people using the data and the fact that these same people who collect the data often have to buy the aggregated data back if they do want to use it for secondary purposes. This was generally condemned. The workgroup also indicated that, much to their displeasure, there is frequently a significant lack of useful feedback to local data collectors.

In terms of current sources of morbidity data that allow cross-country comparisons, the workgroup discussed population-based surveys designed for cross-country comparisons, health interview surveys that use standard definitions, hospitalizations with standard definitions, and provider-based surveys.

Finally, the injury morbidity workshop participants indicated that the following strategies should be carried out in order to facilitate the assimilation of injury morbidity data that is comparable across international borders:

1) Develop standard definitions for injury and injury morbidity as well as standard instruments for measuring and counting injury morbidity.

2) Determine core injury data elements (otherwise known as minimum or uniform data elements).

3) Develop injury morbidity data banks and networks.

4) Provide useful feedback to the collectors of injury data.

5) Add severity to outcome and service utilization as descriptors of morbidity and develop an injury morbidity matrix that allows the use of all three indicators simultaneously.

Table 1. Injury morbidity terms used by ICE speakers

Trauma center admission

Hospital admission

Hospital discharge

Number of care days

Length of stay

Continuous inpatient days

Emergency department visit

Acute visit

Treated by a doctor or nurse

Recent injury

Reported condition

Placement of cast

Restriction of activity

Incidence rate

Mild, moderate, or severe injury

Patient outcome

Doctor consultation

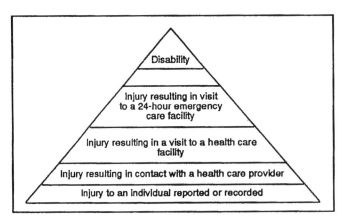

Figure 1. Injury morbidity pyramid

Data Needs for Injury Prevention

Co-chairs: Joseph L. Annest, Ph.D. and Sue Mallonee, M.P.H., R.N.

The purpose of the workshop on data needs for injury prevention was to discuss how to improve the quality, reliability, and comparability of international statistics on injuries relevant to monitoring and evaluating injury prevention programs. The principal questions contemplated and discussion points were:

1) How can public health data systems (e.g., health interview, behavioral risk factor, prehospital, emergency department, hospital, rehabilitation, social services, medical examiner/coroner and vital statistics data systems) be used to provide useful information for monitoring and evaluating injury prevention efforts?

  a) What are the problems?

    - lack of standards and guidelines
    - timeliness of the availability of data
    - lack of population–based data
    - inability to integrate data from different systems
    - inflexibility of data systems for change or modification, e.g., to add new data elements
    - limitation of resources
    - lack of follow–up epidemiologic research, e.g., examining the effects of implementation of new laws, such as those requiring children to wear bicycle helmets
    - lack of data collection by providers

  b) What are the potential solutions?

    - develop internationally accepted guidelines and standards for case definitions and data element definitions
    - automate data collection, data processing and reporting systems
    - develop population–based systems through sampling techniques
    - integrate data systems through data linkage and aggregation of data relevant to injury prevention efforts
    - develop systems that are easily adaptable to change
    - develop mechanisms and allocate resources for timely follow–up of epidemiologic investigations
    - increased emphasis of medical care provider training in the value of injury prevention data collection

2) How can data collection, analysis and reporting methods be standardized to improve data quality and promote comparability of process and outcome data (e.g., changes in knowledge, attitudes, and behaviors, morbidity, disability, and mortality) in relation to injury prevention programs among different countries?

  a) What are the problems?

    - assurance of confidentiality
    - fragmentation/disparity of data systems
    - quality of data sources
    - no uniform quality assurance programs
    - lack of automation data collection and processing procedures
    - long lag time between data collection and the availability of final data for reporting
    - lack of routine data reporting mechanisms
    - lack of public access data tapes
    - poor documentation/no data users manuals

b)   What are the potential solutions?

  – develop guidelines and standards to assure confidentiality
  – conduct an international inventory of injury–related data systems to determine sources, quality, contents, uses, limitations, and accessibility of data
  – develop international standards for guidelines for data collection, analysis and reporting of injury data
  – consider use of an abbreviated ICD coding system that could be mapped back to standard coding

3) What injury data (e.g., circumstances about the injury event, incidence, demographic and socioeconomic factors, interventions (e.g., bicycle helmet laws, DUI laws), behavioral risk factors, morbidity, disability and mortality) are needed for international comparisons of prevention effectiveness?

  a)   What data are needed?

  – incidence of injury
  – characteristics of the population
  – characteristics of injury persons
  – characteristics of high risk subgroups
  – environmental conditions
  – political conditions
  – social conditions
  – risk factors
  – risk behaviors
  – health outcomes
  – cost to society
  – interventions

  b)   What are the problems in making comparisons of what interventions work, assuming high quality data are available?

  – intervention strategies are not clearly defined
  – different priority injury problems among countries and communities within countries
  – different target populations
  – different political, social or environmental influences

  c)   What are the potential solutions?

  – develop a uniform minimum data set for assessment of the effectiveness of injury prevention and control programs
  – conduct a comprehensive, international literature review of all prevention effectiveness studies
  – conduct comparative analysis or meta analysis on selected studies of interventions and their effectiveness among countries
  – publish recommendations for methods to conduct future prevention effectiveness studies that will improve the capacity for international comparisons
  – develop and conduct training courses in surveillance and statistical methods applicable to assessing prevention effectiveness

4) How can those who plan and implement injury prevention programs best communicate their data needs with those responsible for the design, data content and operations of public health systems?

  a)   What are the problems in communicating data needs?

  – data persons are often not involved in the design and implementation of injury prevention program

- program persons are often not involved in the design and implementation of surveillance/data systems

b) <u>What are the potential solutions</u>?

- data and program people need to work together to ensure appropriate high quality data are being obtained for the design and evaluation of injury prevention programs
- statisticians, computer programmers and public health professionals need to use a team approach to establishing public health data systems that are useful for program planning and evaluation

Recommendations

1. Identify a minimum, standardized international injury database with the flexibility to add detailed modules needed to evaluate interventions

   - begin with mortality data
   - standardize groupings of codes
   - standardize how data are reported
   - recommend the use of a narrative variable

2. Develop general guidelines and standards for integrated injury data systems relevant to their use in monitoring and evaluating injury prevention programs.

   - conduct demonstration projects to evaluate the usefulness of these guidelines and standards in several countries with well–developed data systems and injury prevention programs
   - modify the guidelines and standards based on the results of the demonstration projects
   - hold an international consensus conference
   - disseminate guidelines and standards to all countries

3. Increase international collaborative research

   - Produce an international inventory and clearinghouse of available injury–related data and prevention effectiveness research

4. Circulate enhanced ICE mailing list with listing of participant's individual research interests

5. Reconvene ICE participants at the 3rd International Injury Conference in Australia

6. Most of these activities should be coordinated by a subgroup of the WHO International Injury Surveillance Workgroup

Co–chairs: William H. Walsh and Patricia F. Waller, Ph.D.

Issues Addressed

What data systems should be linked?
What is gained from data linkage?
Why conduct international comparisons?
What would we like to see happen?

Data Systems to Be Linked

Non Medical
Crash reports
Vehicle Registration
Driver Licensing
Roadway
Citation

Medical
Emergency medical services
Emergency department
Hospital
Outpatient
Death Certificate

Claim Data
Automobile Insurance
Health Insurance

What Is Gained from Data Linkage

Improved Analytical Capability

Medical and financial outcome linked to crash and exposure
Supports injury control efforts and reduces health costs
Population based data for problem identification

Improves Data Systems

Promotes standardization of data
Expands usefulness of current data at small cost

Supports Policy Making Activities

Promotes collaboration between highway safety and health
Supports investment in prevention activities

With linkage, one can

- Measure the burden of disability on the community

- Set priorities for most effective resource allocation

- Enact/retain effective laws; e.g., motorcycle helmets

- Capitalize on existing data systems

- Identify specific areas from linked data, then conduct more in–depth studies; e.g., studies of seat belt injuries research on design   improved design

- Get people to think beyond their own role, along the Prevention–Treatment–Rehabilitation Continuum

Why Conduct International Comparisons?

- To benefit from experience of others—safety belt laws   reduced injury; bicycle helmet programs

- To identify problem unique to a country and investigate reasons

- To access larger or richer data bases on specific populations; e.g., bicyclists

- To identify potential product safety issues

- To evaluate methodology; e.g., applications of Crash Outcome Data Evaluations Systems (CODES) to data bases with personal identifiers

What Would We like to See Happen?

- Greater standardization of data, including minimum data sets, at national and international levels.

- Improved timeliness and accessibility of data systems

- Improvements in linkage methodology

- Development and support of partnerships among prevention, treatment and rehabilitation   broader vision

- Increased use of linked data by researchers, demonstrating value of linkage

- Routine dissemination of successful strategies where data linkage was effective:

    APHA Electronic Newsletter
    Electronic bulletin board or Internet

- Routine feedback at all levels to:

    Data providers
    Decision makers
    Public

- Data become an integral part of decision making process at all levels

- Linkage with other networks not traditionally identified with injury

Data Linkage--Social and Behavioral Determinants of Injuries

Co–chairs: Yossi Harel, Ph.D. and Mary Overpeck, Dr.P.H.

The goal of this discussion is to identify social and behavioral indicators that should be linked to international injury outcome data so that the analyses of these data can be meaningful. Three main questions guided the workshop discussions:

(1)   What are the most important **social indicators** that may explain the differences in injury rates between populations (e.g., nations)?

(2)   What are the most important **behavioral variables** to be linked to international data on intentional and unintentional injuries?

(3)   What are the possible **data systems** or **data sources** from which we can derive the linkage between information about social and behavioral variables and data on injury outcome?

The discussions led to a distinction between **macro**–level and **micro**–level indicators or variables.   Macro–level variables are social indicator measures at the population level (e.g., country)—measures that might have an effect on the rate of injury in the population. In this case, the unit of analysis is a jurisdiction.

Micro–level variables are social or behavioral determinants of injury liabilities that might effect the probability of injuries in individuals. Micro–level indicators are needed to study cross–national or cross–cultural variation in patterns of risk factors and determinants of injuries. Here the unit of analyses is an individual person stratified within the jurisdiction. This distinction is quite similar to the way numerators and denominators are used to produce sample measures.

The macro analysis is usually used to study differences in population rates and to use those differences as baseline information for further analyses. Then, by using ipsative (relative) scales we are able to look at deviations on individuals from the normative means of their own country or population and then attribute those deviations to the relative risk of injury.

One cannot compare, for example, salaries and income between countries because income is based on very different baseline scales. However, one can compare the deviation or the standardized deviation of a person from the mean income of his or her country and compare those deviations across countries. Using this method, one can then analyze the relation between relative income and the probability of injuries. Such an analysis could not be carried out in the absence of both macro– and micro–level income information. The following discussion describes specific types of indicators recommended by workshop participants.

<u>*Social Indicators*</u>

I.   *Macro Demographics*

Three groups of macro–level social indicators were recommended. Those include (1) age distribution, (2) immigration and ethnic composition, and (3) the structure of the political, health and educational systems.

— *Age distribution*: Injury types and rates are strongly related to age. Populations with different age distributions will produce very different patterns of injury outcomes. To enable unbiased age–adjusted cross–national comparisons, the information on the basic demographic age distribution of participating countries is essential.

— *Immigration and ethnic composition*: Here we recommend that information about the rates of in– and out–migration should be linked together with information about ethnic minorities. What percentage, for example, of a country's population is an ethnic or religious majority and what percentage are regarded as minorities. Are there differences in the definitions of minorities across countries? A sociological measure of the orientation of the country and it's culture towards minority integration could be useful.

— *Structure of political, health and educational systems:* It is recommended that information regarding the structure of the political system (Centralized Democracy, Confederation, etc.), the health care system, including the orientation of the national public health activities, and the structure of the educational system are important as macro–level social indicators to link to injury outcome data. In the educational system, information that might be important is the schooling structure (e.g., K–8,9–12 / K–6,7–9,10–12), the percent of out–of–school children by age group, the percent of public schools vs. private schools, the degree of centralized curriculum, mandatory education by age, and the implementation of national or regional health education curricula.

II.   *Social Inequality*

A great emphasis was placed by the workshop participants on the importance of measures of social inequality. It was agreed that the recommendation is to obtain the most simplified and easily obtained measures to link to injury outcome information. Two concepts on which there was a wide consensus were discussed: (1) the concept of **gradients and steepness** of social inequality and (2) the concept of **variations in indicator definitions**.

Countries differ in their social variations on socioeconomic measures. Some countries, like Norway, have a relatively homogeneous society in which the difference between the top percentile of the population and the bottom percentile is relatively small. In the United States, on the other hand, socioeconomic diversity is much greater, leading to a large gap between the very rich and the very poor populations. The steepness of these differences are important to know on a macro–level to distinguish between types of populations in terms of social inequality.

The main social inequality indicators we recommend include measures of income, education, occupation, housing, and family structure. We still have to determine what dimension of each one of these indicators are the more important and more easily obtained indicators to be linked to injury outcome data.

Concerns were raised regarding comparability of definitions and methodological issues regarding the way in which income, occupation or education are defined and measured in different countries, and how those data can be linked to local sources of information on injury outcome.

There was a wide consensus in each of the workshop regarding our need to obtain the most simplified version of the most meaningful dimension of these indicators. Simplification should increase the probability that we obtain identical and compatible information from as many countries as possible. Measures of education, for example, could include anything from the number of years of education, the number of out of school youth, or mandatory schooling.

Measures of occupation can include a simple scale of 10 or 12 accepted categories that reflect a continuum or white/blue collar. However, there are other dimensions of occupation, not only white/blue collar, that might be important. For example, what percent of the workforce is involved in agriculture or what percent of the workforce is in the service sector as opposed to industry?

It was agreed that there is a need to establish a small working group of social–science injury researchers to look into these measures in greater depth to derive the most important and obtainable measures to indicate the social inequality information that is essential for injury analyses.

In current population surveys, self–reported information is being sought, especially from adolescents and young adults. In these surveys, social inequality is being measured by several simple measures that are common to most societies. In the World Health Organization – Health Behavior in School–age Children cross–national study, social inequality is measured by three indicators that include (1) the number of cars per household, (2) the existence of a phone in the household (if yes, how many lines), and (3) does the respondent have his/her own bedroom. In the United States, a phone in the household is not a useful measure since most people have at least one phone line. Here you might need to ask questions about cellular phones, car phones or faxes.

These sound like very simple measures, whoever, when taken as a whole, we get an indicator of the social and economic quality of life that the respondent is experiencing at home. As simple as it may seem, these indicators provide an instrument to distinguish between variations in social inequality to link to injury outcome information measures in the same survey. Such measures are easily obtained on a self–reported data collection instrument.

One other area of inequality we would like to point out is the area of the **status of women** in the population. Results of many studies have demonstrated relationships between the mother's education, involvement in the workforce and alcohol behavior and the probability of childhood injuries. In the United States, for example, we find a strong correlation between reported aggressiveness by mothers during childhood and the probability of injuries during young adulthood. The findings are consistent across several population studies in that mother indicators affect childhood injuries more strongly than father indicators. We recommend obtaining information on women's education, occupational status and women's health.

III. *Family Structure and Dynamics*

Studies have demonstrated that family or household structure and transitions have a profound effect on the probability of injuries among its members—especially the young ones. Interestingly enough, the findings show that the effects of family indicators on injuries are confounded by the household environment. In fact, children, who experience major disadvantages at home are at higher risk for school injuries and injuries occurring in recreational settings. There is something happening in the home environment that has to do with the family structure and dynamics that predisposes its members to higher probabilities of injuries. These dynamics and effects might differ across countries and should be measured and monitored by linkage to injury outcome information.

Indicators include the number of parents in the household—both on the macro level and on a personal or individual level, whether it is a mother–only household or a father–only household. Other family indicators include the number of children under 18 years of age living in the household, measures of crowding (i.e., rooms per capita), etc. Residential dislocation, as measured by the number of moves a family experiences, or the level of mobility in the country as a whole may also be indicators.

Another family determinant of injuries is family break–up or divorce. Findings from previous studies are quite consistent in the relationship between the breakup of the family structure and the probability of injuries. From an international perspective it is both important and challenging to operationally define and measure family break–up in various populations and societies and link that data to injury outcome information. That is, since divorce rates are very different across countries and cultures, reflecting both a difference in family break–up frequency but also a difference in the social desirability or legality of defining a family break–up as a divorce. In some countries, religious ones in particular, divorce is a non–desired status. Consequently, many families end up with separation that are never registered as divorce. As a result, the official divorce rate might be grossly conservative compared to the actual number of families that broke apart. Therefore, it will be quite a methodological challenge to design an operational definition of family breakup that could be measured across countries and cultures using identical definitions.

IV.   Other Social Indicators

Other relevant and important socioeconomic indicators to be linked to injury outcome data may include: **degree of industrialization, religiosity, urbanization and access to health care.**

Herb Garrison covered some of the issue of access to health care in another workshop presentation. However, since we were talking about information at the macro- and micro-level we ought to point this out again.

At the macro level, we think it is important to obtain information on how people obtain access to health care. Is it direct fee-for-service or a form of health system reimbursements for care through mechanisms such as universal coverage. Does funding for care come from sources such as governmental taxes or combinations of private and public health insurance. Within a reimbursement system, data should include the extent to which the population has health care coverage and the socioeconomic characteristics of the people in that population according to their coverage type.

When talking about the organization of the medical care service resources, we need to know about protocols for access to hospitalization, outpatient care, or emergency systems. What is the organization of those systems? Does organization differ by place of residence, i.e., urban vs. rural sources. At the macro level, information should include the distribution of the population and the case mix at each medical care source. In other words: who isn't getting care? Are we measuring only people who are getting into the system, and what percentage of the population isn't getting care.

This leads to the need to identify access to care at the micro level. Knowing the individual's position in that system in relation to medical care access yields a numerator for the macro level denominator.

Other macro-level indicators that were mentioned include: Exposure to wars or other types of social violence or exposure to natural disasters.

Behavioral Indicators

Most of the workshop time was dedicated to social indicators. Nevertheless, we did identify several areas of risk behaviors that should be collected with injury outcome data due to the central role these behaviors play in the injury matrix.

Injury Risk Behaviors

The main risk behaviors to be included are:

(1)   Use of alcohol and other drugs—especially in conjunction with dangerous activities such as driving or riding cars, high risk sports, etc.

(2)   Use of protective gear such as helmets, seatbelts, safety sport equipment, when engaged in activities that require them.

(3)   Involvement in physical fights and other interpersonal violence, especially physical fights with injuries, which is a more severe behavior.

(4)   Access to and use of weapons—not only handguns which are most important here in the USA, but also weapons like knives and clubs.

(5)   Measures of suicidal ideation and behavior. Four hierarchical measures are used as part of the Youth Risk Behavior Surveillance System here in the United States that are examples of simple measures that can be used to compare suicidal information across countries.

Indicators Related to Risk Behaviors

There are some other personal behaviors that are linked indirectly to injuries. For example, patterns of health risk behaviors such as smoking and sexual habits might be indicative of injury prone lifestyles. Recent findings indicate that early onset of health related risk behaviors are associated with risk for injuries in later adolescent years.

Some participants suggested obtaining information regarding exposure to activities that indirectly relate to injuries. For example, number of hours spent at school, number of working days per week, etc.

On another level, social norms and regulations are related to behaviors. Examples include legislation regarding legal drinking or driving age and the use of mass–media campaigns to reduce specific types of injuries.

Possible Data Systems

This topic was covered quite nicely by previous workshops. However, some additional suggestions that were raised in our discussions. It was suggested that there might be a source of international data, such as the one obtained and maintained at Andre L'Hour's department at the World Health Organization's headquarters in Geneva, that includes most of the macro–level social indicators for many countries around the world.

In addition to the usual existing sources of national data—such as census data, police records, etc.—there was a strong consensus that there is a need for designing and implementing more cross national population surveys. There are several cross–national projects at WHO that are based on population studies in many countries. One of them is MONICA—a study of cardiovascular risk factors in 47(!) countries around the world.

We strongly feel that it is time to develop a population–based survey system focussed on the prevention of injuries and injury–related risk factors. We can not think of a better time than now to begin working on such surveys, especially if we are able to include some longitudinal and cross–national designs. Such a system will enable us to look not only at determinants and predictors of injuries but also at the whole process of the injury matrix, providing us with instruments to evaluate the efficacy of injury prevention strategies across nations.

Coding

Co–Chairs: Gerry Berenholz, R.R.A., M.P.H. and Susan Scavo Gallagher, M.P.H.

Participants Included Clinicians, Coders and Researchers

Lois Fingerhut, Bob Hartford, Rosa Gofin, Jean Langlois, Sue Meads, Donna Pickett, Dan Pollack, Cleone Rooney, Robert Schwartz, Ann Trumble

Workshop Focus

The quality, reliability and comparability of injury and external cause coding at the international level

- A lot of input provided by participants with lively discussion and debate

- Summarized issues that need to be addressed to improve injury data collection, comparison, and analysis and emphasized several specific recommendations

- NOTE: Only two countries outside the U.S. were represented—Israel and the U.K. We need to become aware of coding issues in additional countries. The fact that data maybe collected for different reasons in different countries adds to the comparability problems with injury data across countries.

Method for eliciting discussion: The Co–Chairs developed an outline of talking points around 9 areas:

1. Agencies and personnel responsible for codes, coding, and injury data analysis
2. Sources of coded data
3. Centralization of coded data
4. Comparability of coded data
5. Coding injury diagnoses
6. External cause of injury coding
7. Use of coded data in injury research
8. Training and education
9. Anticipated outcomes and recommendations for next steps

Synthesis of the discussion on issues that need to be addressed to improve coding. These do not appear in any particular order.

1. Improve Communication

   There is insufficient communication between those involved with coding within a given country as well as with counterparts external to the country. Communication must occur across different levels:

   - those organizations that make the rules for coding
   - those who assign the codes
   - those who organize the data bases
   - those who use the data (researchers, health planners. state agencies)

   There is also a great need for understanding **the lengthy process** by which codes are developed and revised.

2. Crosswalks Between Coding Systems

The change from ICD 9 to ICD 10 is an extremely complex process. Crosswalks must be developed to bridge several different coding systems. The WHO will provide the crosswalk between ICD 9 and ICD 10. Should there be an ICD 10 CM version in the U.S., a crosswalk will also be needed between ICD 9 CM and ICD 10 CM. Similarly, a bridge is needed between ICD, NOMESCO, and other coding systems used for injury research.

3.   Training

Training initiatives are a major need. A major educational campaign is required for coding the cause of injury within the ICD scheme.

A.   Expand E–code training in medical record educational programs.

B.   Teach clinicians documentation skills, questions to ask and what information to collect. Do not try to teach them E–coding. Rob Schwartz suggested a method to teach clinicians the information that is necessary to write down for later coding. That is, to use the WHO, WHAT, WHEN, WHERE, WHY and HOW questions used in journalism.

C.   Teach researchers and other end users.

They need a better understanding of the individual codes themselves, the process of coding, and the rules. Example: For ICD 9, some countries only collect one diagnosis code. This has a lot of implications for users.

Where there are multiple codes, what sequencing rules are being followed? Users should not be analyzing only the first listed code. They must look beyond the first code.

4.   Educational Materials

A major issue is the lack of sufficient educational materials for E–coding. There is considerably more information available on how to assign diagnosis codes than cause of injury codes.

A.   Manuals targeted to three different audiences are needed—the coders, clinicians, and researchers and other users.

B.   Data users need to understand coding steps and how they affect research and interpretation of data. This includes the steps in getting from documentation in the record to coding of data to reporting the data to interpretation of the data to publishing the data.

5.   E–Code Guidelines

The lack of comprehensive guidelines for E–codes has been a major impediment to their use in the U.S. The NCHS is currently addressing this problem, but there is a need for other countries to have similar guidelines. Perhaps the U.S. can share the guidelines after they have been finalized and approved.

6.   Standard Reporting Requirements for External Cause of Injury

Reporting requirements are not the same in the states that have mandated E–code reporting in the U.S. The requirements in other countries are unknown.

7.   Multiple Codes

The existing rules and sequencing guidelines for multiple codes need to be widely disseminated. Most researchers and end users are not aware of such rules, nor of the implications of using only one code, nor of the definitions used in different countries for selection of the first listed diagnosis code.

8. Suggested Groupings of Codes for Users

    Using groups of related codes to represent particular injuries or causes of injuries is often done to make it easier to analyze data. Unfortunately, nearly every user seems to come up with their own notion of how to group codes making it nearly impossible to compare studies. In the U.S., this is especially important for comparability of state data.

9. Prompts For Cause of Injury

    Many different paper forms and computer formats are used in different settings (e.g., community health clinics, emergency departments, clinicians offices). A prompt to include the cause of injury would be a helpful reminder. A dedicated, labeled field for cause of injury could be very effective in increasing the use of E–codes for ICD coding.

10. Provision of Routine Feedback to Coders/Clinicians

    To enhance the quality of the data, mechanisms for providing feedback should be instituted in every setting. Newsletters., meetings and grand rounds for clinicians are examples of such mechanisms.

11. Other Incentives

    Additional incentives to improve and maintain the quality of coded data need to be developed.

12. Computer–Based Medical Records

    Although there will always be a need for people, there are some functions that a computer should be able to perform better than a person. For the future, computer–based medical records will improve comparability across countries.

Where Do We Go from Here

A number of excellent ideas were generated to begin the process of improving coding of injury at the international level and create a more collaborative spirit across countries.

- A series of instructional **manuals** for three different audiences should be developed. These could highlight similarities and differences in injury coding and sequencing rules and definitions in different countries.

- Although a structure for sharing coding definitions, process issues and rules across countries and across injury coding schemes exists (e.g., WHO, NCHS, others), a **forum** should be created to improve dissemination of the information.

- An international **directory** of coded data sources, different coding schemes (e.g., ICD, EHLASS, NOMESCO), who is in charge and who does what should be developed.

- Suggested standard **cause of injury groupings** should be developed to improve comparability across studies and countries. This is a project that the National Center for Injury Prevention and Control at the Centers for Disease Control in the U.S. is initiating during 1994.

- A **plan** is required to perform some **evaluation** of comparability of coding across countries. For example, coders in different countries would all be given the same raw data to code and then the results would be analyzed to detect differences in coding. This would also help to assess coding needs.

- Although it may be impossible to gain complete international consensus, **"practice models"** for injury surveillance, injury coding, and injury data analysis should be disseminated (e.g., Australia's efforts and lessons learned). This could be done on a small scale first with others persuaded to join in the effort.

Standard Definitions for Injury Research

Co–Chairs: Vita Barell and Peter Scheidt, M.D., M.P.H.

The questions posed in our group related to the types of data elements which need to be standardized, how they are to be operationalized and implemented.

The methods used were round robin reporting of issues of particular concern, and an active, more focused discussion of the elements raised. We also searched for appropriate processes and strategies by which standardization of these diverse elements might best be implemented within the ICE context. We saw the ICE goal as improving comparability, quality and reliability of international statistics on injury: In addition, relevance and a preventive orientation is required.

A broad spectrum of experts from various backgrounds participated in the two workshop sessions. It was a true learning experience, and much knowledge and insight was gained. I hope the concerns of the workshop participants are fairly presented.

The two major elements discussed are: the need for a standard definition of injury and the need to clarify severity inclusions and exclusions. Definitions must be expanded to include the currently systematically under–reported rural and farm injuries.

We need to include "lost injuries." Ted Miller has estimated that there is a significant percentage of injuries outside N or E codes; for example, musculoskeletal conditions, stress fractures, low back pain, coma. It is estimated that five percent of the motor vehicle accident injuries in California, where E codes are obligatory, are below the 800 codes.

Missing injury data systems, from insurance companies, police, and the military, need to be included, and we need to find out who else is collecting injury data, and get them into the system.

There was some discussion on which injuries are to be included. What is to be done about post–traumatic stress syndrome, where the injury may have occurred to someone else, or food poisoning or stress fractures? How should these definitions be dealt with on the local level.

One of the major concerns was to reconcile the multiplicity of classification schemes, and reduce the proliferation of these systems. The standard approaches, the nature of injury and the external cause codes of ICD–9 and ICD–10, differ from the NOMESCO, NEISS, EHLASS or any number of other systems which have been presented: a frightening number, as a matter of fact. Then there is the question of standardized definitions, categorization, and collapsed coding. Everybody is collapsing their own way.

Coding of severity of injury at entry to care is another very significant issue that was raised: i.e., the appropriateness of coding schemes at different levels of the injury severity scale. ICD–9 and ICD–10 may be suitable for mortality and inpatient morbidity; NOMESCO is more appropriate for milder injury prevention. These two systems are incompatible, and a non–continuous scale has been presented.

The abbreviated injury scale, AIS, is not suitable for mild to moderate injuries. How should these be classified? The whole question of coding the severity of the clinical state at onset of care, which should be used for case–mix evaluation, functional state at outcome, long term consequences, and residual disability—all of these are severity issues.

It was suggested that the design criteria include, first and foremost, usefulness for public health purposes, and the ability to target high risk populations. The hierarchical character of recording was of concern as well as the need for simplicity. Different levels of training of those recording data make it imperative to deal with the simplest tier, yet still maintain compatibility with the major classification systems.

Of course, accuracy and consistency, flexibility and updating, as well as a mechanism for stimulating change in ICD coding practices are necessary. Many of the coding systems are not appropriate in a computer era.

Considerable time was spent considering the data source, whether survey data was being used and, if so, what are the core questions? Who is the respondent? What are the recall times?

Emergency rooms and outpatient departments may be the source of care. Their records, as well as inpatient medical records and mortality data, are post-hoc: they are collected after the event and the nature of the data collected is different.

One important issue raised was the question of gaming the reimbursement system. This may be very different in different states or countries: the way in which coding is systematically done in order to provide the maximum payment for the injured person. What information is selectively omitted from the records?

There was discussion of data elements relating to race, ethnicity and integration, and socioeconomic status. France, for example, restricts the use of race data because of confidentiality laws, and therefore, there is considerable difficulty in identifying the high risk target groups of immigrant children.

The increasing emphasis on confidentiality throughout the world shows a need for some kind of standard method for data linkage, while you strip identifiers off the record. There are a number of these methods which could be investigated.

Proxy data is needed, good proxy data, for socioeconomic status: insurance level or employment status were suggested.

Competing definitions present a problem which make it hard to identify injury types, or activity at time of event. Sports-related injuries are one example: are these sports injuries or school injuries? Occupational injuries are another example: How are motor vehicle accidents en route to work coded? Are they grouped with injuries occurring at the work site? The difficulties of coding farm injuries have already been mentioned. So there is confusion as to type of injury, place and circumstances.

It is often difficult to identify morbidity and mortality data. There are often inadequate descriptors: Army physical training, brought up by one of the session participants, is often very similar to sports activities and the injuries occurring during both are similar.

The circumstances of injury were dealt with, as well as the importance and necessity for narrative. The question remains of how to classify narrative, which is very often the only source for information on personal protective equipment and for consumer products.

The whole question of quantification of data sets might perhaps be jointly addressed by ICE members.

A very interesting point was made by Hank Weiss, and that is that there is probably a trade off somewhere along the line between comparability and information. The more comparability that you have, the more data has been reduced and, often, the less you know. So, this aspect should be dealt with in discussing international or interstate comparisons.

DR. SCHEIDT: Let me also express my thanks to the very active members of the workshop for their valuable contributions.

It is remarkable, how many similarities there are between the reports and recommendations from each of the workshops. May I conclude that great minds think alike, or perhaps it is a matter of sheep, all doing the same thing. I wonder.

In our workshop it was felt that there was a need to pull together specific recommendations that move toward addressing the issues that were outlined above. They included a relatively short list:

–   To establish a clearinghouse function to coordinate and network efforts to increase comparability, as has been mentioned previously.

–   To develop a mechanism to address the multiplicity of classification systems.

–   To utilize consensus development techniques, to promote effective information retrieval and utilization as an ongoing process for change and sharing of information.

–   To develop an international dictionary of health terms and recommendations for data guidelines.

–   To expand and disseminate information on coding. This can be done through the use of ambulatory clinics as well as E–code guidelines and other recommendations.

–   To initiate international, cross–country data collection efforts that use and focus on core variables, that develop and evaluate comparability and define artifacts within the various systems.

–   And finally, a recommendation for a network on an international basis, through newsletters, journals, Internet, that develops, or really provides a home, or various homes, for the distribution of information on the classification issues.

Now, even this short list presents a lot to do, more than one could hope to accomplish, at least in the near future. We thought it was important to identify the highest priorities, We felt the highest priority was to create a mechanism that addresses the classification issues and the importance of standardization with at least a minimum core set of variables, such as the definition of injury itself, as the dependent variable.

We feel that the prime criteria for this is that it be international in scope, and that clearly the field of injury prevention has emerged to a new level that justifies and requires the expansion of structure and resources in order to do this. Such an organization might be, but not necessarily, the World Health Organization (WHO). Clearly, concerning the need for consistent classification of a core set of variables on an international basis, WHO is well positioned to lead the effort. And with that, I will stop, we will take questions.

Minimum Basic Data Set (MBDS), Unintentional Injuries

Co–Chairs: Johan Lund, Yvette Holder, and Richard J. Smith, M.S.

Introduction

Good morning. I was chosen from the group to be the presenter of our discussion and conclusions. I will do my best to give a report from the discussion in these two workshops, which were very creative. Our discussions might be divided into the following topics:

1.   What do we understand with a MBDS

    –   for describing?
    –   for intervention?
    –   for evaluation?

2.   Which severities ought to be surveilled: Deaths, inpatients, handicaps etc.? Which are the data sources?

3.   Which variables belong to the MBDS?

4.   Which event types (accident types) and injury types should be defined for trend analyses which might be utilized in international comparisons?

I noticed, when the group on MBDS for intentional injuries gave their report, they told us that they were driven by the need of which data is desirable to get. In our group, we were also to a great extent driven by the respect about the difficulties in collecting reliable data. A lot of the members in our group had worked with this question for many years, for instance how to collect data in an emergency department. Many of us from the Nordic countries also have presented extensive lists of variables in a MBDS to our health authorities, asking them to collect this MBDS. They then tell us to forget our wishes, because such a list of variables would be impossible to collect in the daily routine in one of our hospitals without special resources in man–power and money. In our group were also representatives from developing countries, some with a rather low level in the infrastructure needed for collecting data in a national health system. Due to this experiences and situation, we need to be realistic about how detailed this MBDS should be and can be in order to be collected in a routine national system for international comparisons.

What Do We Understand With a MBDS?

A figure was presented in the group clarify the difference between a MBDS and other data sets (see figure 1). We might divide the data sets in three groups:

1.   A Minimum Basic Data Set (MBDS), also called a Core Set. The variables in this MBDS ought to be very general case indicators. The purpose for collecting a MBDS as this might be for policy setting, for identifying "hot spots," to follow trends on the main accident/injury types locally, regionally and centrally and for international comparisons. For being able to follow trends, the collection of a MBDS ought to be as close to 100 percent as possible in the group and in the area we want to monitor.

2.   A Standard Data Set (SDS) consists of more detailed indicators, and eventually a free text. The data set collected in most of the existing hospitalbased injury surveillance and registration systems in the world today might be a SDS: NEISS in USA, NOMESCO in the Nordic countries, EHLASS in many European countries, PORS in the Netherlands, HASS in United Kingdom. We might also consider the chapters XIX and XX in the ICD–10 as a SDS, since they are rather detailed. And I have to admit that in my country we doubt that it is possible to collect this information from our hospitals in a routine system, with a quality good enough to enable us to make good and reliable statistics.

A SDS is collected for defining more detailed "hot spots", to identify some preventive means, and for making some research. However, to really get information which makes it possible for you to understand why the accident/injury happened, and hence will give you possibilities to propose efficient preventive means, you have to go to the third level of details:

3. Expanded Data Set (EDS) contains more or less case stories from the different accidents/injuries. There might be modules created for the most important accident/injury types you want to investigate, for instance traffic accidents, burns, occupational accident, spinal cord injuries etc. These modules might contain a set of standardized questions.

**Figure 1. Different data sets for collecting data on unintentional injuries
with regard to the level of detail of the information and
the purpose of collecting the data set**

Level of detail of information	Different data sets	The purpose of collecting the data set
General case indicators	MBDS (A Core Set)	Policy Setting Identify "hot spots" Follow trends International comparisons
More detailed indicators + evt. free text	Standard data set (SDS) ICD – X, chapter XIX, XX NEISS, NOMESCO, EHLASS, HASS, PORS	Identify more detailed "hot spots" Identify preventive means (Research, to some extent)
Case stories	Expanded data sets (EDS) Modules on: Traffic, Burns, Falls, Products etc.	Identify preventive means Research

One very important characteristic of this figure is that the cost for collecting the information will increase the more downwards to the bottom of the figure you get.

Which Severities Ought to Be Surveilled: Deaths, Inpatients, Handicaps Etc.? Which Are the Data Sources?

We put up a list of the different consequences or severities of an accident which we think is important to surveill:

1. Deaths
2. In–patients, number and days
3. Handicaps, impairments, disabilities
4. Rehabilitation, number and days
5. Sick leaves, numbers and days
6. Economic consequences

If we are able to monitor these consequences with a MBDS in a continuously running system, then we really are able to show the burden of accidents and injury to the society, and to monitor how this develops over the years. This will also be very useful for evaluation of preventive efforts.

We identified two main types of data sources. The numbers in the margin show which kind of severities or consequences are found in the different sources:

-       Primary – mostly within the health system

      1.   Death certificates
      2.   Hospital admission and discharge registrations

-       Emergency department registrations
      3–5   Population surveys

-       Family practioners and other primary care providers

-       Secondary, mostly outside the health system:
      3?   Trauma registers
      2   Other surveillance systems
      3–6   Insurance registers
      3–6–   National insurance registers, social security registers

Which Variables Belong to the MBDS?

This question was the most important in our group to discuss. We developed the following list, where the variables are placed in some sort of priority. We think that a surveillance or monitoring system should start on the top and go down as far you get your system to register with the resources available. As one of us said: You will have a meaningful system also when you register just age and sex. But of course, the meaning will increase the longer down you will come on the list (but also the cost)

We have also connected these variables to the important W´s in this business: Who, Where, When and What.

The variable to start with is the *intent*. We have to know if the injury was intentionally or unintentionally.

Who:
Demographic data as: Age, sex, race, residence

For defining main accident type:
Activity when injury occurred (as the fifth digit in ICD–X, chapter XX or one digit in activity code in NOMESCO)

Where:
Place of occurrence (as the sixth digit in ICD–X, chapter XX or one digit in the place of occurrence in NOMESCO) – this is also important for defining main accident type.
Address/municipality where accident happened

When:
Date when injury occurred

Outcome of injury, to measure the consequences:
Type of outcome will depend on your data source: Days in hospital, approx. costs involved, degree of disability etc.

What:
Mechanism of accident/event (as 1–4 digit in ICD–X, chapt XX)
Type of injury/body location (as ICD–10, chapt. XIX)

We think that the activity and place of occurrence are important variables because they will make it possible to define the main accident/event types according to the authorities responsible for the prevention of accident, and those accident types are important to monitor.

Which Event Types (Accident Types) and Injury Types Should Be Followed for Trends Which Might Be Utilized for International Comparison?

In our groups, we also tried to define which event or accident types and injury types we want to register for being able to follow the development of these groups in the different countries, and also for international comparisons. The definition of these types could be a task for this ICE (International Collaborative Effort) or some other group.

There are at least three important variables which enables us to construct or define the main accident/event types and injury types:

–   Activity when accident happened
–   Place of occurrence
–   Nature of injury

Different activities are: Work, education, sport etc.
Places of occurrence are: Home, school, road etc.

A combination of these two variables will create the different main accident/event types as: Occupational accidents, Home accident, School accidents, Sport accidents, Traffic accidents etc. Here international standardization/definition work is necessary.

The nature of injury define important injury types which we should be able to monitor: Burns, drowning, spinal cord injuries etc. Also here international standardization/definition work is necessary.

Well, this was more or less our contribution to answer the question about a minimum basic data set for unintentional injuries. If we are able to define a MBDS which can be used by most countries, and we are able to find some way of reporting the main types, then we would come a great step forward in getting what we all are looking for, a better picture of the situation. Thank you.

Minimum Basic Data Set - Intentional Injuries

Co–Chairs: Ken Powell, M.D. and Jess Kraus, Ph.D.

The following major data elements were recommended as either minimum (core) or optimum in the deliberations on establishing a consistent, uniform, and standardized bases for intentional data collection efforts on intentional injury surveillance or research.

The data elements are not in any particular order but appear as discussed by participants of two workshops.

1)   (MINIMUM) the Intent of Injury

A classification scheme is urged which separates injuries according to intentionality and perpetrator. One possible scheme is:

Perpetrator	Intentionality Intentional	Unintentional	Unknown
Self			
Other			
Unknown			

The issue of intentionality will require some discussion to reach a consensus definition. Illustrations of various types is urged.

2)   (MINIMUM) Place of Occurrence of the Injury Event

Specificity of geographic and/or detail of the event location for descriptive purposes was deemed essential.

3)   (MINIMUM) Time of Event

As recorded by date and hour.

4)   (MINIMUM) Circumstances, Motive, or How the Event Occurred

The workshop addressed several issues on this data variable, including:

 a.   whether the injury arose from an isolated event or multiple connected events
 b.   a need to reconcile criminal justice and public health terminology
 c.   difficulties associated with capturing multiple and not mutually exclusive circumstances (e.g., arguments, alcohol, drugs, and gangs may all be important "circumstances" for a single event
 d.   **optimally**, a narrative field describing the events would aid precision and flexibility

5)   (MINIMUM) Substances Involved: Victim and Perpetrator

A simple dichotomous yes/no is essential. The workshops felt that type of substance, for example, alcoholic beverages, cocaine, heroin, and other drugs would ultimately be desirable for purposes of description and countermeasures development.

6)   (MINIMUM) Data Source

This variable is essential in order to be able to distinguish the source of the information and the nuances or differences in definition from various sources such as police reports, coroner's investigative reports, hospital documents, etc. We want to key all of the variables to a hierarchy of authenticity.

7)   (MINIMUM) Weapon Involved

This important variable is unique, in many respects, to intentional injuries. The variable will need to be operationalized. Methods to record single and multiple weapons, and to encompass the various methods used for self-inflicted injury will be needed. It was judged **optimal** to work toward greater detail on the type of weapon particularly firearms.

8)   (MINIMUM) Relationship of Victim to Perpetrator

9)   (MINIMUM) Demographics of Victim and Perpetrator

FACTOR	VICTIM	PERPETRATOR
Sex	X	X
Age	X	X (interval)
Race/Ethnicity	X	X

The workshop concluded that it would be optimal also to develop some indicator of socio-economic status. Factors such as occupation, census track of residence, employment status, zip code of victim (and event), and a unique identifier were suggested and would need to be operationalized.

10)   (MINIMUM) Injury Factors (of Victim)

The workshops felt that this variable is shared equally with the unintentional minimum data set. It should address factors surrounding severity of the injury, nature/body part involved, post-injury disability, impairment or deficit, expected medical care payer, source of treatment, type of transport, pre-existing medical or emotional/psychiatric questions. These variables would have to be operationalized for factors of accessibility, standardization of terminology, etc.

11)   (OPTIMUM) Elements of Preventive Actions or Countermeasures

The workshop participants felt that it might be important to determine if the violence related injuries occurred in the presence of existing countermeasures, programs, prevention devices, etc.

12)   (OPTIMUM) Prior Events

Among assault victims, prior injury experience associated with the same or similar perpetrators would be an optimal item.

13)   (OPTIMUM) Living Status of the Victim

A classification scheme to record whether the victim was living alone, living with a significant other, living with family, living with a child, etc., at the time of or immediately before the injury would be an optimal item.

Geographic Information Systems

Co-Chairs: Erich M. Daub and Keith D. Harries

In 1853 a massive epidemic of cholera in London killed and disabled thousands of people. Therapy was unavailable; indeed, neither the mode of transmission nor the responsible agent had yet been identified. Despite these limitations, John Snow was able to contain the outbreak. Analyzing data which he carefully collected, Snow mapped the location of every known case; the clustering of cases around one public water pump was obvious. The rest of the story is public health history; the pump handle was removed and the epidemic rapidly subsided.

The story of the Broad Street pump has become a metaphor for public health—sound surveillance and careful epidemiology can often lead to successful prevention even absent a complete understanding of causal relationships. Snow appreciated the value of each of the three now-classic features of epidemiologic investigation: person, place, and time. More than anything else, Snow showed the power of place. Location spoke volumes. Absolute location conferred intrinsic environmental constraints on health; relative location revealed the "activity space" of daily life, with all its unique spatially-dependent risks. Today, after being largely neglected for seven generations, public health is slowly rediscovering the power of place.

Place matters. Geographers have recognized this since the inception of their discipline over two-thousand years ago. Some places are distinguished by their topography, others by their natural resources. Laws and regulations set one place apart from another. Culture, crime, climate, capital, civil unrest—every place has unique features. That these location-specific attributes may influence the incidence of disease and injury—as well as opportunities for intervention—is now awakening the public health community.

If geography has long recognized the importance of spatial variation on the human condition, why has public health taken so long to do the same? Much of the explanation for the current climate favoring a re-awakening to this approach—the "geographic approach"—is the recent proliferation of computer systems and software dedicated to manipulating and mapping spatial data. These systems, called *Geographic Information Systems (GIS)*, are revolutionizing geography. They have the same potential within public health. The advent of these systems effectively puts into the hands of epidemiologists and prevention specialists the power to understand and manipulate "space" and "place". One consequence of this is that public health professionals must now learn to think geographically. As with many school children in the U.S. today, this knowledge is not yet common or easily acquired.

Geography has traditionally had four concerns: the characterization of places, the understanding of man-land relationships, accounting for spatial distributions, and the differentiation of areas and the formation of regions. Geographic analyses usually have one of two aims:

- To account for spatial variation
- To integrate all of the variation at a location so as to explain or characterize a place or region

Public health and injury control can utilize both of these aims to better understand location-specific influences of the environment (natural and built) and behavior, and to determine modifiable features of geographically variable phenomenon. GIS provides an important tool—a window into the geographic world.

GIS software ranges in its capabilities and cost. Some "desk-top" mapping programs are available at no cost, while other full-featured GIS packages cost several thousands of dollars (U.S.) and have long learning curves. Functional mapping and basic spatial analysis programs can be had for between $200 to $2000 (U.S.), and provide accessible methods by which to construct computer-generated maps and moderately sophisticated spatial analyses.

There are three required elements for the application of GIS to public health and injury control. First, a specific GIS software program must be acquired. These are readily available in most Asian and European countries and Australia;

less developed nations have benefited from United Nations-funded GIS software development. Secondly, computer-readable "boundary" files must be acquired. These are digital equivalents of hard copy maps showing various jurisdictional boundaries and perhaps related features (such as streets, topography, etc.). Boundary files will be unique to the GIS user's study area. In the U.S., one might acquire files for census tracts, postal zip-codes, and county or state boundaries, to name but a few. Other nations have their own geographies: postal zones (England), territories (Australia), enumeration districts (Sweden) are examples. These boundary files must be digitally compatible with the specific GIS software product acquired. While there are attempts to standardize spatial data and file structures within the U.S. and internationally, a plethora of frequently incompatible file types presently exists. The most expedient means of acquiring compatible boundary files is to purchase them directly from the manufacturer of the GIS software. Most GIS vendors produce a host of compatible boundary files for use with their product. Boundary files exist for most European and Asian nations; some African and South American countries also have well developed digital maps available. In the U.S. there are wealth of boundaries available for purchase from government and private sources. The third element required to apply GIS to public health and injury control is geographically-referenced attribute data. Attribute data is the raw data describing features of the population and/or "cases" to be mapped. Examples include death certificate files, trauma registries, census data, land and property data, and ambulance/EMS provider data, to name a very few. Such data is said to be "geo-referenced" if it includes at least one data field specifying some location-specific value for each record in the database. This might be a postal code, a county identifier, or (the penultimate geo-reference) a street address. GIS software assigns an X-Y ("latitude" - "longitude") coordinate to every record in the database based on each record's geo-referenced variable. Any record can have more than one geo-referenced variable, making analyses at finer geographic scales possible. The remaining attribute data serves as the basis for relational spatial-analytical operations performed by the GIS. The combination of multiple geo-referenced data sets is the hallmark of GIS. By "layering" data sets over one another, complicated spatial arrangements are easily identified and powerful spatial analyses are possible.

To illustrate these features, consider two examples drawn from work in the Baltimore, Maryland (U.S.A.) metropolitan area. The first concerns an analysis of 2,639 juvenile gun crimes during an 11-year period (190=80-1990) in Baltimore City. U.S. census data was used to develop a social stress index at the census tract-level. The 2,639 juvenile gun crime cases were "geocoded" (assigned x-y coordinates by a GIS system), and evaluated with respect to geographic patterns of social stress and selected demographic attributes. The GIS software was used to layer each of these three elements over one another, and to explore spatial relationships. Spatial patterns of juvenile gun crimes were noted in "high" stress neighborhoods. Other patterns revealed location-specific relationships between stress-intense areas and "victim-perpetrator" ethnicity; most "Black on Black" homicides were confined to "high" stress neighborhoods. Pronounced "edge" or "frontier" effects were seen at margins of differential stress neighborhoods.

A second example of the application of GIS to injury epidemiology and control is the Baltimore County Injury Prevention Program's integration of GIS into their established injury surveillance system. Hard-copy and electronic injury mortality data is obtained from the State Office of the Chief Medical Examiner. This data includes street address-level data relative to three locations for each case: the site of injury, the location of residence, and the location of death. GIS software layers this data with a variety of additional data sets: death certificate data, census data, hospital discharge data, EMS ambulance run reports, zoning data, liquor license data, and other data sets. Maps are constructed and spatial analyses performed to explore absolute and relative relationships of personal, behavioral, environmental, and institutional attributes to injury morbidity and mortality. For example, mapping and locational analyses of three-years of county resident homicide deaths revealed that 25 percent of county residents were injured (mostly with a firearm) outside the county boundary (e.g., within the city of Baltimore). Sixty percent were injured outside their home. The reverse was noted for suicide deaths: 70 percent were injured in their own home; 90 percent of these died there as well. GIS is introducing the "geographic approach" to injury control and public health. This approach re-establishes the importance of place. Geography lends itself especially to answering five types of questions:

1. Why is "X" distributed in a certain way, as opposed to all the other possible ways it could be distributed?

2. Why are there different rates at which "X" spreads over time through an area?

3. Why are there differences in the locational choices we make for our institutions or our interventions?

4. Why are there differences in direction or distance of movements of people, ideas, or phenomena?

5. Why are there differences in the images people hold about their communities and surrounding environment and how does this influence health or the prevention of disease and injury?

Participants in this Workshop deliberated on the accessibility, use, and expansion of GIS and geographic techniques to the study and control of injury. Several recommendations resulted:

- Compile communications illustrating the value and utility of GIS to public health and injury control.

- Make GIS and map analyses accessible to public health workers through training and educational forums.

- Inventory (nationally and internationally) the degree to which existing injury-related data sets contain (and could contain) geo-referenced data.

- Derive consensus and proscribe the acceptable level of spatial data to be captured by injury-related data systems.

- Study and promote ways to safeguard the confidentiality of geo-referenced public health data.

- Promote GIS mapping and analysis projects and sources of experience and guidance.

- Disseminate descriptions of available GIS software, boundary files, and geo-referenced injury-related data sets to national and international audiences.

- Improve the quantity and quality of geographic data available in medical and public health records.

- Create vehicles (task force, E-mail bulletin boards, newsletters, interest groups) to promote and disseminate GIS applications to injury control.

- Work on methods to determine appropriate denominators to use with geo-referenced injury data.

- Expand the querying of "place" to existing data collection mechanisms (e.g., hospital emergency/casualty departments, trauma centers, medical examiners, EMS, police).

- Promote "desk-top" mapping as an introduction to GIS techniques for public health and injury control professionals.

The "invisible college" of public health professionals introducing GIS into their epidemiologic and preventive routine is expanding. Concerted efforts need to focus on infusing GIS into injury prevention. A collection of interested public health professionals is forming to advance these goals and to work toward these recommendations. With the support of colleagues from other disciplines, and through the future efforts of the I.C.E. on Injuries, we hope to see the seeds first sewn almost 150 years ago reap a great harvest.

Closing Remarks

C.J. Romer, M.D.

Let me first express the deep interest and great pleasure I had to participate in the debate which took place this week, and not only share ideas but also concerns with those present.

I wish on behalf of WHO to thank and congratulate the organizers, and particularly, the CDC National Center on Health Statistics, not only for the quality of the organization of this meeting, but also to have taken the initiative to set this International Collaborative effort on injury statistics.

We also deeply appreciate that this International Collaborative Effort was closely associated with the work of the WHO working group on injury surveillance, chaired by Dr Wim Rogmans, Director of the Dutch Consumer Safety Institute, which is also a WHO Collaborating Centre. Indeed, the WHO interest has also been demonstrated to some extent by the fact that 5 WHO Collaborating Centers were participating in addition to Dr L'Hours and myself, from WHO/HQ and Mrs Y. Holder from the CAREC Office.

There has been a wealth of expertise produced during these days. The level of the debate has been very high. We have witnessed enthusiasm, but have also heard a certain dose of skepticism and frustration.

As far as I am concerned, I only wish to stress a few points which "may likely" underline future development of data systems, yet without entering into technical details which have been largely covered.

Health intelligence is the central nervous system of public health. Success achieved for infectious diseases is the best demonstration, particularly when referring to smallpox eradication, yesterday; onchocerciasis, today; poliomyelitis tomorrow, and other diseases the day after tomorrow. In 1993, 143 countries were polio free.

Health intelligence is likely to be even more critical in the future because of the speed of changes societies in the world are facing today. Epidemiological and demographic transition, urbanization, but also rapid democratization processes are causing and reflect a time of changes, which will call for new needs, new information systems management to meeting these needs.

At the same time, new challenges surface because traditional ways of thinking are threatened. Among those is the fact that we, health people and professional have the strong tendency, anchored and rooted in our intellectual mind to think and act very often according to the traditional vertical disease oriented approach. What happens is that each verticality creates its own data system, multiplies them, but usually none of them communicate with the other.

But today, what is at stake is of a totally different nature.

Environmental threats to health, life styles, population issues, social issues and their impact on health call for aggregated, integrated action, in other words for linkages and mechanisms for consolidated decision making. Safety promotion and injury control are certainly today a challenge to health people and others calling for such scientific decision-making and community partnership, with all the consequences it entails on the type of data systems needed.

There is a last point I wish to raise.

We, health professionals, have also thought for a long time that we were the depository of knowledge in health, and consequently, were the only ones to know what to do for the health of people. We have therefore created data systems in isolation of the community which we were supposed to serve, and to a great extent, we have ignored to incorporate in these data systems the indigenous expertise of the community and the potential of the community to be an active partner in the promotion of its own health.
New partnerships have to be created in health to meet new health challenges, violence is a good example, and data systems have also to take this into account.

WHO is going to give stronger attention to data systems development aiming at better serving community needs in the frame of its SAFECOM project coordinated by the Department of Social Medicine of the Karolinska Institute in Stockholm in its capacity of Collaborating Centre on Safety Promotion.

With regard to partnerships, I wish to stress the following. In the area which is of concern today, data generation is one thing, but setting mechanisms so that these data can be used efficiently is another thing. Partnerships with the community including NGOs is a prerequisite and can be an asset not only for collecting data reflecting the situation and needs of the community, but more to ensure these data will be used for action when the community has been convinced it will be for its own benefit.

Concluding Remarks

I am sure we share a common concern, if not frustration, when we consider the weight of injury on the public or the public health agenda when it comes to prioritization of health issues. In general, injury programs are grossly, if not indecently, under-funded in most countries.

To improve the score we must strive to better lighten the burden of injury on health, particularly with regard to the medical, social or individual psychological disablement it entails, burden on the individual's health but also on the family, community and society as a whole. We must do for injury what has been done for more traditional diseases when assessing their impact on society's quality of life. Injury surveillance and data systems are the "big bang" for this chemistry to be initiated.

The global burden of diseases report produced last year by The World Bank, using the DALY index and weighting injury at about 12 percent of the total burden of disease worldwide is an interesting first move in this direction.

Setting objectives and targets and committing ourselves to meet the above needs might be a fundamental step for technical cooperation particularly through this International Collaborative Effort in partnership with NCHS and WHO.

Two other possible grounds for cooperation based on discussions of the ICE group would be:

·   To prepare a glossary of terms used in the injury field. There is still some inconsistency and misunderstanding among safety or injury researchers and practitioners in the use of some terms and concepts. First and not the least, use and translation in non-English languages of the term injury versus the term accident.

·   To establish an international clearing house in the injury field with access to basic information concerning on-going programs and their evaluation, type of institutions and expertise available, etc. This could well be a ground for cooperation between NCHS and the WHO WG on injury surveillance.

Finally, I do think the time is now ripe and needs sufficiently and evidently felt and expressed to consider the possibility of preparing a specific classification on injury as an "epigone" to the ICD. Consultations will be initiated in WHO and ICE and the WHO Working Group on Injury Surveillance should be the key partners in this endeavor.

I now wish to congratulate Lois A. Fingerhut and Bob Hartford the co-chairpersons for the success of the meeting and use this opportunity to call for strengthened cooperation between NCHS and WHO to give as soon as possible, practical application to the recommendations formulated by this group.

Joseph L. Annest, Ph.D.

I appreciate the opportunity to speak on behalf of Dr. Mark Rosenberg, Director, National Center for Injury Prevention and Control (NCIPC) concerning international activities that will stem from this very important ICE conference. NCIPC is committed to working with the National Center for Health Statistics and WHO, and all of you, to accomplish the goal of improved injury data systems and injury statistics throughout the world.

As I reflect on the last couple of days, I see that there is a lot of work to be done, and I think that a lot of you agree.

I recall what Dr. Satcher said to us at the beginning of the conference about the power of high quality data and its influence on decisions regarding public health policy in the area of injury prevention. Most certainly, this potential alone should be the force driving each of us to reconfirm our commitment to the field of injury control and to determine our roles, as individuals, in improving international statistics on injury. Although resources are limited and our schedules are busy, fruitful international collaboration will be necessary to make this effort a success.

As we conduct research to address and overcome problems in injury prevention and surveillance in our own countries, we need to share what we learn with the rest of the international community. Along this line, I would like to briefly describe three injury surveillance projects of international interest that are being conducted by NCIPC. All three of these projects aim to improve data on injury morbidity.

First, we are developing and testing national guidelines for the uniform collection, analysis, and reporting of traumatic brain and spinal cord injuries. In 1992, a draft working group of the Secretary's National Advisory Committee on Injury Prevention and Control assisted CDC in developing guidelines for traumatic and spinal cord injury surveillance. These guidelines were pilot tested at three sites by two state health departments—New York and Rhode Island—and one local health department—Maricopa County, Arizona. The results of these pilot studies have been summarized and used to revise the guidelines, which will soon be reviewed for approval by the National Advisory Committee for Injury Prevention and Control. The final guidelines are expected to be disseminated later this year and will be made available to federal, state, and local officials and health departments in this country, as well as internationally. Also, recently, the Traumatic Brain Injury Act of 1990 passed the U.S. Senate and is now pending in the U.S. House of Representatives. We hope this will provide additional resources to develop a uniform national reporting system to determine the incidence, severity, and magnitude of traumatic brain injury in the United States.

Second, NCIPC is working toward establishing a uniform data set for emergency department surveillance. This effort is a public/private partnership, coordinated by Dr. Dan Pollock, Acute Care Team Leader of our Division of Acute Care, Rehabilitation Research, and Disability Prevention, who has been participating in this symposium. Currently, we are exploring groups that can serve as planners and cosponsors for this activity. We will conduct a conference patterned after the 1988 consensus conference that led to the development of uniform case criteria and standardized data elements for trauma registries. These trauma registry guidelines have been disseminated around the world. In addition to data standards, the upcoming ED surveillance conference will address important issues concerning linkage of data systems for pre–hospital, hospital, and rehabilitation services. Linking these data systems to provide information on the circumstances, risk factors and behaviors, treatment, and health outcomes related to injury is essential to assessing quality of care issues and to carrying out injury surveillance, research and prevention activities.

Third, NCIPC is addressing the growing epidemic of firearm–related injury in the United States. This epidemic needs close attention and scrutiny. What we are learning about monitoring and preventing firearm–related injuries may have important international implications if, at some point, the epidemic spreads to other countries.

In the United States, firearms are the weapons used in approximately 68 percent of homicides and 60 percent of suicides. In 1991, firearm–related injuries accounted for over 38,000 deaths in the United States. As Lois Fingerhut mentioned in her talk, if trends continue as they have in the past 15 years or so, firearm–related injuries will soon surpass motor–vehicle–related injuries as the leading cause of death from injury in our country.

We know remarkably little about the patterns and causes of nonfatal firearm–related injury. NCIPC has been involved in several projects that will help us to understand better the magnitude and impact of firearm–related injuries and to evaluate the effectiveness of prevention programs that address firearm–related injuries as a major cause of morbidity, disability, and death in the United States.

Currently, through an interagency agreement with the U.S. Consumer Product Safety Commission, we are collecting data through the National Electronic Injury Surveillance System for use in computing national estimate of nonfatal firearm injuries. Preliminary estimates indicate that there are about 2.5 times as many nonfatal gunshot wounds as there are firearm–related deaths in the United States. My colleagues and I are currently preparing manuscripts to summarize our findings, based on the first full year of data collection—June 1, 1992 through May 31, 1993.

We also have two cooperative agreements, one with the Massachusetts Department of Public Health, working on a statewide injury emergency–department–based surveillance system for weapon–related injury, and the other with the New York City Department of Health, establishing an emergency–department–based surveillance system for weapon–related injury in Harlem, New York.

We are exploring mechanisms for establishing a national information database on fatal and nonfatal firearm–related injuries, that will enable us to monitor trends, examine risk factors, and evaluate interventions. Also, state–based behavioral risk factor survey systems are currently being used to assess risk behaviors for firearm–related injuries. Our intent is to share with all of you our experience in developing and improving surveillance systems useful for designing, monitoring, and evaluating prevention programs aimed at reducing firearm–related injuries in the United States.

In closing, I would like to thank Lois Fingerhut, Bob Hartford, and other NCHS staff for hosting an outstanding ICE symposium. It has been very informative and insightful. It has been a real privilege to attend this symposium and brainstorm about how to improve injury data systems and injury statistics with some of the most talented health professionals in the world. My hope is for success, and I look forward to future collaborations with all of you.

Robert Israel

You have all been participating here for a little over 2½ days now, and I am sure that you have been stimulated and found the proceedings of relevance and interest. But I am also sure that you are tired and would like to get up and stretch and go on about your business and, for many of you, to go home. Some of you have been away from home for a long time. So, I promise that I will not spend too much time in making just a few concluding remarks.

Let me start out by saying that one of the primary themes of the International Collaborative Effort on Injury Statistics should be described by paraphrasing the well known admonition by Socrates, "know thyself" . . . "know thy data."

And in that spirit, the objectives of this collaboration include learning more about national injury data through comparisons, through improvement of comparability and of data quality, and strengthening international systems for data collection and analysis, through in–depth understanding of a selected set of national practices for defining and measuring injury morbidity and mortality, leading to a better understanding of the causes of injury and the means of effective prevention.

A sub–objective of these activities is to develop, on the basis of our mutual experiences, input into the various coding systems, including the new ICD–10, future revisions of ICD, the development of new systems, the modification of other existing systems, and especially, as I have heard from several speakers today, the development and enhancement of potential members of the ICD family of classifications to focus on the more specific and detailed needs in the injury data area.

Now, the content and accomplishments at this symposium can be described as having covered a broad range of issues, including recommendations described in the workshop reports. That leaves us with a large number of problems and issues, as well as recommendations. At the same time we have, through this symposium, I think, strengthened the networking on a personal basis, on an institutional basis, and on national and international levels as well, which should lead to better collaboration within and among nations, including the strengthening of multinational efforts with the leadership of such organizations as the injury surveillance working group, and directly with WHO and its collaborating centers, and the Pan American Health Organization in this region of the world.

In that connection, I say, Dr. Romer, we accept your invitation with great pleasure, to work together, because none of us singly or individually, regardless of the size of our agency, can tackle all of the many facets of the problems of injury prevention and control.

While this particular collaborative effort is, by design, focused mainly on certain aspects of the overall problem, we feel that the pooling together of talents and interests can significantly overcome some of the stated and unstated resource concerns that we all share.

There are some next steps that we hope will flow from this symposium. I can't elaborate on them in great detail because we are going to have to sit down quietly and think about all of the exciting things that have come out in these last 2½ days, but we certainly will try to capture the momentum that has developed here by establishing an international Collaborative Effort Working Group. We will set it up and we will convene a somewhat smaller group later this year. We hope this smaller group can take all of the inputs and ideas from this meeting and integrate the data needs of injury prevention programs with the congressionally mandated responsibility for the National Center for Health Statistics to be the nation's health statistics focal point.

We will try to work with all of our colleagues to define an ongoing activity that will be do–able—what that turns out to be remains to be seen. But certainly, on the basis of our experience with international collaborative efforts of this type, we feel quite confident that if each participating organization and country puts a bit of effort into the overall activity, we will reach a critical mass that will have an impact on the improvement of injury data, which then hopefully will also result in stronger and more effective injury prevention programs.

So, let me thank you. You, the participants, are the leaders on my list to be thanked, because without your hard work these few days, and all of the preparatory work leading up to these few days, we would not have had a successful and useful symposium.

Secondly, I would like to thank our cosponsors, the National Institute for Child Health and Human Development, in helping us to bring this symposium about.

And next, I would like to specifically thank our CDC colleagues. The National Center for Health Statistics is one of a number of components of the Centers for Disease Control and Prevention, particularly working on this activity with our colleagues in the National Center for Injury Prevention and Control, the National Center for Environmental Health, and the National Institute of Occupational Safety and Health.

And I certainly would be remiss in not thanking the ICE Steering Committee, which has put many hours into the planning of this symposium.

I also would like to thank the support staff from the National Center for Health Statistics, especially Ms. Linda McCleary and Ms. Ginger Richards who did a lot of the staffing of the front desk and photocopying for you and made numerous telephone calls and ticket reconfirmations on your behalf. They are probably not here now, but I will extend our thanks to them later.

Finally, I want to give my own personal, deep appreciation of the co–chairs of this whole effort—Bob Hartford, who is my deputy and so I can attest to how many hours he put in on this—and to Lois Fingerhut, who is special Assistant for Injury Epidemiology in the Division of Analysis at the National Center for Health Statistics. Lois and Bob, you have done a very fine job, if I must say so myself. I appreciate it. I think all of the participants appreciate it and I just know that you will feel that all of the hard work that you have done leading to this point is but a prelude to more hard work.

So, in closing, let me remind you that you are about to embark upon a hazardous portion of your day, so let me wish you all a very, very safe journey back home, wherever that may be, and we look forward to seeing you all again another day. Thank you very much.